Resource Manual to Accompany

Nursing Research

GENERATING AND ASSESSING EVIDENCE FOR NURSING PRACTICE

EIGHTH EDITION

Denise F. Polit, PhD
President
Humanalysis, Inc.
Saratoga Springs, New York, *and*
Adjunct Professor
Griffith University School of Nursing,
Research Centre for Clinical Practice Innovation
Gold Coast, Australia
(www.denisepolit.com)

Cheryl Tatano Beck, DNSc, CNM, FAAN
Professor
School of Nursing
University of Connecticut
Storrs, Connecticut

Wolters Kluwer Health | Lippincott Williams & Wilkins
Philadelphia • Baltimore • New York • London
Buenos Aires • Hong Kong • Sydney • Tokyo

Acquisitions Editor: Audrey Lickwar
Managing Editor: Mary Kinsella
Director of Nursing Production: Helen Ewan
Senior Managing Editor / Production: Erika Kors
Manufacturing Coordinator: Karin Duffield
Senior Manufacturing Manager: William Alberti
Compositor: Aptara, Inc.
Printer: R. R. Donnelley, Crawfordsville

ISBN-10: 0-7817-7052-1
ISBN-13: 978-0-7817-7052-1

9 8 7 6 5 4 3 2 1

LWW.com

Preface

This *Resource Manual* for the 8th edition of *Nursing Research: Generating and Assessing Evidence for Nursing Practice* complements and strengthens the textbook in important new ways. The manual provides opportunities to reinforce the acquisition of basic research skills through systematic learning exercises, and in this edition we have placed particular emphasis on exercises that involve careful reading and critiquing of actual studies. We have moved in this direction because critiquing skills are increasingly important in an environment that promotes evidence-based nursing practice. Moreover, the ability to think critically about research decisions is fundamental to being able to design and plan one's own study.

Full research reports and a grant application are included in 12 appendices to this *Resource Manual*. These reports, which represent a rich array of research endeavors, form the basis for exercises in each chapter. There are reports of quantitative and qualitative studies, an instrument development paper, a meta-analysis, and a metasynthesis. We are particularly excited about being able to include a full grant application that was funded by the National Institute of Nursing Research, together with the Study Section's summary sheet. We firmly believe that nothing is more illuminating than a good model when it comes to research communication.

The most important new feature of this *Resource Manual* is the Toolkit, which offers important research resources to beginning and advanced researchers, and is provided on an accompanying CD-ROM. Our mission was to include easily adaptable tools for a broad range of research situations. In our own careers as researchers, we have found that adapting existing forms, manuals, or protocols is far more efficient and productive than "starting from scratch." By making these tools available as Word files, we have made it possible for you to adapt tools to meet your specific needs, without the tedium of having to re-type basic information. We wish we had had this Toolkit in our early years as researchers! We think seasoned researchers are likely to find parts of the Toolkit useful as well.

The *Resource Manual* consists of 27 chapters—one chapter corresponding to every chapter in the textbook. Each chapter has relevant resources and exercises, and answers to exercises for which there are objective answers are included at the back of the book in Appendix M. Each of the 27 chapters consists of four components:

- *A Crossword Puzzle*. Terms and concepts presented in the textbook are reinforced in an entertaining and challenging fashion through crossword puzzles.
- *Study Questions*. Each chapter contains three to six short individual exercises relevant to the materials in the textbook.
- *Application Exercises*. These exercises are geared to helping you to read, comprehend, and critique nursing studies. These exercises focus on studies in the appendices and ask questions that are relevant to the content covered in the textbook. There are two

sets of questions—*Questions of Fact* and *Questions for Discussion.* The Questions of Fact will help you to read the report and find specific types of information related to the content covered in the textbook. For these questions, there are "right" and "wrong" answers. For example, for the chapter on sampling, a question might ask: How many people participated in this study? The Questions for Discussion, by contrast, require an assessment of the merits of various features of the study. For example, a question might ask: Was there a *sufficient number* of study participants in this study? The second set of questions can be the basis for classroom discussions.

- ***Toolkit*** . This section, on the accompanying CD-ROM, includes tools and resources that can save you time—and that will hopefully result in higher-quality tools than might otherwise have been the case. Each chapter has tools appropriate for the content covered in the textbook.

We hope that you will find these resources rewarding, enjoyable, and useful in your effort to develop and hone skills needed in critiquing and doing research.

Contents

PART 1

Foundations of Nursing Research and Evidence-Based Practice

CHAPTER 1

Introduction to Nursing Research in an Evidence-Based Practice Environment

■ A. Crossword Puzzle

Complete the crossword puzzle below, which uses terms and concepts presented in Chapter 1. (Puzzles may be removed for easier viewing.)

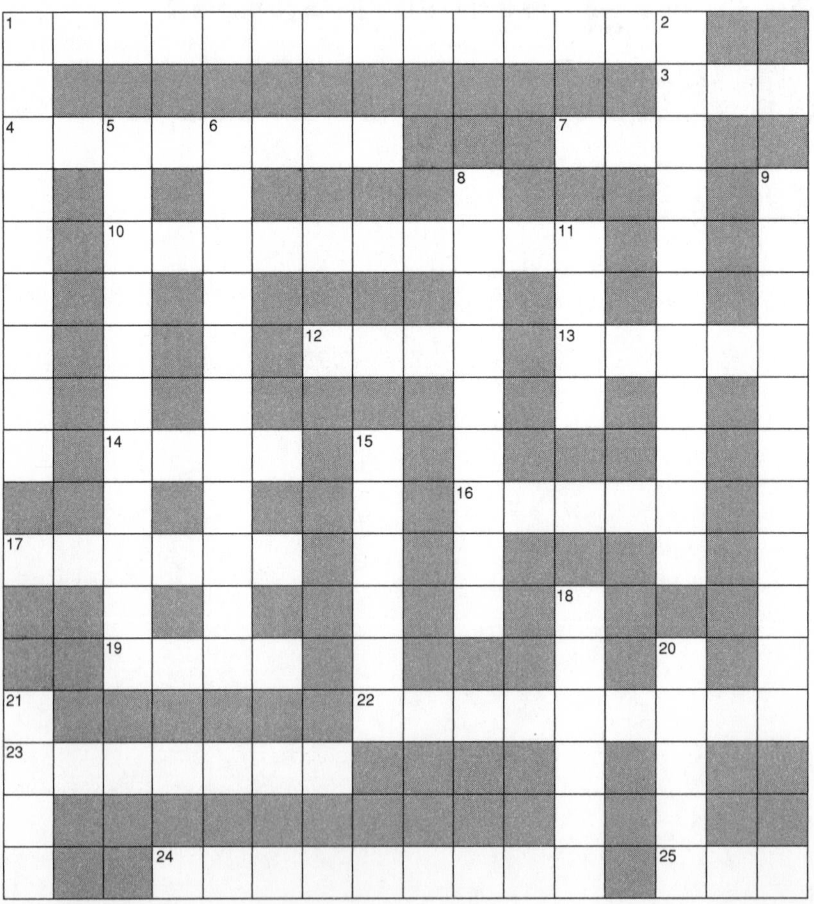

Note that there is a crossword puzzle in each chapter of this *Resource Manual.* We hope they will be a "fun" way for you to review key terms used in each chapter. However, we are not professional puzzle designers, and so there are some oddities about the puzzles. These oddities are not intended to be trick questions, but rather represent liberties we took in trying to get as many terms as possible into the puzzle. So, for example, there are a lot of acronyms (e.g., evidence-based practice = EBP) and abbreviations (e.g., evidence = evid), and even a few words that are written backwards (e.g., evidence = ecnedive). Two-word answers sometimes appear with a space (e.g., evidence-based), and sometimes they are just run together (e.g., evidencebased). The crossword puzzle answers are at the back of this *Resource Manual,* in case our intent is too obscure!

ACROSS

1. Nurses are increasingly encouraged to develop a practice that is ________ (hyphenated).
3. The clinical learning strategy developed at the McMaster School of Medicine (acronym)
4. A world view, a way of looking at natural phenomena
7. The world view that holds that there are multiple interpretations of reality (abbr.)
10. The world view that assumes that there is an orderly reality that can be studied objectively
12. The precursor to the National Institute of Nursing Research (acronym)
13. Successively trying alternative solutions is known as ________ and error
14. Research designed to solve a pressing practical problem is ________ research (abbr.).
16. Nurses get together in practice settings to critique studies in the context of journal ________.
17. Research designed to guide nursing practice is referred to as ________ nursing research (abbr.).
19. The U.S. agency that promotes and sponsors nursing research (acronym)
22. A source of evidence reflecting ingrained customs
23. The ________ of nursing research began with Florence Nightingale.
24. The degree to which research findings can be applied to people who did not participate in a study (abbr.)
25. The type of reasoning that involves developing specific predictions from general principles (abbr.)

DOWN

1. Evidence that is rooted in objective reality and gathered through the senses
2. The assumption that phenomena are not random, but rather have antecedent causes
5. The repeating of a study to determine whether findings can be upheld with a new group of people

6. A purpose of doing research, involving a portrayal of phenomena as they exist
8. A scheme for ordering the utility of evidence for practice is an evidence ________.
9. A purpose of doing research, often linked to theory in quantitative studies
11. The techniques used by researchers to structure a study are called research ________ (abbr.).
15. The type of research that analyzes narrative, subjective materials is ________ research (abbr.).
18. The use of findings from research in a practice setting is called research ________ (abbr.).
20. Naturalistic inquiry typically takes place in the ________.
21. The U.S. agency charged with supporting research designed to improve the quality of health care and reduce health costs (acronym)

■ B. Study Questions

1. Why is it important for nurses who will never conduct their own research to understand research methods?

2. What are some potential consequences to the nursing profession if nurses stopped conducting their own research?

3. What are some of the current changes occurring in the health care delivery system, and how could these changes influence nursing research and the use of research findings?

4. Below are descriptions of several research problems. Indicate whether you think the problem is best suited to a qualitative or quantitative approach, and explain your rationale.

   a. What is the decision-making process of AIDS patients seeking treatment?
   b. What effect does room temperature have on the colonization rate of bacteria in urinary catheters?
   c. What are sources of stress among nursing home residents?
   d. Does therapeutic touch affect the vital signs of hospitalized patients?
   e. What is the meaning of *hope* among stage IV cancer patients?
   f. What are the effects of prenatal instruction on the labor and delivery outcomes of pregnant women?
   g. What are the health care needs of the homeless, and what barriers do they face in having those needs met?

5. What are some of the limitations of quantitative research? What are some of the limitations of qualitative research? Which approach seems best suited to address problems in which you might be interested? Why is that?

6. Scan the titles in the table of contents of a recent issue of a nursing research journal (e.g., *Nursing Research, Research in Nursing & Health, Journal of Advanced Nursing)*. Find the title of a study that you think is basic research and another that you think is applied research. Read the abstracts for these studies to see if you can determine whether your original supposition was correct.
7. Apply the questions from Box 1.1 of the textbook (available as a Word document in the Toolkit on the accompanying CD-ROM) to one or both of the following studies:
   - Ryan, S., Hassell, A. B., Lewis, M., & Farrell, A. (2006). Impact of a rheumatology expert nurse on the wellbeing of patients attending a drug monitoring clinic. *Journal of Advanced Nursing, 53*(3), 277–286.
   - Bailey, P., Jones, L., & Way, D. (2006). Family physician/nurse practitioner: Stories of collaboration. *Journal of Advanced Nursing, 53*(4), 381–391.

■ C. Application Exercises

EXERCISE 1: STUDY IN APPENDIX A

Read the abstract and introduction to the report by Hill and colleagues ("Chronically ill rural women") in Appendix A. Then answer the following questions:

Questions of Fact

a. Is this report an example of "disciplined research"?
b. Is this a qualitative or quantitative study?
c. What is the underlying paradigm of the study?
d. Does the study involve the collection of empirical evidence?
e. Is the purpose of this study identification, description, exploration, explanation, and/or prediction and control?
f. Is this study applied or basic research?
g. Does this study address an EBP-focused question, such as a question about treatment, diagnosis, prognosis, etc.?

Questions for Discussion

a. How relevant is this study to the actual practice of nursing?
b. Could this study have been conducted as *either* a quantitative or qualitative study? Why or why not?

EXERCISE 2: STUDY IN APPENDIX B

Read the abstract and introduction to the report by Rew ("Homeless youth") in Appendix B. Then answer the following questions:

Questions of Fact

a. Is this report an example of "disciplined research"?
b. Is this a qualitative or quantitative study?
c. What is the underlying paradigm of the research?
d. Does the study involve the collection of empirical evidence?
e. Is the purpose of this study identification, description, exploration, explanation, and/or prediction and control?
f. Is this study applied or basic research?
g. Does this study address an EBP-focused question, such as a question about treatment, diagnosis, prognosis, etc.?

Questions for Discussion

a. How relevant is this study to the actual practice of nursing?
b. Could this study have been conducted as *either* a quantitative or qualitative study? Why or why not?
c. Which of the two studies cited in these exercises (the one in Appendix A or Appendix B) is of greater interest and/or relevance to you personally? Why?

Note: Appendix M contains answers to selected exercises from each chapter in this resource manual. It also includes the solutions to the crossword puzzles.

■ D. The Toolkit

For Chapter 1, the Toolkit on the CD-ROM provided with this Resource Manual contains the following:

- Questions for a Preliminary Overview of a Research Report (Box 1.1 of the textbook)*

---

*In the Toolkit lists throughout this Resource Manual, items are either identified by their textbook reference or do not appear in the textbook at all.

CHAPTER 2

Translating Research Evidence Into Nursing Practice: Evidence-Based Nursing

■ A. Crossword Puzzle

Complete the crossword puzzle below, which uses terms and concepts presented in Chapter 2. (Puzzles may be removed for easier viewing.)

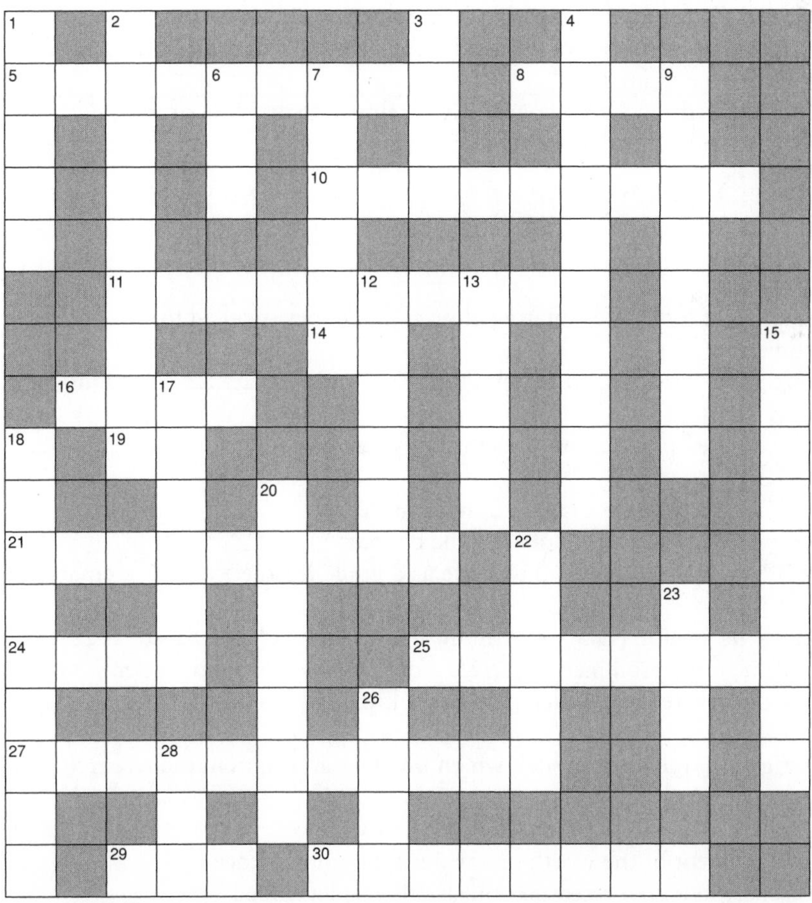

ACROSS

5. A clinical practice ________ based on rigorous systematic evidence is an important tool for evidence-based care.
8. An important database for finding clinical guidelines (UK-based) is the ________ database.
10. Environmental readiness for an innovation often involves assessments of implementation ________ in a given setting.
11. ________ reviews of RCTs are at the pinnacle of most evidence hierarchies.
14. The Cochrane Collaboration is a cornerstone of the EBP _ _ vement.
16 _ _ _ _ ground questions are ones that can be answered based on current best research evidence.
19. Are case reports of individual patients at the top of the evidence hierarchy?
21. Evidence-based decision making should integrate best research evidence with clinical ________.
24. Researchers can compute indices called ________ as estimates of the absolute magnitude of an effect.
25. ________ questions are foundational questions for a clinical problem, answers to which may be found, for example, in textbooks (abbr.).
27. In assessing whether an innovation is appropriate in a given setting, a ________ ratio should be estimated.
29. An index called ________ concerns the relative magnitude of an effect.
30. There is abundant evidence that nurses face several ________ to using research in their practice.

DOWN

1. An important tool for evaluating clinical guidelines is called the ________ instrument.
2. An important model for research utilization is called ________ of Innovations Theory.
3. Evidence-based practice involves the conscientious use of current ________ evidence.
4. CAT is an acronym for ________ appraised topic.
6. Acronym describing main focus of the chapter
7. RU/EBP models are intended to serve as a guide for the _ _ _ _ _ _ entation of an innovation.
9. Research utilization is narrower in meaning than evidence-based ________.
12. Two of the most prominent ________ of EBP are Iowa and Stetler.
13. In a systematic review, evidence from multiple studies on the same ________ is integrated.
15. One trigger in the Iowa model, which involves an origin in the research literature, is called ________-focused.
17. The originator of a prominent theory on how new ideas are diffused and adopted.
18. An arrangement of the worth of various types of evidence
20. The earliest model of research utilization was developed by _______.

22. Acronym for the 5-component scheme for asking EBP questions
23. One trigger in the Iowa model, stemming from practice issues, is called ____-focused (abbr.).
26. A statistical method of combining evidence in a systematic review is ____-analysis.
28. The type of study at the second level of an evidence hierarchy focusing on intervention questions (abbr. and backwards)

■ B. Study Questions

1. Identify the factors in your own practice setting that you think facilitate or inhibit research utilization and evidence-based practice (or, in an educational setting, the factors that promote or inhibit a climate in which RU/EBP is valued).
2. Think about a nursing procedure that you have learned. What is the basis for this procedure? Determine whether the procedure is based on scientific evidence indicating that the procedure is effective. If it is not based on scientific evidence, on what is it based, and why do you think scientific evidence was not used?
3. Read either Brett's (1987) article regarding the adoption of 14 nursing innovations ("Use of nursing practice research findings," *Nursing Research, 36*, pp. 344–349) or the more recent (1990) replication study based on the same 14 innovations by Coyle and Sokop ("Innovation adoption behavior among nurses," *Nursing Research, 39*, pp. 176–180). For each of the 14 innovations, indicate whether you are aware of the findings, are persuaded that the findings should be used, use the findings sometimes in a clinical situation, or use the findings always in a clinical situation.
4. Read one of the following articles and identify the steps of the Iowa model (or an alternative model of EBP) that are represented in the RU/EBP projects described.
   a. Clarke, H. F., Bradley, C., Whytock, S., Handfield, S., van der Wal, R., & Gundry, S. (2005). Pressure ulcers: Implementation of evidence-based nursing practice. *Journal of Advanced Nursing, 49*(6), 578–590.
   b. Robinson, C. B., Fritch, M., Hullett, L., Peterson, M. A., Siikena, S., Theuninck, L., & Timmer, K. (2000). Development of a protocol to prevent opioid-induced constipation with cancer: A research utilization project. *Clinical Journal of Oncology Nursing, 4*, 79–84.
   c. Samselle, C. M., Wyman, J. F., Thomas, K. K., Newman, D. K., Gray, M., Dougherty, M., & Burns, P. A. (2000). Continence for women: Evaluation of AWHONN's third research utilization project. *Journal of Obstetric, Gynecologic, & Neonatal Nursing, 29*, 9–17.
5. Select a clinical study from the nursing research literature. Using the criteria indicated in Box 2.1 of the textbook (available as a Word document in the Toolkit in the accompanying CD-ROM), assess the potential for using the study results in your practice setting. If the study meets the three major classes of criteria for implementation potential, develop a utilization plan.

■ C. Application Exercises

EXERCISE 1: STUDY IN APPENDIX C

Read the abstract and introduction to the report by Wang and Chan ("Culturally tailored diabetes education") in Appendix C. Then answer the following questions:

Questions of Fact

a. Is this report an example of "disciplined research"?
b. Is this a qualitative or quantitative study?
c. What is the underlying paradigm of the study?
d. Does the study involve the collection of empirical evidence?
e. Does this study address an EBP-focused question, such as a question about treatment, diagnosis, prognosis, etc.?
f. Is this an example of pre-appraised evidence?

Questions for Discussion

a. Could a clinical practice guideline be developed based on the findings from this study? Why or why not?
b. Where on the evidence hierarchy (Figure 2.1 of the textbook) do you think this study would fall?
c. Articulate a clinical foreground question that this study could be used to address, and identify components of your question (e.g., population, intervention, etc.).
d. If you read this study and found it relevant to your practice setting, and then used information in it to plan an EBP project, would you say the project had a knowledge-focused or problem-focused trigger?
e. What steps would you need to undertake if you were interested in using this study as a basis for an EBP project in your own practice setting?

EXERCISE 2: STUDY IN APPENDIX F

Read the abstract and introduction to the report by Giddings ("Health disparities") in Appendix F. Then answer the following questions:

Questions of Fact

a. Is this report an example of "disciplined research"?
b. Is this a qualitative or quantitative study?
c. What is the underlying paradigm of the research?
d. Does the study involve the collection of empirical evidence?
e. Does this study address an EBP-focused question, such as a question about treatment, diagnosis, prognosis, etc.?
f. Is this an example of pre-appraised evidence?

Questions for Discussion

a. Could a clinical practice guideline be developed based on the findings from this study? Why or why not?
b. Where on the evidence hierarchy (Figure 2.1 of the textbook) do you think this study would fall?
c. Articulate a clinical foreground question that this study could be used to address, and identify components of your question (e.g., population, intervention, etc.).
d. If you read this study and found it relevant to your practice setting, and then used information in it to plan an EBP project, would you say the project had a knowledge-focused or problem-focused trigger?
e. What steps would you need to undertake if you were interested in using this study as a basis for an EBP project in your own practice setting?

■ D. The Toolkit

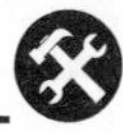

For Chapter 2, the Toolkit on the CD-ROM provided with this Resource Manual contains the following:

- **Question Templates for Selected Clinical Foreground Questions** (Table 2.1 of the textbook)
- Questions for Appraising the Evidence (Box 2.1 of the textbook)
- Criteria for Evaluating the Implementation Potential of an Innovation Under Scrutiny (Box 2.2 of the textbook)

CHAPTER 3

Generating Evidence: Key Concepts and Steps in Qualitative and Quantitative Research

■ A. Crossword Puzzle

Complete the crossword puzzle below, which uses terms and concepts presented in Chapter 3. (Puzzles may be removed for easier viewing.)

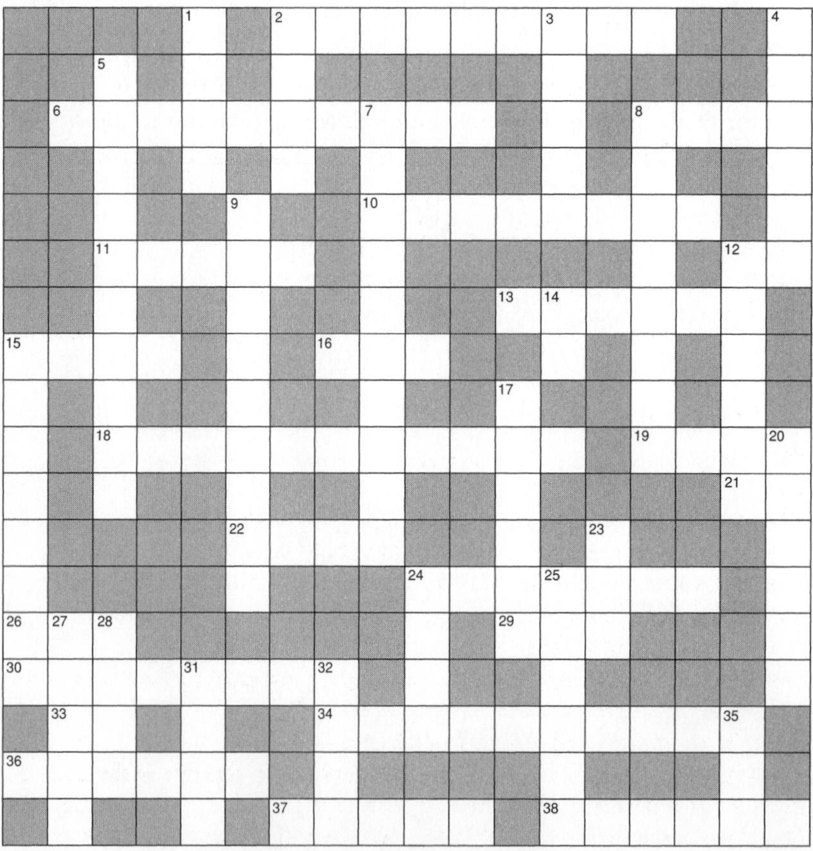

ACROSS

2. Another name for outcome variable is ________ variable.
6. An individual with whom a researcher must negotiate to gain entrée into a site
8. Two operationalizations of weight involve the pound system and the ________ system.
10. A step in experimental research involves the development of an intervention ________.
11. In "What is the effect of radon on health?" the independent variable is ________.
13. If the probability of a statistical test were .001, the results would be highly ________ (abbr.).
15. Pieces of information gathered in a study
16. Data that are in the exact same form as when they were collected are ________ data.
18. The ________ definition indicates how a variable will be measured or observed.
19. A variable that has only two values or categories (abbr.)
21. A systematic, abstract explanation of phenomena (first & last letter)
22. A type of fieldwork done to enhance the value of a study for practicing nurses (abbr.)
24. The type of tests used by quantitative researchers to assess the reliability of their results (abbr.)
26. One ________ offered in the textbook was to always select a research problem in which there is a strong personal interest.
29. Some qualitative researchers do not undertake an up-front ________ review to avoid having their conceptualization influenced by the work of others (abbr.)
30. The type of design used in qualitative studies
33. A bond or connection between phenomena (first two letters)
34. The type of research that involved an intervention
36. Technical terminology that often makes research reports difficult to read
37. A research investigation
38. The procedure of translating data into numeric values (backwards!)

DOWN

1. The qualitative research tradition that focuses on lived experiences (abbr.)
2. In "What is the effect of diet on cancer?" the independent variable
3. The qualitative tradition that focuses on the study of cultures (abbr.)
4. In a qualitative analysis, researchers search for these (backwards).
5. A principle used to decide when to stop sampling in a qualitative study
7. The entire aggregate of units in which a researcher is interested
8. A qualitative tradition that focuses on social psychological processes within a social setting is ________ theory.
9. A somewhat more complex abstraction than a concept
12. If the independent variable is the cause, the dependent variable is the ________.
14. The cause of another variable (acronym)
15. A variable with a finite number of values between two points

17. A relationship in which one variable directly results in changes in another is a ________ relationship.
20. Quantitative researchers formulate ________, which state expectations about how variables are related (abbr.).
23. Quantitative researchers develop a knowledge context by doing a ________ review early in the project (abbr.).
24. The first ________ in a project involves formulating a research problem.
25. In terms of ________, the independent variable occurs before the dependent variable.
27. The type of format used to structure most research reports (acronym)
28. The type of reviewers who typically make recommendations about reports published in journals
31. A sample that is representative of the population is a ________ sample.
32. Quantitative researchers use a statistics ________ to analyze their data and test their hypotheses.
35. A relationship expresses a bond between at least ________ variables.

■ B. Study Questions

1. Suggest operational definitions for the following concepts.
   a. Stress
   b. Prematurity of infants
   c. Fatigue
   d. Pain
   e. Obesity
   f. Prolonged labor
   g. Smoking behavior

2. In each of the following research questions, identify the independent and dependent variables.
   a. Does assertiveness training improve the effectiveness of psychiatric nurses?
   b. Does the postural positioning of patients affect their respiratory function?
   c. Is the psychological well-being of patients affected by the amount of touch received from nursing staff?
   d. Is the incidence of decubitus reduced by more frequent turnings of patients?
   e. Are people who were abused as children more likely than others to abuse their own children?
   f. Is tolerance for pain related to a patient's age and gender?
   g. Are the number of prenatal visits of pregnant women associated with labor and delivery outcomes?
   h. Are levels of depression higher among children who experience the death of a sibling than among other children?
   i. Is compliance with a medical regimen higher among women than among men?

j. Does participating in a support group enhance coping among family caregivers of AIDS patients?
k. Is hearing acuity of the elderly affected by the time of day?
l. Does home birth affect the parents' satisfaction with the childbirth experience?
m. Does a neutropenic diet in the outpatient setting decrease the positive blood cultures associated with chemotherapy-induced neutropenia?

3. Below is a list of variables. For each, think of a research question for which the variable would be the independent variable, and a second for which it would be the dependent variable. For example, take the variable "birth weight of infants." We might ask, "Does the age of the mother affect the birth weight of her infant?" (dependent variable). Alternatively, our research question might be, "Does the birth weight of infants (independent variable) affect their sensorimotor development at 6 months of age?" HINT: For the dependent variable problem, ask yourself, What factors might affect, influence, or cause this variable? For the independent variable, ask yourself, What factors does this variable influence, cause, or affect?
   a. Body temperature
   b. Amount of sleep
   c. Frequency of practicing breast self-examination
   d. Level of hopefulness in cancer patients
   e. Stress among victims of domestic violence
4. Look at the table of contents of a recent issue of *Nursing Research* (available at *http://www.nursingcenter.com/library*) or *Research in Nursing & Health* (available at *http://www.interscience.wiley.com*). Pick out a study title (not looking at the abstract) that implies that a relationship between variables was studied. Indicate what you think the independent and dependent variable might be, and what the title suggests about the nature of the relationship (i.e., causal or not).
5. Describe what is wrong with the following statements:
   a. Opitz's experimental study was conducted within the ethnographic tradition.
   b. Brusser's experimental study examined the effect of relaxation therapy (the dependent variable) on pain (the independent variable) in cancer patients.
   c. Ball's grounded theory study of the caregiving process for caretakers of patients with dementia controlled for the confounding variables of patient age and gender.
   d. In Walsh's phenomenological study of the meaning of futility among AIDS patients, subjects received an intervention designed to sustain hope.
   e. In her experimental study, Gabris developed her data collection plan after she introduced her intervention to a group of patients.
6. Read the following report of a qualitative study and identify segments of *raw data*. Describe the effect that removal of the raw data would have on the report.
   - Sullivan-Boyai, S., et al. (2006). Reflections on parenting young children with type 1 diabetes. *MCN: The American Journal of Maternal/Child Nursing, 31*, 24–31.
7. Apply the questions from Box 3.3 of the textbook (available as a Word document in the Toolkit on the accompanying CD-ROM) to one or both of the following studies:

a. Thompson, G., McClement, S., & Daeninck, P. (2006). Nurses' perceptions of quality end-of-life care on an acute medical ward. *Journal of Advanced Nursing, 5392,* 169–177.
b. Gary, R. (2006). Self-care practices in women with diastolic heart failure. *Heart & Lung, 35*(1), 9–19.

▪ C. Application Exercises

EXERCISE 1: STUDY IN APPENDIX E

Read the abstract and introduction (before the methods section) to the report by Loeb ("Older men's health") in Appendix E. Then answer the following questions:

Questions of Fact

a. Who was the researcher and what are her credentials and affiliation?
b. Who were the study participants?
c. What is the independent variable (or variables) in this study? Is this variable *inherently* an independent variable?
d. What is the dependent variable (or variables) in this study? Is this variable *inherently* a dependent variable?
e. Did the introduction actually use the term "independent variable" or "dependent variable"?
f. Were the data in this study quantitative or qualitative?
g. Were any relationships under investigation? What type of relationship?
h. Is this an experimental or nonexperimental study?
i. Was there any intervention? If so, what is it?
j. Did the study involve statistical analysis of data? Did it involve the qualitative analysis of data?
k. Does the report follow the IMRAD format?

Questions for Discussion

a. How relevant is this study to the actual practice of nursing?
b. Could this study have been conducted as *either* a quantitative or qualitative study? Why or why not?
c. How good a job did the researcher do in summarizing her study in the abstract?
d. How long do you estimate it took for this study to be completed?

EXERCISE 2: STUDY IN APPENDIX D

Read the abstract and introduction to the report by Beck ("Post-traumatic stress disorder") in Appendix D. Then answer the following questions:

Questions of Fact

a. Who was the researcher and what are her credentials and affiliation?
b. Did the researcher receive funding that supported this research?
c. Who were the study participants?
d. What were the key concepts in this study?
e. Were the data in this study quantitative or qualitative?
f. In what type of setting did the study take place?
g. Were any relationships under investigation?
h. Could the study be described as an ethnographic, phenomenological, or grounded theory study?
i. Is this an experimental or nonexperimental study?
j. Does the report describe an intervention? If so, what is it?
k. Did the report provide information about how key study variables were measured?
l. Did the study involve statistical analysis of data? Did the study involve qualitative analysis of data?
m. Does the report follow the IMRAD format?

Questions for Discussion

a. How relevant is this study to the actual practice of nursing?
b. Could this study have been conducted as *either* a quantitative or qualitative study? Why or why not?
c. How good a job did the researcher do in summarizing her study in the abstract?
d. How long do you estimate it took for this study to be completed?
e. Which of the two studies cited in these exercises (the one in Appendix E or Appendix D) is of greater interest and/or relevance to you personally? Why?

EXERCISE 3: TRANSLATION EXERCISE

Below is an example of a summary of a fictitious study, written in the style typically found in research journal articles. Terms that can be looked up in the glossary of the textbook are underlined. Then, a "translation" of this summary is presented, recasting the research information into language that is more digestible. Study this example and then use it as a model for "translating" the abstracts of one of the studies in the appendices of this book.

Summary of Fictitious Study. The potentially negative sequelae of having an abortion on the psychological adjustment of adolescents have not been adequately studied. The present study sought to determine whether alternative pregnancy resolution decisions have different long-term effects on the psychological functioning of young women.

Three groups of low-income pregnant teenagers attending an inner-city clinic were the subjects in this study: Those who delivered and kept the baby; those who delivered and relinquished the baby for adoption; and those who had an abortion. There were 25 subjects in each group. The study instruments included a self-administered questionnaire and a battery of psychological tests measuring depression, anxiety, and psychosomatic symptoms. The instruments were administered upon entry into the study (when the subjects first came to the clinic) and then 1 year after termination of the pregnancy.

The data were analyzed using analysis of variance (ANOVA). The ANOVA tests indicated that the three groups did not differ significantly in terms of depression, anxiety, or psychosomatic symptoms at the initial testing. At the posttest, however, the abortion group had significantly higher scores on the depression scale, and these girls were significantly more likely than the two delivery groups to report severe tension headaches. There were no significant differences on any of the dependent variables for the two delivery groups.

The results of this study suggest that young women who elect to have an abortion may experience a number of long-term negative consequences. It would appear that appropriate efforts should be made to follow-up abortion patients to determine their need for suitable treatment.

Translated Version. As researchers, we wondered whether young women who had an abortion had any emotional problems in the long run. It seemed to us that not enough research had been done to know whether any psychological harm resulted from an abortion.

We decided to study this question ourselves by comparing the experiences of three types of teenager who became pregnant—first, girls who delivered and kept their babies; second, those who delivered the babies but gave them up for adoption; and third, those who elected to have an abortion. All teenagers in the sample were poor, and all were patients at an inner-city clinic. Altogether, we studied 75 girls—25 in each of the three groups. We evaluated the teenagers' emotional states by asking them to fill out a questionnaire and to take several psychological tests. These tests allowed us to assess things such as the girls' degree of depression and anxiety and whether they had any complaints of a psychosomatic nature. We asked them to fill out the forms twice: once when they came into the clinic, and then again a year after the abortion or the delivery.

We learned that the three groups of teenagers looked pretty much alike in terms of their emotional states when they first filled out the forms. But when we compared how the three groups looked a year later, we found that the teenagers who had abortions were more depressed and were more likely to say they had severe tension headaches than teenagers in the other two groups. The teenagers who kept their babies and those who gave their babies up for adoption looked pretty similar 1 year after their babies were born, at least in terms of depression, anxiety, and psychosomatic complaints.

Thus, it seems that we might be right in having some concerns about the emotional effects of having an abortion. Nurses should be aware of these long-term emotional effects, and it even may be advisable to institute some type of follow-up procedure to find out if these young women need additional help.

■ D. The Toolkit

For Chapter 3, the Toolkit on the CD-ROM provided with this Resource Manual contains the following:

- Additional Questions for a Preliminary Review of a Study (Box 3.3 of the textbook)

PART 2

Conceptualizing a Study to Generate Evidence for Nursing

CHAPTER 4

Conceptualizing Research Problems, Research Questions, and Hypotheses

■ A. Crossword Puzzle

Complete the crossword puzzle below, which uses terms and concepts presented in Chapter 4. (Puzzles may be removed for easier viewing.)

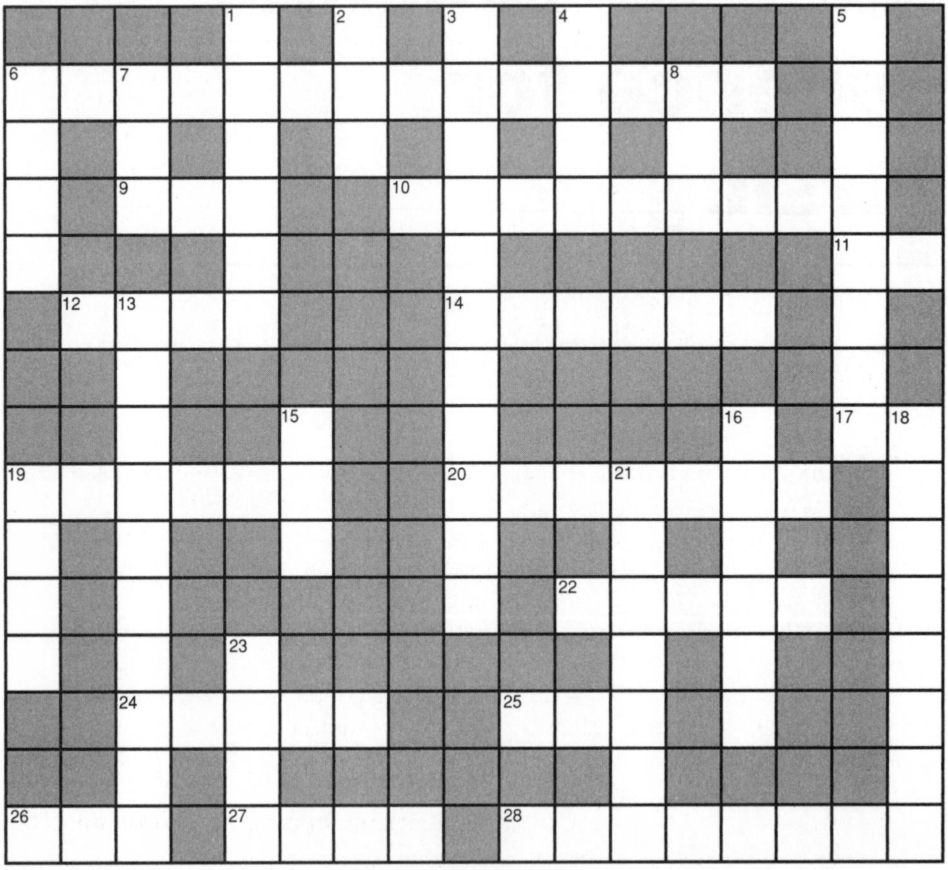

ACROSS

6. A hypothesis in which the specific nature of the predicted relationship is not stipulated.
9. A statement of purpose in a quantitative study indicates the key study variables and the ________ of interest (abbr.).
10. Researchers express the disturbing situation in need of study in their problem ________.
11. A hypothesis stipulates the expected relationship between an ________ and a DV (abbr.).
12. One phrase that indicates the relational aspect of a hypothesis is: ________ than.
14. A topic for a research problem might arise from global ________ or political issues.
17. The name of a popular television series based on a hospital drama.
19. One source of research problems, especially for hypothesis-testing research.
20. A hypothesis with two or more independent and/or dependent variables.
22. The results of hypothesis testing never constitute ________ that the hypotheses are or are not correct.
24. The purpose of a study is often conveyed through the judicious choice of ________.
25. A hypothesis must always involve at least ________ variables.
26. In the question, "What is the effect of daily exercise on mood and weight?" mood and weight are the ________ (acronym).
27. A statement of purpose indicating that the intent of the study was to *prove* or *demonstrate* something suggests a ________.
28. A research ________ is what researchers wish to answer through systematic study.

DOWN

1. A hypothesis with one independent and one dependent variable.
2. The *actual* hypothesis of an investigator is the ________ hypothesis (abbr.).
3. Another name for *null* hypothesis
4. A practical consideration in assessing feasibility concerns the ________ of undertaking the study.
5. In complex hypotheses, there are ________ independent or dependent variables.
6. The hypothesis that posits no relationship between variables.
7. In the research question, "Does a mid-afternoon ________ improve evening mood state in the elderly?" the independent variable
8. A desired accomplishment in conducting a study.
13. The researcher's overall goals of undertaking a study.
15. A statement of the researcher's prediction about variables in the study (abbr.).
16. The study hypotheses should be stated ________ collecting the research data.
18. Hypotheses must predict a ________ between the independent and dependent variables (abbr.).
19. Hypotheses are typically put to a statistical ________.
21. A statement of ________ is a declaration that captures the general direction of the inquiry.
23. A research ________ is an enigmatic or troubling condition (abbr.)

■ B. Study Questions

1. Below is a list of general topics that could be investigated. Develop at least one research question for each, making sure that some are questions that could be addressed through qualitative research and others are ones that could be addressed through quantitative research. It will probably be helpful to use the question template in the accompanying Toolkit. (HINT: For quantitative research questions, think of these concepts as potential independent or dependent variables, then ask, "What might cause or affect this variable?" and "What might be the consequences or effects of this variable?" This should lead to some ideas for research questions.)
   a. Patient comfort
   b. Psychiatric patients' readmission rates
   c. Anxiety in hospitalized children
   d. Elevated blood pressure
   e. Incidence of sexually transmitted diseases (STDs)
   f. Patient cooperativeness in the recovery room
   g. Caregiver stress
   h. Mother–infant bonding
   i. Menstrual irregularities
2. Below are five nondirectional hypotheses. Restate each one as a directional hypothesis.
   a. Tactile stimulation is associated with comparable physiologic arousal as verbal stimulation among infants with congenital heart disease.
   b. The risk for hypoglycemia in term newborns is related to the infant's birth weight.
   c. The use of isotonic sodium chloride solution before endotracheal suctioning is related to oxygen saturation.
   d. Fluid balance is related to degree of success in weaning older adults from mechanical ventilation.
   e. Nurses administer the same amount of narcotic analgesics to male and female patients.
3. Below are five simple hypotheses. Change each one to a complex hypothesis by adding either a dependent or independent variable.
   a. First-time blood donors experience greater stress during the donation than donors who have given blood previously.
   b. Nurses who initiate more conversation with patients are rated as more effective in their nursing care by patients than those who initiate less conversation.
   c. Surgical patients who give high ratings to the informativeness of nursing communications experience less preoperative stress than do patients who give low ratings.
   d. Appendectomy patients whose peritoneum is drained with a Jackson-Pratt drain will experience more peritoneal infection than patients who are not drained.
   e. Women who give birth by cesarean delivery are more likely to experience postpartum depression than women who give birth vaginally.
4. In study questions 2 and 3 above, 10 research hypotheses were provided. Identify the independent and dependent variables in each.

5. Below are five statements that are *not* research hypotheses as currently stated. Suggest modifications to these statements that would make them testable research hypotheses.
   a. Relaxation therapy is effective in reducing hypertension.
   b. The use of bilingual health care staff produces high utilization rates of health care facilities by ethnic minorities.
   c. Nursing students are affected in their choice of clinical specialization by interactions with nursing faculty.
   d. Sexually active teenagers have a high rate of using male methods of contraception.
   e. In-use intravenous solutions become contaminated within 48 hours.
6. Read the introduction of one of the following reports. Use the critiquing guidelines in Box 4.3 of the textbook (available as a Word document in the Toolkit) to assess the study's problem statement, purpose statement, research questions, and/or hypotheses:
   - Jurgens, C. Y. (2006). Somatic awareness, uncertainty, and delay in care-seeking in acute heart failure. *Research in Nursing & Health, 29*(2), 74–86.
   - Strang, V. R., et al. (2006). Family caregivers and transition to long-term care. *Clinical Nursing Research, 15*(1), 27–45.

■ C. Application Exercises

EXERCISE 1: STUDY IN APPENDIX A

Read the abstract and introduction to the report by Hill and colleagues ("Chronically ill rural women") in Appendix A. Then answer the following questions:

Questions of Fact

a. In which paragraph of this report is the research problem stated?
b. Does this report present a statement of purpose? If so, what *verb* do the researchers use in the statement, and is that verb consistent with the type of research that was undertaken?
c. Does the report specify a research question? If so, was it well-stated? If not, state what the question was.
d. Does the report specify hypotheses? If there are hypotheses, were they appropriately worded? Are they directional or nondirectional? Simple or complex? Research or null?
e. If no hypotheses were stated, what would one be?
f. Were hypotheses tested?

Questions for Discussion

a. Did the researchers do an adequate job of describing the research problem? Describe in two or three sentences what the problem is.
b. Comment on the significance of the study's research problem for nursing.
c. Did the researchers do an adequate job of explaining the study purpose, research questions, and/or hypotheses?

EXERCISE 2: STUDY IN APPENDIX F

Read the abstract and introduction to the report by Giddings ("Health disparities") in Appendix F. Then answer the following questions:

Questions of Fact

a. In which paragraph of this report is the research problem stated?
b. Does this report present a statement of purpose? If so, what *verb* do the researchers use in the statement, and is that verb consistent with the type of research that was undertaken?
c. Does the report specify a research question? If so, was it well-stated? If not, state what the question was.
d. Does the report specify hypotheses? If there are hypotheses, were they appropriately worded? Are they directional or nondirectional? Simple or complex? Research or null?
e. Were hypotheses tested?

Questions for Discussion

a. Did the researcher do an adequate job of describing the research problem? Describe in two or three sentences what the problem is.
b. Comment on the significance of the study's research problem for nursing.
c. Did the researcher do an adequate job of explaining the study purpose, research questions, and/or hypotheses?

■ D. The Toolkit

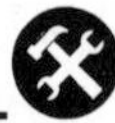

For Chapter 4, the Toolkit on the CD-ROM provided with this Resource Manual contains the following:

- Research Question Templates for Selected Clinical Problems
- Worksheet: Key Components of a Problem Statement
- Guidelines for Critiquing Research Problems, Research Questions, and Hypotheses (Box 4.3 of the textbook)

CHAPTER 5

Finding and Critiquing Evidence: Research Literature Reviews

■ A. Crossword Puzzle

Complete the crossword puzzle below, which uses terms and concepts presented in Chapter 5. (Puzzles may be removed for easier viewing.)

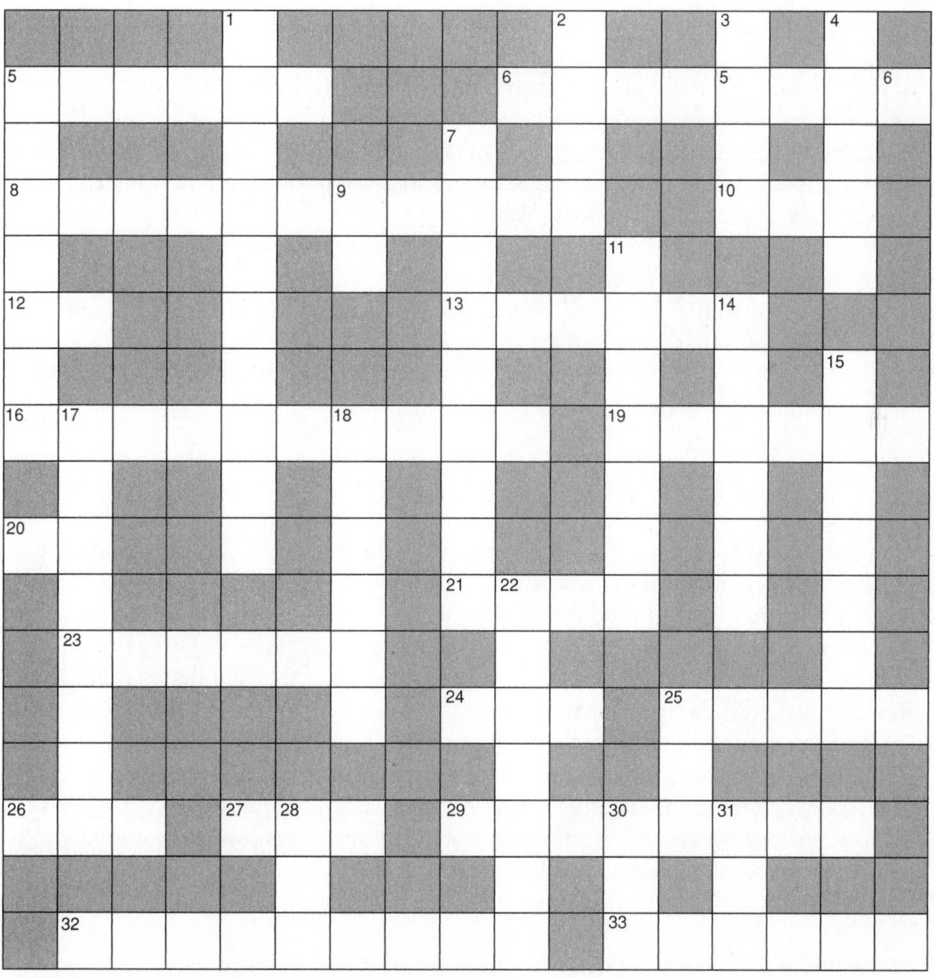

ACROSS

5. A good way to organize information when doing a complex literature review is to use one or more ________.
6. A careful appraisal of the strengths and weaknesses of a study
8. A search strategy that involves finding a pivotal early study and then searching for subsequent citations to it is the ________ approach.
10. A common abbreviation for "literature"
12. In a Results Matrix, the columns could be the ________s (acronym).
13. The most important bibliographic database for nurses
16. The matrix to record assessments about prior studies is the ________ matrix.
19. The MEDLINE database can be accessed for free through ________.
20. A Boolean operator
21. In summarizing the literature, it is important to point out the ________ in the research literature that suggest the need for further research (backwards!).
23. If a researcher has been prominent in an area, it is useful to do a(n)________search.
24. In doing a computerized search, a match between a bibliographic entry and your search criteria is sometimes called a "________."
25. In most databases, there are "wildcard codes" that can be used to extend and search for truncated ________.
26. A written lit ________ usually appears in the introduction of a research report (abbr.).
27. It is wise to ________ your search activities in a log book or a notebook to avoid unnecessary duplication of effort (abbr.).
29. The Cochrane ________ of Systematic Reviews is an excellent resource for locating earlier research reviews (secondary sources).
32. Descriptions of studies prepared by someone other than the investigators are ________ sources.
33. A ________ system that categorizes results in a systematic fashion is a good tool for better organizing research results.

DOWN

1. Qualitative researchers do not all agree about whether the ________ should be reviewed before undertaking a study.
2. Research reports with limited distribution is sometimes called the ________ literature.
3. A major resource for finding research reports are ________ databases (abbr.).
4. Reviewers should paraphrase and avoid a ________ from the literature if possible.
5. A very important bibliographic database for health care professionals
7. Research literature reviews contain few (if any) clinical ________.
9. In a Results Matrix, the columns could be the ________s (acronym).
11. A mechanism through which computer software translates topics into appropriate subject terms for a computerized literature search.
14. Literature searches can be done on one's own or with the assistance of a(n) ________ (abbr.).
15. When doing a database search, one often begins with one or more ________.

17. In launching a search, it might be best to conceptualize key ________s broadly, to avoid missing an important study.
18. An up-front literature review may not be undertaken by researchers doing a study within the grounded ________ tradition.
22. Findings from a report written by researchers who conducted a study are a ______ source in a research review.
25. The ________ of Knowledge is an important database, especially for its citation indexes.
28. In writing a review, reviewers should paraphrase information in their ________ words.
30. A search strategy sometimes called "footnote chasing" is the ________ approach (abbr.).
31. A Boolean operator

■ B. Study Questions

1. Below are several research questions. Indicate one or more keywords that you would use to begin a literature search on this topic.
   a. What is the lived experience of being a survivor of a suicide attempt?
   b. Does contingency contracting improve patient compliance with a treatment regimen?
   c. What is the decision-making process for a woman considering having an abortion?
   d. Is a special intervention for spinal cord injury patients effective in reducing the risk for pressure ulcers?
   e. Do children raised on vegetarian diets have different growth patterns than other children?
   f. What is the course of appetite loss among cancer patients undergoing chemotherapy?
   g. What is the effect of alcohol skin preparation before insulin injection on the incidence of local and systemic infection?
   h. Are bottle-fed babies introduced to solid foods sooner than breastfed babies?
2. Below are fictitious excerpts from research literature reviews. Each excerpt has a stylistic problem. Change each sentence to make it acceptable stylistically.
   a. Most elderly people do not eat a balanced diet.
   b. Patient characteristics have a significant impact on nursing workload.
   c. A child's conception of appropriate sick role behavior changes as the child grows older.
   d. Home birth poses many potential dangers.
   e. Multiple sclerosis results in considerable anxiety to the family of the patients.
   f. Studies have proved that most nurses prefer not to work the night shift.
   g. Life changes are the major cause of stress in adults.
   h. Stroke rehabilitation programs are most effective when they involve the patients' families.
   i. It has been proved that psychiatric outpatients have higher-than-average rates of accidental deaths and suicides.

Questions for Discussion

a. Did Swartz do an adequate job of explaining the problem and the study purpose?
b. Did she appear to do a thorough job in her search for relevant studies?

EXERCISE 3: STUDY IN APPENDIX G

Read the article by Forchuk and colleagues ("Postoperative arm massage") in Appendix G and use the critiquing guidelines for a quantitative research report in Box 5.2 of the textbook (also in the accompanying Toolkit) to answer as many questions as you can. Then read the critique of the study that is also included in Appendix G, making note of issues that are absent in your critique (or in ours!).

EXERCISE 4: STUDY IN APPENDIX H

Read the article by Walsh ("Traditional birth attendant practices") in Appendix H and use the critiquing guidelines for a qualitative research report in Box 5.3 of the textbook (also in the accompanying Toolkit) to answer as many questions as you can. Then read the critique of the study that is also included in Appendix H, making note of issues that are absent in your critique (or in ours!).

■ D. The Toolkit

For Chapter 5, the Toolkit on the CD-ROM provided with this Resource Manual contains the following:

- Guide to an Overall Critique of a Quantitative Research Report (Box 5.2 of the textbook)
- Guide to an Overall Critique of a Qualitative Research Report (Box 5.3 of the textbook)
- Guidelines for Critiquing Literature Reviews (Box 5.4 of the textbook)
- Literature Review Protocol (Figure 5.5 of the textbook)
- Methodologic Matrix for Recording Key Methodologic Features of Studies for a Literature Review (Figure 5.6 of the textbook)
- Two Results Matrices for Recording Key Findings for a Literature Review (Figure 5.7 of the textbook)
- Evaluation Matrix for Recording Strengths and Weaknesses of Studies for a Literature Review (Figure 5.8 of the textbook)
- Log of Literature Search Activities in Bibliographic Databases (not in textbook)

CHAPTER 6

Developing a Theoretical or Conceptual Context

■ A. Crossword Puzzle

Complete the crossword puzzle below, which uses terms and concepts presented in Chapter 6. (Puzzles may be removed for easier viewing.)

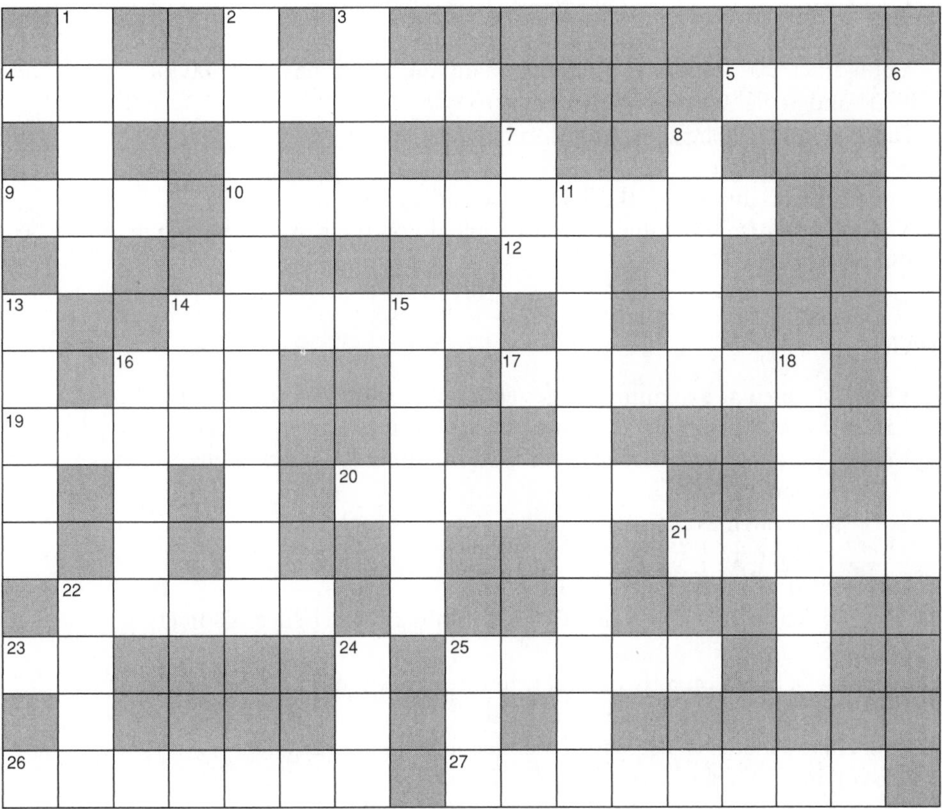

ACROSS

4. The conceptual underpinnings of a study
5. The originator of the Health Promotion Model (abbr.)
9. One of the four elements in conceptual models of nursing (abbr.)
10. Abstractions assembled because of their relevance to a core theme form a ________ model.
12. Psychiatric nurse researchers sometimes obtain funding from an institute within the National Institutes of Health (NIH) with the acronym NI __ __.
14. A theory that focuses on a piece of human experience is sometimes called ________ -range.
16. Another term for a schematic model is conceptual ________.
17. The originator of the Science of Unitary Human Beings
19. Roy's conceptualized the ________ Model of nursing (abbr.).
20. The originator of the Theory of Uncertainty in Illness
21. The originator of the Theory of Human Becoming
22. A schematic ________ is a mechanism for representing concepts with a minimal use of words.
23. A construct that is a key mediator in many models of health behavior, such as the HPM and Social Cognitive Theory (acronym)
25. The mutually beneficial relationship between theory and research has been described as ________ (abbr.).
26. One of the originators of the Theory of Stress and Coping
27. A model of nursing involving what people do on their own behalf to maintain health and well-being.

DOWN

1. A theory aimed at explaining large segments of behavior or other phenomena.
2. A theory that thoroughly accounts for or describes a phenomenon
3. A social psychological theory often used in nursing research is the Social ________ Theory (abbr.).
6. As classically defined, theories consist of concepts arranged in a logically interrelated ________ system.
7. The acronym for Pender's model
8. A theory that focuses on a single piece of human experience is sometimes called middle-________.
11. If a study is based on a theory, its framework is called the ________ framework.
13. The Stages of Change Model is also called the _ _ _ _ _ theoretical Model.
14. A schematic model is also called a conceptual ________.
15. The originator of the Conservation Model of nursing
16. Another name for a grand theory is a ________ theory.
18. A type of theory originally from another discipline used productively by nurse researchers
22. The originator of the Model of Self-Care (backwards!)
24. The originator of the social psychological theory focusing on a person's outcome expectations was _ _ _ dura.

25. Theories are built inductively from observations, which are often from disciplined ________ (abbr.).

■ B. Study Questions

1. Read some recent issues of a nursing research journal. Identify at least three different theories cited by nurse researchers in these research reports.
2. Choose one of the conceptual frameworks of nursing that were described in this chapter. Develop a research hypothesis based on this framework.
3. Select one of the research questions/problems listed below. Could the selected problem be developed within one of the models or theories discussed in this chapter? Defend your answer.
   a. How do men cope with a diagnosis of prostate cancer?
   b. What are the factors contributing to perceptions of fatigue among patients with congestive heart failure?
   c. What effect does the presence of the father in the delivery room have on the mother's satisfaction with the childbirth experience?
   d. The purpose of the study is to explore why some women fail to perform breast self-examination regularly.
   e. What are the factors that lead to poorer health among low-income children than higher-income children?
4. Suggest an important outcome that could be studied using the Health Promotion Model. Identify another theory described in this chapter that could be used to explain or predict the same outcome. Which theory or model do you think would do a better job? Why?
5. Read one of the following articles, and then apply the criteria in Box 6.2 (available as a Word document in the Toolkit on the accompanying CD-ROM) to make a judgment about whether the study involved a *test* of a model or theory.
   - Cook, A., Pierce, L., Hicks, B., & Steiner, C. (2006). Self-care needs of caregivers dealing with stroke. *Journal of Neuroscience Nursing, 38*(1), 31–36.
   - Davis, B. (2005). Mediators of the relationship between hope and well-being in older adults. *Clinical Nursing Research, 14*(3), 253–272.
   - Shyu, Y., Liang, J., Lu, J., & Wu, C. (2004). Environmental barriers and mobility in Taiwan: Is the Roy Adaptation Model applicable? *Nursing Science Quarterly, 17,* 165–170.
6. Read one of the following articles, and then apply the critiquing criteria in Box 6.3 (available as a Word document in the Toolkit on the accompanying CD-ROM) to evaluate the conceptual basis of the study.
   - Andenaes, R., Kalfoss, M., & Wahl, A. (2006). Coping and psychological distress in hospitalized patients with chronic obstructive pulmonary disease. *Heart & Lung, 35*(1), 46–57.
   - Montgomery, P., Tomkins, C., Forchuk, C., & French, S. (2006). Keeping close: Mothering with serious mental illness. *Journal of Advanced Nursing, 54*(1), 20–28.

- Russell, K., Perkins, S., Zollinger, T., & Champion, V. (2006). Sociocultural context of mammography screening use. *Oncology Nursing Forum, 33*(1), 105–112.

7. Read the following article, and then address these two questions: (a) What evidence does the researcher offer to substantiate that her grounded theory is a good fit with her data? and (b) To what extent is it clear or unclear in the article that symbolic interactionism was the theoretical underpinning of the study?
   - George, L. (2005). Lack of preparedness: Experiences of first-time mothers. *MCN: The American Journal of Maternal/Child Nursing, 30*(4), 251–255.

■ C. Application Exercises

EXERCISE 1: STUDY IN APPENDIX E

Read the abstract and introduction of the report by Loeb ("Older men's health") in Appendix E. Then answer the following questions:

Questions of Fact

a. Does Loeb's study involve a conceptual or theoretical framework? What is it called?
b. Is this framework one of the models of nursing cited in the textbook? Is it related to one of those models?
c. Does the report include a schematic model?
d. What are the key concepts in the model?
e. According to the framework, what factors *directly* affect the exercise of self-care agency?
f. According to the framework, what factors *directly* affect health outcomes? And what factors *indirectly* affect health outcomes?
g. Based on information in the abstract, did the study include a measure of a variable within the "Health-promoting self-care" construct block of the framework (Figure 1)?
h. Did the report present conceptual definitions of key concepts?
i. Did the report explicitly present hypotheses deduced from the framework?

Questions for Discussion

a. Do the research problem and hypotheses (if any) naturally flow from the framework? Does the link between the problem and the framework seem contrived?
b. Do you think any aspects of the research would have been different without the framework?
c. Could the study have been undertaken using Pender's Health Promotion Model as its framework (see Figure 6.1 in the textbook)? Why or why not?
d. Would you describe this study as a model-testing inquiry, or do you think the model was used more as an organizing framework?

EXERCISE 2: STUDY IN APPENDIX B

Read the abstract and introduction to the report by Rew ("Homeless youth") in Appendix B. Then answer the following questions:

Questions of Fact

a. Does Rew's study involve a conceptual or theoretical framework? What is it called?
b. Is this framework one of the models of nursing cited in the textbook? Is it related to one of those models?
c. Does the report include a schematic model?
d. What are the key concepts in the framework?
e. Did the report explicitly present hypotheses deduced from the framework?

Questions for Discussion

a. Does the research problem naturally flow from the framework? Does the link between the problem and the framework seem contrived?
b. Do you think any aspects of the research would have been different without the framework?
c. How helpful was the schematic model in communicating important features of the grounded theory?
d. On the basis of your own personal and professional experience, how would you characterize the resulting grounded theory, in terms of its descriptive power and accuracy?

■ D. The Toolkit

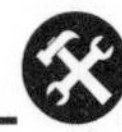

For Chapter 6, the Toolkit on the CD-ROM provided with this Resource Manual contains the following:

- Some Questions for a Preliminary Assessment of a Model of Theory (Box 6.1 of the textbook)
- Criteria to Determine Whether a Theory/Model Is Being Tested in a Study (Box 6.2 of the textbook)
- Guidelines for Critiquing Theoretical and Conceptual Frameworks (Box 6.3 of the textbook)

CHAPTER 7

Generating Research Evidence Ethically

■ A. Crossword Puzzle

Complete the crossword puzzle below, which uses terms and concepts presented in Chapter 7. (Puzzles may be removed for easier viewing.)

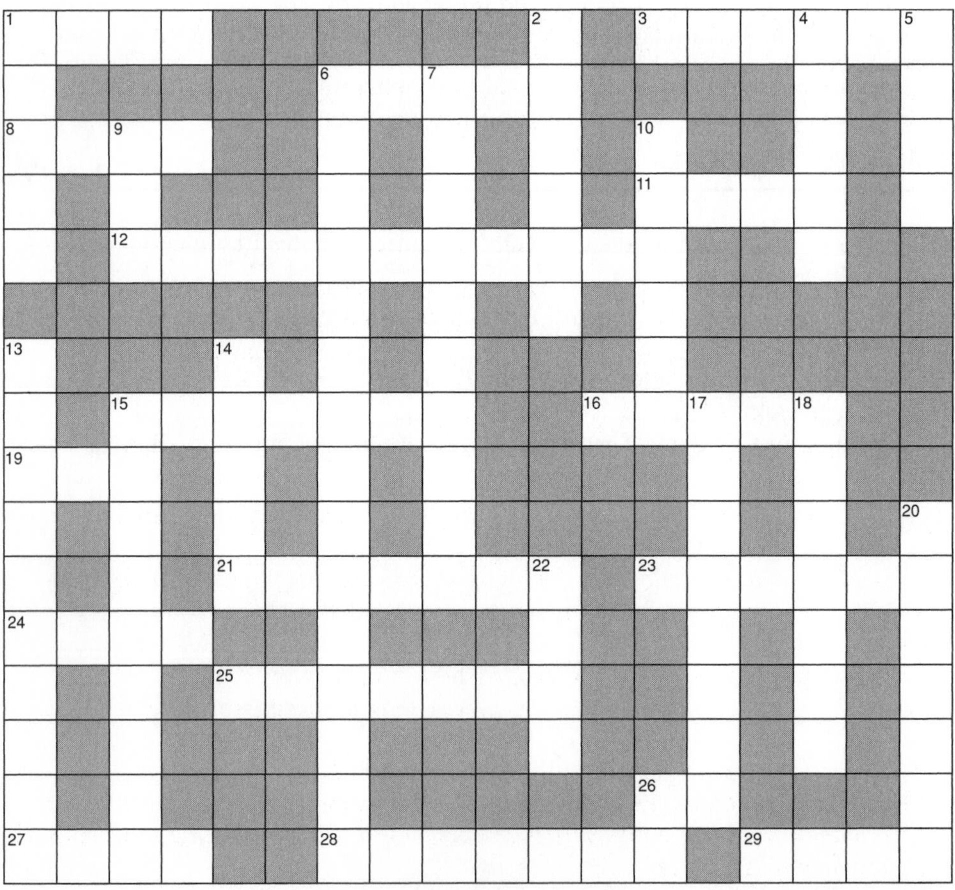

ACROSS

1. A fundamental right for study participants is freedom from ________.
3. Involves changing or omitting data or distorting results (abbr.)
6. Most disciplines have developed ________ of ethics.
8. Anonymity is a method of protecting this (abbr.).
11. Researchers should conduct a ________-benefit assessment.
12. A major ethical principle concerning maximizing benefits of research
15. The type of consent procedure that may be required in qualitative research
16. A young ________ is usually considered a vulnerable subject
19. Debriefings give participants an opportunity to ________ complaints.
21. A payment sometimes offered to participants as an incentive to take part in a study
23. Data collection without participants' awareness, using concealment
24. A procedure for collecting data without linking them to individual participants (abbr.)
25. The report that is the basis for ethical regulations for studies funded by the U.S. government
26. Numbers used in place of names to protect individual identities (abbr.)
27. Fraud and misrepresentations are examples of research ________ (abbr.).
28. A major ethical principle involves respect for human ________ (reversed!).
29. The return of a questionnaire is often assumed to demonstrate _ _ _ _ ied consent (abbr.).

DOWN

1. Legislation passed in the U.S. in 1996 concerning privacy (acronym)
2. Informal agreement to participate in a study (e.g., by minors)
4. The Declaration of Hel________ , the code of ethics of the World Medical Association
5. The ethical principle of *justice* includes the right to ________ treatment.
6. Participants' privacy is often protected by these procedures, even though the researchers know participants' identities.
7. People can make informed decisions about research participation when there is full ________.
9. A committee (in the U.S.) that reviews the ethical aspects of a study (acronym).
10. A situation in which private information is divulged is a ________ of confidentiality.
13. The appropriation of someone's ideas without proper credit
14. When short ________ are used to document consent, third-party witnesses are needed.
15. A vulnerable, institutionalized group with diminished autonomy
17. Most studies adhere to the practice of obtaining written ________ consent.
18. A conflict between the rights of participants and the demands for rigorous research creates an ethical ________.
20. Research that adheres to ________ guidelines is designed to protect participants' rights.

22. Mismanagement of _______ can result in a type of research misconduct.
26. Numbers used in place of names to protect individual identities (abbr.)

■ B. Study Questions

1. Below are brief descriptions of several research studies. Suggest some ethical dilemmas that are likely to emerge for each.
   a. A study of coping behaviors among rape victims
   b. An unobtrusive observational study of fathers' behaviors in the delivery room
   c. An interview study of the determinants of heroin addiction
   d. A study of dependence among mentally retarded children
   e. An investigation of verbal interactions among schizophrenic patients
   f. A study of the effects of a new drug on humans
   g. A study of the relationship between sleeping patterns and acting-out behaviors in hospitalized psychiatric patients
2. Evaluate the ethical aspects of one or more of the following studies using the critiquing guidelines in Box 7.3 of the textbook (available as a Word document in the Toolkit of the accompanying CD-ROM), paying special attention (if relevant) to the manner in which the subjects' heightened vulnerability was handled.
   - Hinck, S. (2004). The lived experience of the oldest-old rural adults. *Qualitative Health Research, 14*(6), 779–791.
   - McFarlane, J., Groff, J., O'Brien, J., & Watson, K. (2006). Behaviors of children following a randomized controlled treatment program for their abused mothers. *Issues in Comprehensive Pediatric Nursing, 28*(4), 195–211.
   - Wise, B. V. (2002). In their own words: The lived experience of pediatric liver transplantation. *Qualitative Health Research, 12*, 74–90.
   - Zieber, C., Hagen, B., Armstrong-Esther, C., & Alo, M. (2005). Pain and agitation in long-term care residents with dementia: Use of the Pittsburgh Agitation Scale. *International Journal of Palliative Nursing, 11*(2), 71–78.
3. In the textbook, two actual studies with ethical problems are described (the study of syphilis among black men and the study in which live cancer cells were injected in elderly patients). Identify which ethical principles were transgressed in these studies.
4. In the following study, the authors indicated that informed consent was not required because there was "no deviation from the standard of care or risk to the subjects" (p. 108). Skim the introduction and method section of this paper and comment on the researchers' decision to not obtain informed consent:
   - Byers, J. F., et al. (2006). A quasi-experimental trial on individualized, developmentally supportive family-centered care. *Journal of Obstetric, Gynecologic, & Neonatal Nursing, 35*(1), 105–115.
5. Below is a brief description of the ethical aspects of a fictitious study, followed by a critique. Do you agree with the critique? Can you add other comments relevant to the ethical dimensions of the study?

Fictitious Study. Fortune conducted an in-depth study of nursing home patients to determine whether their perceptions about personal control over decision making differed from the perceptions of the nursing staff. The investigator studied 25 nurse–patient dyads to determine whether there were differing perceptions and experiences regarding control over activities of daily living, such as arising, eating, and dressing. All of the nurses in the study were employed by the nursing home in which the patients resided. Because the nursing home had no IRB, and because Fortune's study was not funded by an organization that required IRB approval, the project was not formally reviewed. Fortune sought permission to conduct the study from the nursing home administrator. She also obtained the consent of the legal guardian or responsible family member of each patient. All study participants were fully informed about the nature of the study. The researcher assured the nurses and the legal guardians and family members of the patients of the confidentiality of the information and obtained their consent in writing. Data were gathered primarily through in-depth interviews with the patients and the nurses, at separate times. The researcher also observed interactions between the patients and nurses. The findings from the study showed that patients perceived that they had more control over all aspects of the activities of daily living (except eating) than the nurses perceived that they had. Excerpts from the interviews were used verbatim in the research report, but Fortune did not divulge the location of the nursing home, and she used fictitious names for all participants.

Critique. Fortune did a reasonably good job of adhering to basic ethical principles in the conduct of her research. She obtained written permission to conduct the study from the nursing home administrator, and she obtained informed consent from the nurse participants and the legal guardians or family members of the patients. The study participants were not put at risk in any way, and the patients who participated may actually have enjoyed the opportunity to have a conversation with the researcher. Fortune also took appropriate steps to maintain the confidentiality of participants. It is still unclear, however, whether the patients knowingly and willingly participated in the research. Nursing home residents are a vulnerable group. They may not have been aware of their right to refuse to be interviewed without fear of repercussion. Fortune could have enhanced the ethical aspects of the study by taking more vigorous steps to obtain the informed, voluntary consent of the nursing home residents or to exclude patients who could not reasonably be expected to understand the researcher's request. Given the vulnerability of the group, Fortune might also have established her own review panel composed of peers and interested lay people to review the ethical dimensions of her project. Debriefing sessions with study participants would also have been appropriate.

■ C. Application Exercises

EXERCISE 1: STUDY IN APPENDIX C

Read the procedures subsection in the method section of the report by Wang and Chan ("Culturally tailored diabetes education") in Appendix C. Then answer the following questions:

[illegible]. Do you consider that the researchers took adequate steps to [illegible]? If not, what else should they have done?

[illegible]. The report [illegible] whether [illegible]

[illegible]

For [illegible] following:

- [illegible]
- [illegible]
- [illegible]
- [illegible]
- [illegible]
- [illegible]
- [illegible]

PART 3

Designing a Study to Generate Evidence for Nursing

CHAPTER 8

Planning a Nursing Study

■ A. Crossword Puzzle

Complete the crossword puzzle below, which uses terms and concepts presented in Chapter 8. (Puzzles may be removed for easier viewing.)

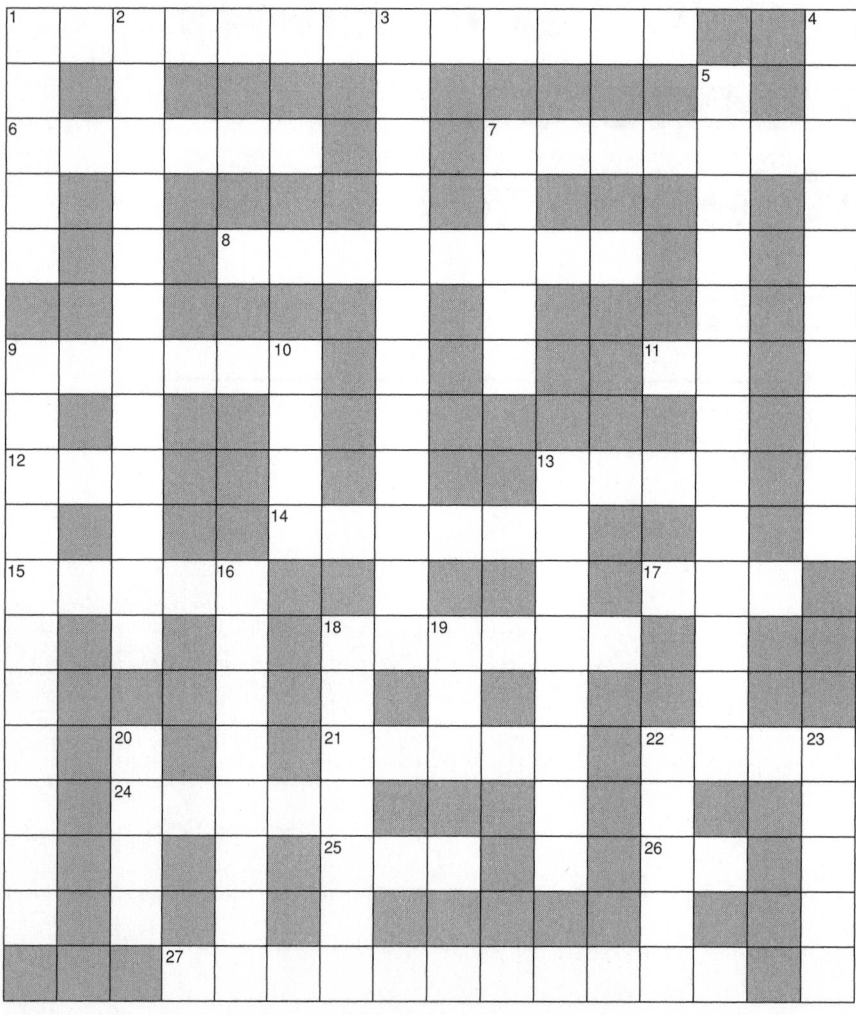

ACROSS

1. The use of multiple sources or referents to draw conclusions about what constitutes the truth
6. Quantitative researchers aim to control ________ variables (abbr.).
7. The type of design in which different people are compared is a ________-subjects design.
8. An important criterion for evaluating quantitative studies, referring broadly to the soundness of evidence
9. The extent to which qualitative study methods engender confidence in the truth of the data and interpretations (abbr.)
11. A type of study in which data are collected at a single point in time (acronym)
12. A bias that is ________ systematic is random bias.
13. One purpose of a pilot study of an intervention is to determine how large a(n) "________" of the intervention is appropriate
14. When masking is used only for study participants (not researchers), the study is ________ blind.
15. A design involving comparisons of multiple age groups is a c _ _ _ _ _ comparison design.
17. Loss of participants from a study over time (abbr.)
18. A study in which masking (blinding) has been used
21. When reflexivity is rigorously pursued, reflections and personal values are ________ in a diary or in memos.
22. A pilot study is undertaken to ________ the methods and procedures that would be used in a larger study.
24. A ________ study is sometimes called a feasibility study.
25. The accuracy and consistency of information obtained in a study (abbr.)
26. One type of longitudinal study is a follow-________ study.
27. The process of reflecting critically on the self

DOWN

1. A ________ study involves multiple points of data collection with different samples from the same population to detect patterns of change over time.
2. One critical design decision involves whether or not there will be a(n) ________, or whether the study will be nonexperimental.
3. The type of study that involves multiple points of data collection
4. The concept of ________ involves having certain features of the study established by chance.
5. A ________ design involves looking backward in time for a cause of or antecedent to a present outcome.
7. A strategy for minimizing the effects of *awareness* is to ________ researchers and/or participants.
9. Another term for *extraneous* variable
10. An influence that distorts study results

13. In qualitative studies, a quality criterion that concerns whether evidence is believable and stable over time (abbr.).
16. In planning a study, it is useful to develop a ________ for major tasks.
18. Research ________ is used to hold constant extraneous influences on the dependent variable.
19. Attrition is problematic because those who drop ________ of a study are rarely a random subset of all participants.
20. When there is no masking, the study may be described as ________.
22. For gaining entrée, the establishment of ________ is a central issue.
23. Transferability is enhanced when qualitative researchers use ________ description in their reports.

■ B. Study Questions

1. A team of nurses wanted to assess whether a special intervention would lower the risk for bone mineral density loss among women undergoing chemotherapy for breast cancer. Think of how a study could be designed. Could the study be designed as any of the following—if yes, provide examples of how this could be designed:
   a. A within-group study?
   b. A between-group study?
   c. A cross-sectional study?
   d. A longitudinal study?
   e. A retrospective study?
   f. A prospective study?

2. Read one of the following studies. Point out instances of what you consider to be *thick description.*
   - Cannaerts, N., de Casterle, B., & Grypdonck, M. (2004). Palliative care, care for life. *Qualitative Health Research, 14*(6), 816–835.
   - Cricco-Lizza, R. (2005). The milk of human kindness: Environmental and human interactions in a WIC clinic that influence infant-feeding decisions of black women. *Qualitative Health Research, 15*(4), 525–538.

3. Read one of the following studies. Point out instances of what you consider to be *reflexivity.*
   - Evans, M. K., & O'Brien, B. (2005). Gestational diabetes: The meaning of an at-risk pregnancy. *Qualitative Health Research, 15*(1), 66–81.
   - Ransom, J. E., Siler, B., Peters, R., & Maurer, M. J. (2005). Worry: Women's experience of HIV testing. *Qualitative Health Research, 15*(3), 382–393.

4. Read one of the following studies and try to estimate what a timeline for the study might have looked like (If useful, use the timeline in Figure 8.3 in the Toolkit ⊗ on the accompanying CD-ROM):
   - Lee, P., Chang, W., Liou, T., & Chang, P. (2006). Stage of exercise and health-related quality of life among overweight and obese adults. *Journal of Advanced Nursing, 53*(3), 295–303.
   - Renker, P., & Ronkin, P. (2006). Women's views of prenatal violence screening. *Obstetrics & Gynecology, 107*(2), 348–354.

■ C. Application Exercises

EXERCISE 1: STUDY IN APPENDIX C

Read the introduction and method section of the report by Wang and Chan ("Culturally tailored diabetes") education in Appendix C. Then answer the following questions:

Questions of Fact

a. Did this study involve an intervention?
b. Was this designed to make any comparisons? If so, what type of comparison was made?
c. Did this study use a within-subjects or between-subjects design?
d. Was the study cross-sectional or longitudinal? How many times were data collected from study participants?
e. Was the study prospective or retrospective?
f. Was masking (blinding) used with study participants or with research personnel?
g. What was the location for this study?

Questions for Discussion

a. This study was described as a pilot study. Discuss some of the elements of the study that support (or undermine) this description.
b. Over how many months do you think this study was conducted?
c. Find at least one example of how the researchers controlled extraneous variables by "holding constant" possible confounding influences.
d. Describe some of the things you might recommend doing in a larger-scale study designed to assess the intervention. Do you think the intervention merits a larger, more rigorous study?

EXERCISE 2: STUDY IN APPENDIX D

Read the introduction and method section of the report by Beck ("Post-traumatic stress disorder") in Appendix D. Then answer the following questions:

Questions of Fact

a. Did this study involve an intervention?
b. Was this designed to make any comparisons? If so, what type of comparison was made?
c. Was the study cross-sectional or longitudinal? How many times were data collected from study participants?
d. Was the study prospective or retrospective?
e. Was masking (blinding) used with study participants or with research personnel?
f. What was the location for this study?

Questions for Discussion

a. Discuss how Beck addressed reflexivity in this study.
b. Discuss aspects of this study that might bear on the issue of transferability.
c. Try to develop a timeline for the major activities in this study.

■ D. The Toolkit

For Chapter 8, the Toolkit on the accompanying CD-ROM contains the following:

- Sample Letter of Inquiry for Gaining Entrée into a Research Site (Figure 8.2 of the textbook)
- Project Timeline, in Calendar Months (for a 24-Month Project) (Figure 8.3 of the textbook)
- Worksheet for Documenting Design Decisions

CHAPTER 9

Developing an Approach for a Qualitative Study

■ A. Crossword Puzzle

Complete the crossword puzzle below, which uses terms and concepts presented in Chapter 9. (Puzzles may be removed for easier viewing.)

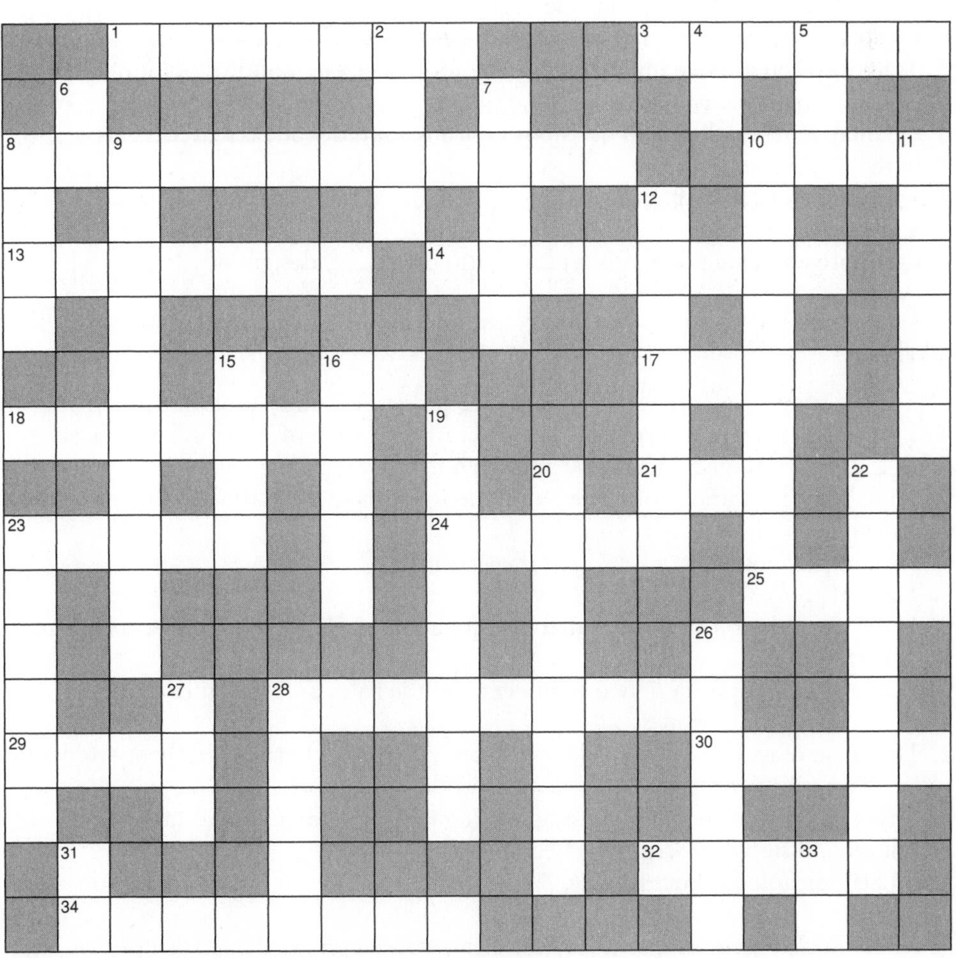

ACROSS

1. A(n) ________ aid is a resource that tells researchers what is in an archive.
2. A(n) ________ case study design is appropriate when an exemplar represents an extreme or unique case.
8. Leininger's phrase for research at the interface between culture and nursing
10. The type of phenomenology that includes the step of bracketing (abbr.)
13. Another term for auto-ethnography is ________ ethnography.
14. Research that focuses on gender domination
16. _ _ ternal criticism concerns the authenticity of historical evidence.
17. A type of psychological research that studies the environment's influence on behavior (abbr.)
18. One of the two originators of grounded theory
21. A type of action research (acronym)
23. Knowledge that is so embedded in a culture that people do not talk about it
24. A type of phenomenology sometimes called hermeneutics (abbr.)
25. The perspective that is the outsider's view
28. Qualitative researchers' ability to derive information from a wide array of sources
29. Traditional qualitative research does not adopt a strong political point of view or ________ perspective (abbr.).
30. Qualitative research design decisions typically unfold while researchers are in the ________.
32. Qualitative research that is not done within any specific tradition is typically called ________ (abbr.).
34. Qualitative research design is typically a(n) ________ design.

DOWN

2. ________ analysis focuses on *story* as the object of inquiry (abbr.).
4. _ _ternal criticism concerns an assessment of the worth of historical evidence.
5. ________ developed a linguistic approach for narrative analysis.
6. A qualitative tradition concerned with theory development about social processes (acronym)
7. Phenomenologists study ________ experiences.
8. The perspective that is the insider's view
9. The systematic collection and analysis of materials relating to the past is ________ research.
10. The type of analysis designed to understand the rules and structure of conversations
11. The nurse researcher who worked with an originator of grounded theory to develop an alternative approach
12. A type of phenomenology focusing on the *meaning* of experiences (abbr.)
15. The second step in descriptive phenomenology is to in_ _ _ _.
16. A phenomenological question is: What is the ________ of this phenomenon? (abbr.).
19. Research that involves a critique of society is based on ________ theory.

20. The biology of human behavior
22. An aspect of experience that phenomenologists study is relationality or lived human ________ (backwards!).
23. An approach to classifying qualitative research design is according to a qualitative ________ (abbr.).
26. Qualitative researchers often maintain this type of journal to record their own presuppositions and biases (abbr.).
27. Qualitative designs are ________ experimental.
28. The phenomenological concept ________-in-the-world acknowledges people's physical ties to their world.
31. Another term for insider ethnography (abbr.)
33. A procedure in grounded theory research used to develop and refine categories (acronym)

■ B. Study Questions

1. For each of the research questions below, indicate what type of qualitative research tradition would likely guide the inquiry, and why you think that would be the case.
   a. What is the social psychological process through which couples deal with the sudden loss of an infant through SIDS?
   b. How does the culture of a suicide survivors' self-help group adapt to a successful suicide attempt by a former member?
   c. What are the power dynamics that arise in conversations between nurses and bed-ridden nursing home patients?
   d. What is the lived experience of the spousal caretaker of an Alzheimer patient?

2. Skim the following two studies, which are examples of ethnographic and phenomenological studies. What were the central phenomena under investigation? Compare and contrast the methods used in these two studies (e.g., How were data collected? How many study participants were there? To what extent did the design unfold while the researchers were in the field?)
   - *Ethnographic study:* Tutton, E., & Seers, K. (2004). Comfort on a ward for older people. *Journal of Advanced Nursing, 46,* 380–389.
   - *Phenomenological study:* Enriquez, M., Lackey, N., O'Connor, M., & McKinsey, D. (2004). Successful adherence after multiple HIV treatments. *Journal of Advanced Nursing, 45,* 438–446.

3. Skim one of the following participatory action research studies and comment on the roles of participants and researchers. In what ways might the study have been different if a participatory approach had not been used?
   - Brackley, M., Davila, Y., Thornton, J., Leal, C., Mudd, G., Shafer, J., Castillo, P., & Spears, W. (2003). Community readiness to prevent intimate partner violence in Bexar County, Texas. *Journal of Transcultural Nursing, 14,* 227–236.

- Choudhry, U. K., Jandu, S., Mahal, J., Singh, R., Sohi-Pabla, H., & Mutta, B. (2002). Health promotion and participatory action research with South Asian women. *Journal of Nursing Scholarship, 34*, 75–81.
- vanLoon, A., Koch, T., & Kralik, D. (2004). Care for female survivors of child sexual abuse in emergency departments. *Accident and Emergency Nursing, 12*(4), 208–214.

4. Read one of the case studies suggested below and evaluate the extent to which the case study approach was appropriate. What were the drawbacks and benefits of using this approach? Was this a single or multiple case study? Would the design best be described as holistic or embedded?
   - Pepler, C. J., et al. (2005). Unit culture and research-based nursing practice in acute care. *Canadian Journal of Nursing Research, 37*(3), 66–85.
   - Kavanaugh, K., et al. (2005). Life support decisions for extremely premature infants: Report of a pilot study. *Journal of Pediatric Nursing, 20*(5), 347–359.

5. Read one of the studies below, and evaluate the extent to which the problem was amenable to the grounded theory research tradition. Which of the two schools of grounded theory thought was followed in this study? Does the report explicitly discuss how the constant comparative method was used?
   - Brink, E., Karlson, B., & Hallberg, L. (2006). Readjustment 5 months after a first-time myocardial infarction: Reorienting the active self. *Journal of Advanced Nursing, 53*(4), 403–411.
   - Nelson, A., & Sethi, S. (2005). The breastfeeding experiences of Canadian teenage mothers. *Journal of Obstetric, Gynecologic, & Neonatal Nursing, 34*(5), 615–624.

6. Read one of the studies below, and think about how the researcher could have adopted a critical theory or feminist perspective. In what way would the methods for such a modification differ from the methods used?
   - Forchuk, C., Nelson, G., & Hall, G. (2006). "It's important to be proud of the place you live in": Housing problems and preferences of psychiatric survivors. *Perspectives in Psychiatric Care, 42*(1), 42–52.
   - Haglund, K. (2006). Understanding sexual abstinence in African American teens. *MCN: The American Journal of Maternal/Child Nursing, 31*(2), 86–92.
   - Webb. M., & Gonzalez, L. (2006). The burden of hypertension: Mental representations of African American women. *Issues in Mental Health Nursing, 27*(3), 249–271.

■ C. Application Exercises

EXERCISE 1: STUDY IN APPENDIX B

Read the procedures subsection in the method section of the report by Rew ("Homeless youth") in Appendix B. Then answer the following questions:

Questions of Fact

a. In which tradition was this study based? Did this study have an ideological perspective?
b. Which specific approach was used—that of Glaser and Strauss, or that or Strauss and Corbin?
c. What is the central phenomenon under study?
d. Was the study longitudinal?
e. What was the setting for this research?
f. Did the report indicate or suggest that constant comparison was used?
g. Is the research question congruent with a qualitative approach and with the specific research tradition? Is the domain of inquiry for the study congruent with the domain encompassed by the tradition?

Questions for Discussion

a. How well is the research design described in the report? Are design decisions explained and justified?
b. Does it appear that Rew made all design decisions up-front, or did the design emerge during data collection, allowing her to capitalize on early information?
c. Were there any elements of the design or methods that appear to be more appropriate for a qualitative tradition other than the one Rew identified as the underlying tradition?
d. Could this study have been undertaken within an ideological framework? If so, what changes to the research methods would be necessary?

EXERCISE 2: STUDY IN APPENDIX D

Read the abstract and introduction to the report by Beck ("Post-traumatic stress disorder") in Appendix D. Then answer the following questions:

Questions of Fact

a. In which tradition was this study based? Did this study have an ideological perspective?
b. Was this a descriptive or interpretive study?
c. What is the central phenomenon under study?
d. Was the study longitudinal?
e. Is there evidence of bracketing?
f. Is the research question congruent with a qualitative approach and with the specific research tradition (i.e., is the domain of inquiry for the study congruent with the domain encompassed by the tradition)?

Questions for Discussion

a. How well is the research design described in the report? Are design decisions explained and justified?

b. Does it appear that Beck made all design decisions up front, or did the design emerge during data collection, allowing her to capitalize on early information?
c. Were there any elements of the design or methods that appear to be more appropriate for a qualitative tradition other than the one Beck identified as the underlying tradition?
d. Could this study have been undertaken within an ideological framework? If so, what changes to the research methods would be necessary?

EXERCISE 3: STUDY IN APPENDIX F

Read the introduction and method section of the report by Giddings ("Health disparities") in Appendix F. Then answer the following questions:

Questions of Fact

a. In which tradition was this study based? Did this study have an ideological perspective?
b. What is the central phenomenon under study?
c. Was the study longitudinal?
d. What was the setting for this research?
e. Is the research question congruent with a qualitative approach and with the specific research tradition (i.e., is the domain of inquiry for the study congruent with the domain encompassed by the tradition)?

Questions for Discussion

a. How well is the research design described? Are design decisions explained and justified?
b. Does it appear that the researcher made all design decisions up front, or did the design emerge during data collection, allowing researchers to capitalize on early information?
c. Is there evidence that ideological methods and goals were achieved? (e.g., was there evidence of full collaboration between researchers and participants? Did the research have the power to be transformative, or is there evidence that a transformative process occurred?)

■ D. The Toolkit

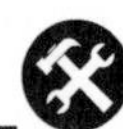

For Chapter 9, the Toolkit on the accompanying CD-ROM contains a Word file with the following:

- Guidelines for Critiquing Qualitative Designs (Box 9.1 of the textbook)

CHAPTER 10

Designing Quantitative Studies

■ A. Crossword Puzzle

Complete the crossword puzzle below, which uses terms and concepts presented in Chapter 10. (Puzzles may be removed for easier viewing.)

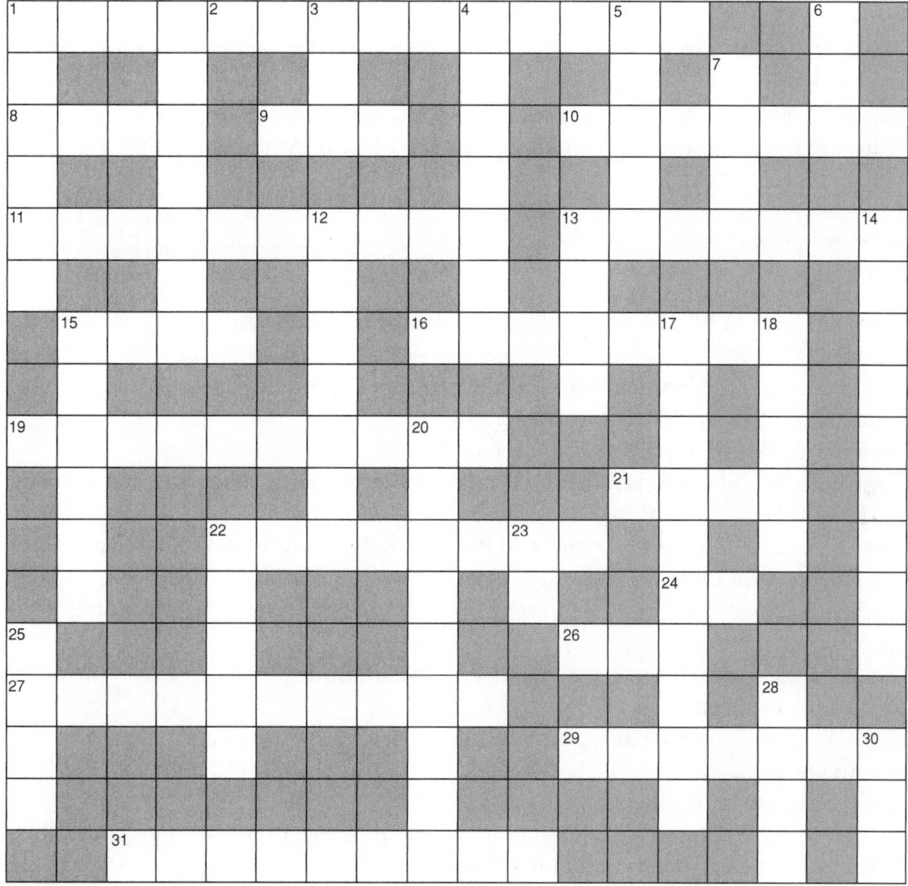

ACROSS

1. That against which the outcomes for an experimental group are compared
8. A type of control group in a quasi-experiment, using data from an earlier point in time (abbr.)

9. A type of control group used to offset the effect of special care to the experimental group (abbr.)
10. Randomization of subjects within specified subgroups (abbr.)
11. A design that begins with the effect and looks back in time for a cause (abbr.)
13. Another name for the "before" (preintervention) measures of the outcome variables
15. A major bias in research that does not involve random assignment is ________ selection.
16. A design that begins with the cause and looks forward to an effect (abbr.)
19. The number with a condition or disease at a fixed point, based on cross-sectional data from the population at risk
21. A box in a diagram of a factorial design.
22. One criterion for causality is ________ plausibility.
24. The rate of new cases with a condition or disease for a fixed period of time (abbr.)
26. In the medical literature, the term sometimes used for *group* or *condition*
27. To protect from possible bias, ________ concealment is recommended during randomization.
29. Randomized ________ is often referred to as the Zelen design.
31. A bias that can arise from people's awareness of being studied is called the ________ effect.

DOWN

1. A(n) ________ design is the term used in the medical literature for a nonexperimental prospective study.
2. A(n) ________ experiment looks at the effects of an event that transpires in a fairly random fashion, such as a hurricane.
3. Another name for an experiment (acronym)
4. The type of randomization involving assignment of larger units than individual subjects
5. The ________-only design collects data from subjects following administration of the intervention only.
6. A type of intervention that is tailored to particular characteristics of people (acronym)
7. A ________-listed control group gets delayed treatment.
12. A pseudo-intervention
13. A ________ test is a measure of an outcome after the intervention has been administered.
14. Another term for an intervention
15. A type of quasi-experimental design involving multiple points of data collection before and after an intervention is a time ________.
17. The gold standard for inferring cause-and-effect relationships
18. One method of randomization involves use of a ________ of random numbers.
20. A type of design in which subjects serve as their own controls
22. When stratification is used before randomization, the design is called a randomized ________ design.

23. In an experiment, that which is manipulated (acronym)
25. Nonexperimental studies that test theory-driven causal linkages use ________ analysis.
28. Randomization of multiple groups of a small number of subjects is called ________ block randomization (abbr.).
30. A factorial study involves at least ________ independent, manipulated variables.

■ B. Study Questions

1. Suppose you wanted to study self-efficacy among successful dieters who lost 20 or more pounds and maintained their weight loss for at least 6 months. Specify at least two different types of comparison strategies that might provide a useful comparative context for this study. Do your strategies lend themselves to experimental manipulation? If not, why not?

2. Below are 20 subjects who have volunteered for a study of the effects of noise on pulse rate. Ten must be assigned to the low-volume group and 10 to a high-volume group. Use the table of random numbers in Table 10.2 of the textbook to randomly assign subjects to groups.

L. Bentley	M. McGowan
L. Boehm	A. Messenger
D. Chorna	U. Moore
H. Dann	P. Morrill
L. Dansker	C. O'Dea
E. Gordon	A. Petty
R. Greenberg	D. Roberts
J. Harte	V. Rotan
S. Kulli	H. Seidler
P. Labovitz	R. Smalling

Assume all participants in the first column above are in their 20s and all those in the second column are in their 30s. How good a job did your randomization do in terms of equalizing the two groups according to age? Add 10 more names to each age group and assign these additional 20 subjects. Now compare the low-volume and high-volume groups in terms of the age distribution. Did doubling the sample size improve the distribution of subjects' ages within the two volume-level groups?

3. A nurse researcher found a relationship between teenagers' level of knowledge about birth control and their level of sexual activity. That is, teenagers with higher levels of sexual activity knew more about birth control than teenagers with less sexual activity. Suggest at least three interpretations for this finding. Is this a research problem that is *inherently* nonexperimental? Why or why not?

4. The following study was described a double-blind experiment. Review the design for this study, and comment on the appropriateness of the masking procedures. What biases were the researchers trying to avoid? Were they successful?

- Schmelzer, M., Schiller, L., Meyer, R., Rugari, S., & Case, P. (2004). Safety and effectiveness of large-volume enema solutions. *Applied Nursing Research, 17*(4), 265–274.

5. Suppose that you were interested in testing the hypothesis that regular ingestion of aspirin reduced the risk for colon cancer. Describe how such a hypothesis could be tested using a retrospective case-control design. Now describe a prospective cohort design for the same study. Compare the strengths and weaknesses of the two approaches.

6. Read the introduction and method sections of one of the following reports. Use the critiquing guidelines in Box 10.1 of the textbook (available as a Word document in the Toolkit) to evaluate features of the research design:
   - Groth, S. (2006). Adolescent gestational weight gain: Does it contribute to obesity? *MCN: The American Journal of Maternal/Child Nursing, 31*(2), 101–105.
   - Scisney-Matlock, M., Glazewki, L., McClerking, C., & Kachorek, L. (2006). Development and evaluation of DASH diet tailored messages for hypertension treatment. *Applied Nursing Research, 19*(2), 78–87.
   - Wyman, L. L. (2005). Comparing the number of ill or injured students who are released early from school by school nursing and nonnursing personnel. *Journal of School Nursing, 21*(6), 350–355.

■ C. Application Exercises

EXERCISE 1: STUDY IN APPENDIX A

Read the method section of the report by Hill and colleagues ("Chronically ill rural women") in Appendix A. Then answer the following questions:

Questions of Fact

a. Was there an intervention in this study?
b. Is the design for this study experimental, quasi-experimental, or nonexperimental?
c. What were the independent and dependent variables?
d. Was randomization used? If yes, what method was used to assign subjects to groups?
e. In terms of the counterfactual strategies described in the textbook, what approach did the researchers use?
f. What is the specific name of the research design used in this study?
g. Is the overall design a within-subjects or between-subjects design?
h. Was any masking/blinding used in this study?
i. Would this study be described as longitudinal?
j. Was this study based on an earlier pilot study?

Questions for Discussion

a. What was the intervention? Comment on how well the intervention was described, including a description of how it was developed and refined.

b. Comment on the researchers' counterfactual strategy. Could a more powerful or effective strategy have been used?
c. Discuss ways in which this study achieved or failed to achieve the criteria for making causal inferences.
d. Comment on the researchers' masking strategy.
e. Comment on the timing of postintervention data collection.

EXERCISE 2: STUDY IN APPENDIX E

Read the method section of the report by Loeb ("Older men's health") in Appendix E. Then answer the following questions:

Questions of Fact

a. Was there an intervention in this study?
b. Is the design for this study experimental, quasi-experimental, or nonexperimental?
c. What were the independent and dependent variables in this study?
d. Was the independent variable amenable to manipulation?
e. Was randomization used? If yes, what method was used to assign subjects to groups?
f. What is the specific name of the research design used in this study?
g. Was any masking/blinding used in this study?
h. Would this study be described as longitudinal?

Questions for Discussion

a. Comment on the researchers' comparison. Could a more powerful or effective strategy have been used?
b. Discuss ways in which this study achieved or failed to achieve the criteria for making causal inferences.
c. Comment on the researchers' masking strategy.
d. Comment on the timing of data collection.

■ D. The Toolkit

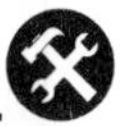

For Chapter 10, the Toolkit on the CD-ROM provided with this Resource Manual contains the following:

- Guidelines for Critiquing Research Designs in Quantitative Studies (Box 10.1 of the textbook)

7. One method of statistically controlling extraneous variables is through analysis of ________ (abbr.).
9. If a control group member receives the intervention, this is ________ of treatments (abbr.).
10. A hybrid design is often used in ________ clinical trials in real-world clinical settings (abbr.).
11. The "R" in the RE-AIM framework stands for this.
12. A threat to internal validity is temporal ________, questions about which came first, the independent or dependent variable.
14. Effectiveness trials focus on external validity issues, whereas ________ trials are more concerned with internal validity.
21. The "M" in the RE-AIM framework stands for this (abbr.).
22. A threat to internal validity concerning the occurrence of events external to an independent variable that could affect outcomes
25. The bias that is of concern in crossover designs
27. Concerns inferences from the particular exemplars of a study to higher order constructs (acronym)
28. A ________ check evaluates whether the treatment was in place as intended (abbr.).
31. A ________ of enhancements to internal validity is that external validity often is lowered.
32. ________ matching involves individualized efforts to make subjects in different groups equivalent with regard to key extraneous variables.
33. The best mechanism for controlling extraneous subject characteristics is ________ (acronym).
36. A(n) _ _-protocol analysis involves analyzing outcomes only for those who received their assigned condition.

■ B. Study Questions

1. Suppose you wanted to compare the growth of infants whose mothers were heroin addicts with that of infants of nonaddicted mothers. Describe how you would design such a study, being careful to indicate what confounding variables you would need to control and how you would control them. Identify the major threats to the internal validity of your design.

2. A nurse researcher is interested in testing the effect of a special high-fiber diet on cardiovascular risk factors (e.g., cholesterol level) in adults with a family history of cardiovascular disease. Describe a design you would recommend for this problem, being careful to indicate what confounding variables you would need to control and how you would control them. Suggest methods of strengthening the power of the design. Identify possible threats to the internal validity of your design.

3. Read the method section of one of the following quasi-experimental studies. Identify one or more threats to the internal validity of the study. Then describe strategies that could be used to strengthen the study's internal validity.

- Creedon, S. A. (2006). Health care workers' hand decontamination practices: An Irish study. *Clinical Nursing Research, 15*(1), 6–26.
- Horodynski, M. A., & Stommel, M. (2005). Nutrition education aimed at toddlers: An intervention study. *Pediatric Nursing, 31*(5), 364–372.
- Sinclair, V., & Scroggie, J. (2005). Effects of a cognitive-behavioral program for women with multiple sclerosis. *Journal of Neuroscience Nursing, 37*(5), 249–257.

4. Suppose you were studying the effects of range-of-motion exercises on radical mastectomy patients. You start your experiment with 50 experimental subjects and 50 control subjects. Your intervention requires experimental subjects to come for daily sessions over a 2-week period, whereas control subjects come only once at the end of 2 weeks. Your final group sizes are 40 for the experimental group and 49 for the control group. The results of your study indicate that the experimental group did better in raising the arm of the affected side above head level. What effects, if any, do you think the subject attrition might have on the internal validity of your study?
5. For each of the following research questions, indicate the type of design you could use to best address it; indicate confounding variables that should be controlled and how your design would control them:
   - What effect does the presence of the newborn's father in the delivery room have on the mother's subjective report of pain?
   - What is the effect of different types of bowel evacuation regimes for quadriplegic patients?
   - Does the inability to speak and understand English affect a person's access to hospice services?
6. Read the introduction and method section of one of the following reports. Use the critiquing guidelines in Box 11.1 of the textbook (available as a Word document in the Toolkit) to assess the study's validity:
   - Bakas, T., et al. (2006). Outcomes among family caregivers of aphasic versus nonaphasic stroke survivors. *Rehabilitation Nursing, 31*(1), 33–42.
   - Brewer, S., et al. (2006). Pediatric anxiety: Child life intervention in day surgery. *Journal of Pediatric Nursing, 21*(1), 13–22.
   - McMillan, S. C., et al. (2006). Impact of coping skills intervention with family caregivers of hospice patients with cancer. *Cancer, 106*(1), 214–222.

■ C. Application Exercises

EXERCISE 1: STUDY IN APPENDIX A

Read the method section of the report by Hill and colleagues ("Chronically ill rural women") in Appendix A. Then answer the following questions:

Questions of Fact

a. Which of the methods of research control described in this chapter were used to control confounding variables?

b. What confounding variables were controlled?
c. Was there any attrition in this study?
d. Is there evidence that constancy of conditions was implemented?
e. Were group treatments as distinct as possible to maximize power? If not, why not?

Questions for Discussion

a. Does this study seem strong in terms of statistical conclusion validity? How could statistical conclusion validity have been strengthened?
b. Discuss issues relating to the intervention fidelity in this study.
c. Is this study strong in internal validity? What, if any, are the threats to the internal validity of this study?
d. Is this study strong in construct validity? What, if any, are the threats to the construct validity of this study?
e. Is this study strong in external validity? What, if any, are the threats to the external validity of this study?
f. Consider the pros and cons of adding an attention control group in this study. What type of *attention* condition could have been used?

EXERCISE 2: STUDY IN APPENDIX C

Read the method section of the report by Wang and Chan ("Culturally tailored diabetes education") in Appendix C. Then answer the following questions:

Questions of Fact

a. Is the design for this study experimental, quasi-experimental, or nonexperimental?
b. What were the independent and dependent variables in this study?
c. Was randomization used? If no, would it have been possible to randomize?
d. In terms of the counterfactual strategies described in the previous chapter of the textbook, what approach did the researchers use?
e. What is the specific name of the research design used in this study?
f. Which of the methods of research control described in this chapter were used to control confounding variables?
g. What confounding variables were controlled?
h. Is there evidence that attention was paid to maintaining constancy of conditions?
i. Was there any attrition in this study?

Questions for Discussion

a. What was the intervention? Comment on how well the intervention was described, including the description of how it was developed and refined.
b. Comment on the researchers' counterfactual strategy. Could a more powerful or effective strategy have been used?
c. Discuss ways in which this study achieved or failed to achieve the criteria for making causal inferences.

d. Does this study seem strong in terms of statistical conclusion validity? How could statistical conclusion validity have been strengthened?
e. Discuss issues relating to intervention fidelity in this study.
f. Is this study strong in internal validity? What, if any, are the threats to the internal validity of this study?
g. Is this study strong in construct validity? What, if any, are the threats to the construct validity of this study?
h. Is this study strong in external validity? What, if any, are the threats to the external validity of this study?

■ D. The Toolkit

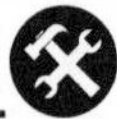

For Chapter 11, the Toolkit on the accompanying CD-ROM contains a Word file with the following:

- Guidelines for Critiquing Design Elements and Study Validity in Quantitative Studies (Box 11.1 of the textbook)
- Example of a Table of Contents for a Procedures Manual for an Intervention Study
- Example of an Observational Checklist for Monitoring Delivery of an Intervention
- Example of a Contact Information Form for Longitudinal Studies
- Examples of Methods to Enhance External Validity, and Potential Associated Costs to Internal (or Other) Validity
- Matrix for Design Decisions and Possible Effects on Study Validity

CHAPTER 12

Undertaking Research for Specific Purposes

■ A. Crossword Puzzle

Complete the crossword puzzle below, which uses terms and concepts presented in Chapter 12. (Puzzles may be removed for easier viewing.)

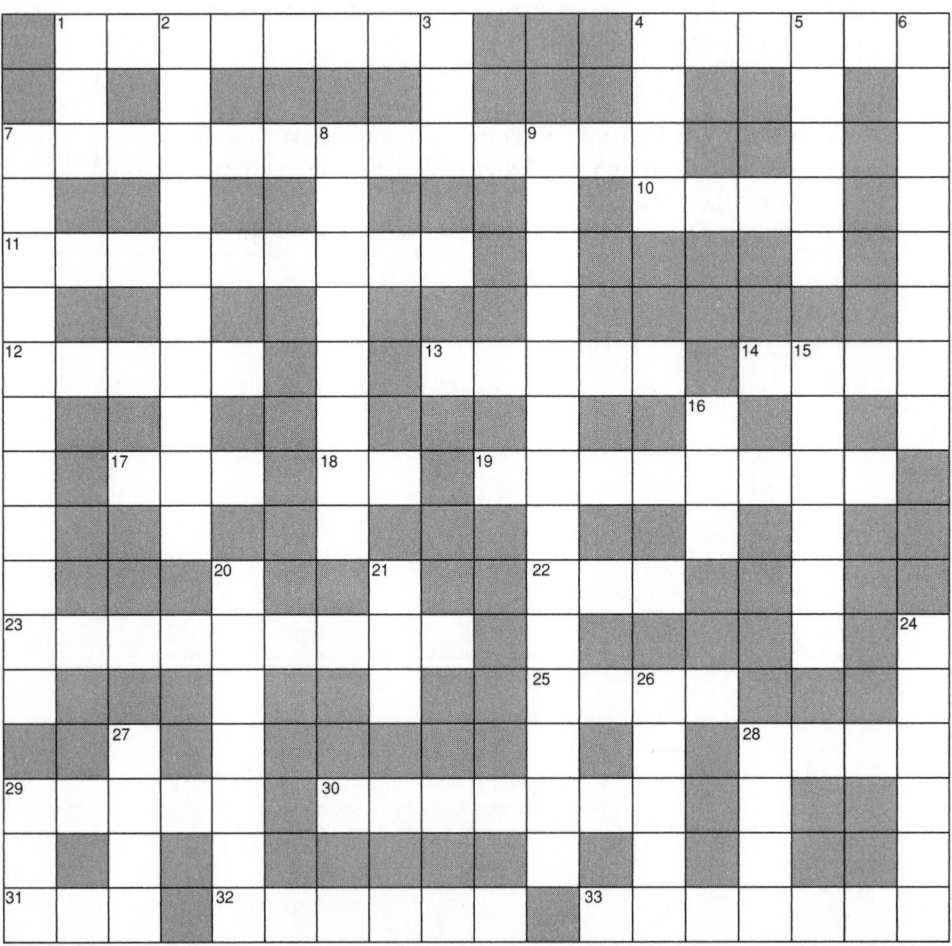

ACROSS

1. Interviews that are done face to face
4. An evaluation of the worth of a program or policy (abbr.)
7. A multiphase effort to refine and test the effectiveness of a clinical treatment (two words)
10. Another term for interviews done in person is ________ to ________.
11. An analysis of data done with an existing data set
12. In nursing intervention research, work may ________ with developmental qualitative research.
13. Surveys can be done by distributing these by mail (abbr.).
14. A ________ design is an effort to bridge the gap between efficacy and effectiveness studies (abbr.).
17. An impact analysis provides information about the ________ effects of a program.
18. In a clinical trial, phase ________ is sometimes called effectiveness research.
19. This type of research focuses on improving research strategies (abbr.).
22. An alternative to in-person interviews is interviews by ________ (abbr.).
23. A method of collecting self-report data
25. A Phase II trial often involves a pilot ________ of a new treatment.
28. A mixed method design involving discrete segments of an overall inquiry (abbr.)
29. In clinical trials, an efficacy study is the third ________.
30. In evaluations, a(n) ________ analysis describes the extent to which a program is achieving certain goals.
31. The phase of a clinical trial that is an RCT
32. A Gallup poll is one of these.
33. An approach to needs assessments that involves organizing existing information (abbr.)

DOWN

1. Findings from evaluations and outcomes research can be used in the formulation of local and national ________ (abbr.).
2. A Phase III clinical trial is ________.
3. Personal interviews are an expensive approach to surveys because they require a ________ of personnel time.
4. Data collected by asking people questions in a survey is via ________ reports.
5. Researchers use both qualitative and quantitative approaches in ________ method research.
6. In the Donabedian framework, the three key factors are process, outcomes, and s________.
7. One type of evaluation of the economic effects of an intervention
8. In a cost utility ________, quality-adjusted life year is often an important outcome.
9. An evaluation of the process of putting a new intervention into place is a(n) ________ analysis.
15. An especially ambitious application of mixed method research involves the building of ________ (backwards!).

20. Another name for an implementation analysis
21. Sometimes surveys can be administered over the Inter ________.
24. The type of evaluation that uses an experimental design is a(n) ________ analysis.
26. A ________ assessment can use a survey or key informant approach (backwards!).
27. A new survey technology that gives respondents privacy in answering questions is audio-________.
28. Large-scale telephone surveys increasingly rely on ________ technology.
29. The Del ________ technique involves multiple rounds of questioning to achieve consensus.

■ B. Study Questions

1. Read one of the following studies, in which quantitative data were gathered and analyzed to address a research question. Suggest ways in which the collection of qualitative data might have enriched the study, strengthened its validity, or enhanced its interpretability:
   - Hollman, G., Olsson, A., & Ek, A. (2006). Disease knowledge and adherence to treatment in patients with familial hypercholesterolemia. *Journal of Cardiovascular Nursing, 21*(2), 103–108.
   - Kozachik, S., Wyatt, G., Given, C., & Given, B. (2006). Patterns of use of complementary therapies among cancer patients and their family caregivers. *Cancer Nursing, 29*(2), 84–94.
   - McCurry, S. M., Gibbons, L. E., Logsdon, R. G., & Teri, L. (2004). Anxiety and nighttime behavioral disturbances: Awakenings in patients with Alzheimer's disease. *Journal of Gerontological Nursing, 30*, 12–20.
2. Read one of the following qualitative studies. Suggest ways that the findings could have been validated or the emergent hypotheses could have been tested by adding a quantitative component:
   - Gould, D., & Fontenla, M. (2006). Commitment to nursing: Results of a qualitative interview study. *Journal of Nursing Management, 14*(3), 213–221.
   - Logan, J., Hackbusch-Pinto, R., & DeGrasse, C. (2006), Women undergoing breast diagnostics: The lived experience of spirituality. *Oncology Nursing Forum, 33*(1), 121–126.
   - Milne, J., & Moore, K. (2006). Factors impacting self-care for urinary incontinence. *Urologic Nursing, 26*(1), 41–51.
3. Suppose you were interested in studying the research questions below by conducting a survey. For each, indicate whether you would recommend using a personal interview, a telephone interview, or a self-administered questionnaire to collect the data. What is your rationale?
   a. What are the coping strategies of newly widowed individuals?
   b. What strategies do emergency department nurses use to identify and correct medical errors?
   c. What type of nursing communications do presurgical patients find most helpful?

d. What is the relationship between a teenager's health-risk appraisal and his/her risk-taking behavior (e.g., smoking, unprotected sex, drug use, etc.)?
e. What are the health-promoting activities pursued by inner-city single mothers?
f. How is employment of parents affected by the health problems or disability of their child?

4. Below is a brief description of a mixed method study, followed by a critique. Do you agree with this critique? Can you add other comments regarding the study design?

Fictitious Study. Krout conducted a study designed to examine the emotional well-being of women who had a mastectomy. Krout wanted to develop an in-depth understanding of the emotional experiences of women as they recovered from their surgery, including the process by which they handled their fears, their concerns about their sexuality, their levels of anxiety and depression, their methods of coping, and their social supports.

Krout's basic study design was a descriptive qualitative study. She gathered information from a sample of 26 women, primarily by means of in-depth interviews with the women on two occasions. The first interviews were scheduled within 1 month after the surgery. Follow-up interviews were conducted about 12 months later. Several women in the sample participated in a support group, and Krout attended and made observations at several meetings. Additionally, Krout decided to interview the "significant other" (usually the women's husbands) of most of the women, when it became clear that the women's emotional well-being was linked to the manner in which the significant other was reacting to the surgery.

In addition to the rich, in-depth information she gathered, Krout wanted to be able to better interpret the emotional status of the women. Therefore, at both the original and follow-up interview with the women, she administered a psychological scale known as the Center for Epidemiological Studies Depression Scale (CES-D), a quantitative measure that has scores that can range from 0 to 60. This scale has been widely used in community populations, and has cut-off scores designating when a person is at risk for clinical depression (i.e., a score of 16 and above).

Krout's qualitative analysis showed that the basic process underlying psychological recovery from the mastectomy was something she labeled "Gaining by Losing," a process that involved heightened self-awareness and self-respect after an initial period of despair and self-pity. The process also involved, for some, a strengthening of personal relationships with significant others, whereas for others, it resulted in the birth of awareness of fundamental deficiencies in their relationships. The quantitative findings confirmed that a very high percentage of women were at risk for being depressed 1 month after the mastectomy, but after 12 months, the average level of depression was actually modestly lower than in the general population of women.

Critique. In her study, Krout embedded a quantitative measure into her fieldwork in an interesting manner. The bulk of data were qualitative—in-depth interviews and in-depth observations. However, she also opted to include a well-known measure of depression, which provided her with an important context for interpreting her data. A major advantage of using the CES-D is that this scale has known characteristics in the general population, and therefore provided a built-in "comparison group."

Krout used a flexible design that allowed her to use her initial data to guide her inquiry. For example, she decided to conduct in-depth interviews with significant others when she learned their importance to the women's process of emotional recovery. Krout did do some advance planning, however, that provided loose guidance. For example, although her questioning undoubtedly evolved while in the field, she had the foresight to realize that to capture a process as it evolved, she would need to collect data longitudinally. She also made the up-front decision to use the CES-D to supplement the in-depth interviews.

In this study, the findings from the qualitative and quantitative portions of the study were complementary. Both portions of the study confirmed that the women initially had emotional "losses," but eventually they recovered and "gained" in terms of their emotional well-being and their self-awareness. This example illustrates how the validity of study findings can be enhanced by the blending of qualitative and quantitative data. If the qualitative data alone had been gathered, Krout might not have gotten a good handle on the degree to which the women had actually "recovered" (*vis-à-vis* women who had never had a mastectomy). Conversely, if she had collected only the CES-D data, she would have had no insights into the process by which the recovery occurred.

6. Read the introduction and methods section of one of the following reports. Use the critiquing guidelines in Box 12.1 of the textbook (available as a Word document in the Toolkit ⊗) to critique the study:
   - Kovner, C., Brewer, C., Wu, Y., Cheng, Y., & Suzuki, M. (2006). Factors associated with work satisfaction of registered nurses. *Journal of Nursing Scholarship, 38*(1), 71–79.
   - Lee, V., Cohen, S., Edgar, L., Laizner, A., & Gagnon, A. (2006). Meaning-making and psychological adjustment to cancer: Development of an intervention and pilot results. *Oncology Nursing Forum, 33*(2), 291–302.
   - Robins, J., McCain, N., Gray, D., Elswick, R., Walter, J., & McDade, E. (2006). Research on pyschoneuroimmunology: Tai chi as a stress management approach for individuals with HIV disease. *Applied Nursing Research, 19*(1), 2–9.

■ C. Application Exercises

EXERCISE 1: ALL STUDIES IN APPENDICES

Which of the studies in the appendices of this Resource Manual (if any) could be considered:

a. mixed method research?
b. a clinical trial?
c. outcomes research?
d. survey research?

EXERCISE 2: STUDY IN APPENDIX I

Read the first few sections before the data analysis section of the report by Johnson and Rogers ("Medication-taking questionnaire") in Appendix I. Then answer the following questions:

Questions of Fact

a. Was this study a clinical trial or nursing intervention research? If yes, what phase would this most likely be?
b. Was this study an evaluation? If yes, what type (process analysis, etc.)?
c. Was this outcomes research?
d. Was this study a survey?
e. Was this study an example of methodologic research?
f. What is the basic research design for this study (i.e., experimental, nonexperimental, etc.)?
g. Was this a mixed method study? If yes, what strategy of integration was used?

Questions for Discussion

a. Comment on the adequacy and appropriateness of the use of various types of data in this study.
b. What are some of the uses to which the findings and product of this study could be put?

■ D. The Toolkit

For Chapter 12, the Toolkit on the CD-ROM provided with this Resource Manual contains a Word file with the following:

- Some Guidelines for Critiquing Studies Described in Chapter 12 (Box 12.1 of the textbook)
- Guidelines for Critiquing Cost/Economic Analyses
- Examples of Strategies for Designing an Evidence-Based Intervention
- Common Pitfalls in Intervention Research

■ B. Study Questions

1. Draw a simple random sample of 15 people from the sampling frame of Table 13.3 of the textbook, using the table of random numbers that appears in Table 10.2. Begin your selection by blindly placing your finger at some point on the table.
2. Suppose you have decided to use a systematic sampling design for a study. The known population size is 5000, and the sample size desired is 250. What is the sampling interval? If the first element selected is 23, what would be the second, third, and fourth elements selected?
3. Suppose you were interested in studying the attitude of clinical specialists toward autonomy in work situations. Suggest a possible target and accessible population. What strata might be identified if quota sampling were used?
4. Identify the type of quantitative sampling design used in the following examples:
   a. One hundred inmates randomly sampled from a random selection of five federal penitentiaries
   b. All the oncology nurses participating in a continuing education seminar
   c. Every 20th patient admitted to the emergency room between January and June
   d. The first 20 male and the first 20 female patients admitted to the hospital with hypothermia
   e. A sample of 250 members randomly selected from a roster of American Nurses' Association members
   f. 25 experts in critical care nursing
5. Nurse A is planning to study the effects of maternal stress, maternal depression, maternal age, and family economic resources on a child's socioemotional development among both intact and mother-headed families. Nurse B is planning to study body position on patients' respiratory functioning. Describe the kinds of samples that the two nurses would need to use. Which nurse would need the larger sample? Defend your answer.
6. Suppose a qualitative researcher wanted to study the life quality of cancer survivors. Suggest what the researcher might do to obtain a maximum variation sample; a typical case sample; a homogeneous sample; and an extreme case sample.
7. Read the introduction and methods section of one of the following quantitative reports. Use the guidelines in Box 13.1 of the textbook (available as a Word document in the Toolkit ⊗) to critique the sampling plan:
   - Froman, R., & Owen, S. (2005). Randomized study of stability and change in patients' advance directives. *Research in Nursing & Health, 28*, 398–407.
   - Roelands, M., Van Oost, P., Depoorter, A., Buysse, A., & Stevens, V. (2006). Introduction of assistive devices: Home nurses' practices and beliefs. *Journal of Advanced Nursing, 54*(2), 180–199.
   - Yousey, Y. (2006). Household characteristics, smoking bans, and passive smoke exposure in young children. *Journal of Pediatric Health Care, 20*(2), 98–105.

8. Read the introduction and method section of one of the following qualitative reports. Use the guidelines in Box 13.2 of the textbook (available as a Word document in the Toolkit ⊗) to critique the sampling plan:
   - Drew, D., & Hewitt, H. (2006). A qualitative approach to understanding patients' diagnosis of Lyme disease. *Public Health Nursing, 23*(1), 20–26.
   - Hopkinson, J., Wright, D., & Corner, J. (2006). Exploring the experience of weight loss in people with advanced cancer. *Journal of Advanced Nursing, 54*(3), 304–312.
   - Montgomery, P., Tompkins, C., Forchuk, C., & French, S. (2006). Keeping close: Mothering with serious mental illness. *Journal of Advanced Nursing, 54*(1), 20–28.

■ C. Application Exercises

EXERCISE 1: ALL STUDIES IN APPENDICES

Which of the studies in Appendices A through I of this Resource Manual (if any) used

a. a probability sample?
b. convenience sampling?
c. quota sampling?

EXERCISE 2: STUDY IN APPENDIX E

Read the method sections of the report by Loeb ("Older men's health") in Appendix E. Then answer the following questions:

Questions of Fact

a. What was the target population of Loeb's study? How would you describe the accessible population?
b. What were the eligibility criteria for the study?
c. Was the sampling method probability or nonprobability? What specific sampling method was used?
d. How were study participants recruited?
e. What efforts did Loeb make to ensure a diverse (and hence more representative) sample?
f. What was the sample size that Loeb achieved?
g. Was a power analysis used to determine sample size needs? If yes, what number of subjects did the power analysis estimate as the minimum needed number?

Questions for Discussion

a. Comment on the adequacy of Loeb's sampling plan and recruitment strategy. How representativeness was the sample of the target population? What types of sampling biases might be of special concern?
b. Do you think Loeb's sample size was adequate? Why or why not?

EXERCISE 3: STUDY IN APPENDIX B

Read the method section of the report by Rew ("Homeless youth") in Appendix B. Then answer the following questions:

Questions of Fact

a. What were the eligibility criteria for this study?
b. How were study participants recruited?
c. What type of sampling approach was used?
d. How many study participants comprised the sample?
e. Was data saturation achieved?
f. Did Rew's sampling strategy include confirming and disconfirming cases?

Questions for Discussion

a. Comment on the adequacy of Rew's sampling plan and recruitment strategy for achieving the goals of a grounded theory study.
b. Do you think Rew's sample size was adequate? Why or why not?

■ D. The Toolkit

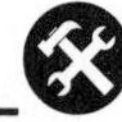

For Chapter 13, the Toolkit on the accompanying CD-ROM contains a Word file with the following:

- Guidelines for Critiquing Quantitative Sampling Designs (Box 13.1 of the textbook)
- Guidelines for Critiquing Qualitative Sampling Designs (Box 13.2 of the textbook)

PART 4

Collecting Research Data

CHAPTER 14

Designing and Implementing a Data Collection Plan

■ A. Crossword Puzzle

Complete the crossword puzzle below, which uses terms and concepts presented in Chapter 14. (Puzzles may be removed for easier viewing.)

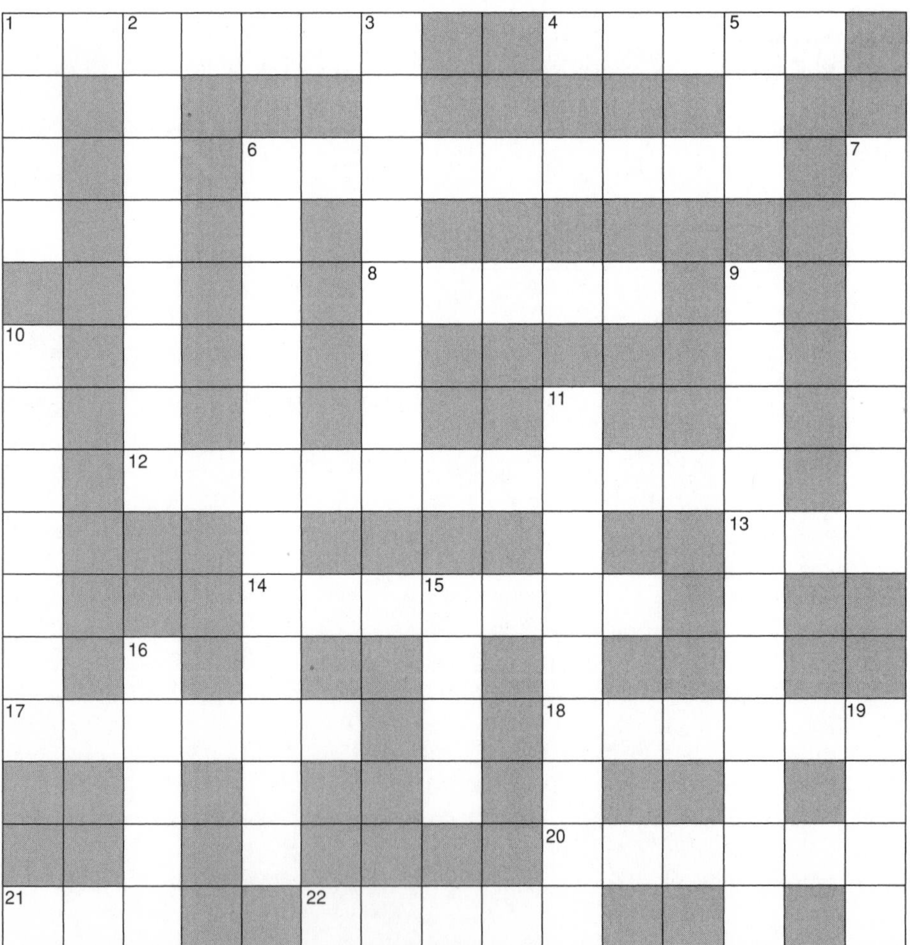

ACROSS

1. The full instrument package should undergo a ________ before being used in the full study.
4. In qualitative studies, various issues arise in the ________ during data collection, such as emotional involvement with study participants.
6. Sometime researchers ________ their quantitative data by reading through and reporting on the responses of individual participants.
8. The normal values for standardized instruments applied to a specified population
12. A pitfall that can occur in qualitative research when data collectors get too close to participants (two words)
13. In selecting instruments, researchers may need to consider if their financial ________ are adequate to pay for all associated costs (abbr.).
14. Structured data collection usually involves the use of a formal ________ (abbr.).
17. Qualitative researchers who tape their interviews usually then tran________ them.
18. If participants have low literacy levels, the readability of the instruments should be ________ before proceeding with the study.
20. The most commonly used data collection method is self-________.
21. One consideration in selecting an instrument is its ________ with experts in the field (abbr.).
22. An issue that qualitative researchers face is how to ________ their data while they are still in the field.

DOWN

1. Qualitative researchers may need to ensure that the ________ of data collection is not too intense.
2. Researchers must decide whether to use ________ data or collect new data.
3. In many studies, the people collecting data must undergo rigorous ________ before they can begin their work.
5. One of the drawbacks of self-reports is that respondents may ________ or distort the truth so as to "look good."
6. One of the dimensions along which data can vary is the extent to which they are ________.
7. With increased emphasis on clinical issues, ________ measures are playing an increasing role as outcomes in nursing research (abbr.).
9. The major way to obtain data about people's behavior is through ________.
10. Nurses often use existing ________ from hospitals or other health settings in their research.
11. A key dimension along which data vary is ________.
15. The best way to record qualitative interviews is to ________ them.
16. In thinking about data needs, it may be important to consider analyses of sub________ effects.
19. The collection of research ________ is typically a time-consuming step in the study.

■ B. Study Questions

1. Below are several research questions. Indicate what method or methods of data collection (self-report, observation, biophysiologic measures) you would recommend using to address each. Defend your response.
   a. How does an elderly patient manage the transition from hospital to home?
   b. What are the predictors of intravenous site symptoms?
   c. What are the factors associated with smoking during pregnancy?
   d. To what extent and in what manner do nurses interact differently with male and female patients?
   e. What are the coping mechanisms of parents whose infants are long-term patients in neonatal intensive care units?
2. For each of the research problems in Question B.1, indicate where on the four dimensions discussed in this chapter (structure, quantifiability, researcher obtrusiveness, and objectivity) you would recommend that data should lie.
3. Read one of the following articles, which relied exclusively on self-report, and identify concepts/variables that *could* have been captured with an alternative approach (also: *Should* they have been?):
   - Primomo, J., Johnston, S., Dibiase, F., Nodolf, J., & Noren, L. (2006). Evaluation of a community-based Outreach worker program for children with asthma. *Public Health Nursing, 23*(3), 234–241.
   - Shaughnessy, M., Resnick, B., & Macko, F. (2006). Testing a model of post-stroke exercise behavior. *Rehabilitation Nursing, 31*(1), 15–21.
   - Small, J., & Montoro-Rodriguez, J. (2006). Conflict resolution styles: A comparison of assisted living and nursing home facilities. *Journal of Gerontological Nursing, 32*(1), 39–45.
4. Read one of the following articles, and indicate how, if at all, you might modify the study to triangulate data collection methods:
   - McGrath, P. (2006). Exploring Aboriginal people's experience of relocation for treatment during end-of-life care. *International Journal of Palliative Nursing, 12*(3), 102–108.
   - Barnason, S., Zimmerman, L., Brey, B., Catlin, S., & Nieveen, J. (2006). Patterns of recovery following percutaneous coronary intervention. *Applied Nursing Research, 19,* 31–37.
5. Read the introduction and method sections of one of the following reports. Use the critiquing guidelines in Box 14.1 of the textbook (available as a Word document in the Toolkit ⊗) to critique the data collection aspects of the study:
   - DeSanto-Madeya, S. (2006). The meaning of living with spinal cord injury 5 to 10 years after the injury. *Western Journal of Nursing Research, 28*(3), 265–289.
   - Jesse, D. E., Graham, M., & Swanson, M. (2006). Psychosocial and spiritual factors associated with smoking and substance use during pregnancy in African American and white low-income women. *Journal of Obstetric, Gynecologic, & Neonatal Nursing, 35*(1), 68–77.

- Li, H., & Lopez, V. (2006). Assessing children's emotional responses to surgery. *Journal of Advanced Nursing, 53*(5), 543–550.

■ C. Application Exercises

EXERCISE 1: ALL STUDIES IN APPENDICES

Which of the studies in Appendices A through I of this Resource Manual (if any) used the following:

a. existing data from records?
b. biophysiologic data?
c. observational data?

EXERCISE 2: STUDY IN APPENDIX A

Read the method section of the report by Hill and co-researchers ("Chronically ill rural women") in Appendix A—paying special attention to the design and measures subsections. Then answer the following questions:

Questions of Fact

a. How would you rate the data collection methods of this study in terms of structure, quantifiability, obtrusiveness, and objectivity?
b. Did the researchers develop their own measures, or did they use instruments or scales that had been developed by others?
c. Did this study use any self-report measures? If no, could they have been used to measure key concepts? How were self-report data recorded? What variables were measured by self-report?
d. Did this study collect any data through observation? If no, could observation have been used to measure key concepts? If yes, what variables were measured through observation? How were data obtained and recorded?
e. Did this study collect any biophysiologic measures? If no, could such measures have been used to capture key concepts? If yes, what variables were measured through biophysiologic methods? How were the measurements made?
f. Were records used in this study? If no, could records have been used to measure key concepts? If yes, what records were used and what variables were captured?
g. Did the researchers describe the criteria they used in selecting instruments? If so, what were they?
h. Who gathered the data in this study? How were the data collectors trained?

Questions for Discussion

a. Comment on the adequacy of the data collection approaches used in this study. Did Hill and colleagues operationalize their outcome measures in the best possible manner?

b. Comment on the procedures used to collect data in this study. Were adequate steps taken to ensure the highest possible quality data?

EXERCISE 3: STUDY IN APPENDIX D

Read the method section of the report by Beck ("Post-traumatic stress disorder") in Appendix D—specifically the research design and procedure subsections. Then answer the following questions:

Questions of Fact

a. How would you rate the data collection methods of this study in terms of structure, quantifiability, obtrusiveness, and objectivity?
b. Did this study collect any self-report data? If no, could self-reports have been used? If yes, what concepts were captured by self-report? How were self-report data recorded?
c. Did this study collect any data through observation? If no, could observation have been used? If yes, what concepts were captured through observation? How were data obtained and recorded?
d. Did this study collect any biophysiologic measures? If no, could such measures have been used to capture important concepts? If yes, what variables were measured through biophysiologic methods? How were the measurements made?
e. Were records, documents, or artifacts used in this study? If no, could they have been used? If yes, what records were used and what concepts were captured?
f. Who collected the data in this study? How were data collectors trained?

Questions for Discussion

a. Comment on the adequacy of the data collection approaches used in this study. Did Beck fully capture the concepts of interest in the best possible manner?
b. Comment on the procedures used to collect data in this study. Were adequate steps taken to ensure the highest possible quality data?

■ D. The Toolkit

For Chapter 14, the Toolkit on the accompanying CD-ROM contains a Word file with the following:

- Guidelines for Critiquing Data Collection Plans (Box 14.1 of the textbook)
- Example of a Data Matrix for Recording Data Decisions (adapted from Figure 14.2 of the textbook)
- Example of a Table of Contents for an Interviewer Training Manual (Table 14.1 of the textbook)

- Model Sections for an Interviewer Training Manual
  - Answering Respondents' Questions
  - Avoiding Interviewer Bias
  - Probing and Obtaining Full Responses
- Annotated Guidelines Relating to Key Demographic Questions
- Example of a Basic Demographic Questionnaire
- Example of a Letter Requesting Permission to Use an Instrument

CHAPTER **15**

Collecting Unstructured Data

■ A. Crossword Puzzle

Complete the crossword puzzle below, which uses terms and concepts presented in Chapter 15. (Puzzles may be removed for easier viewing.)

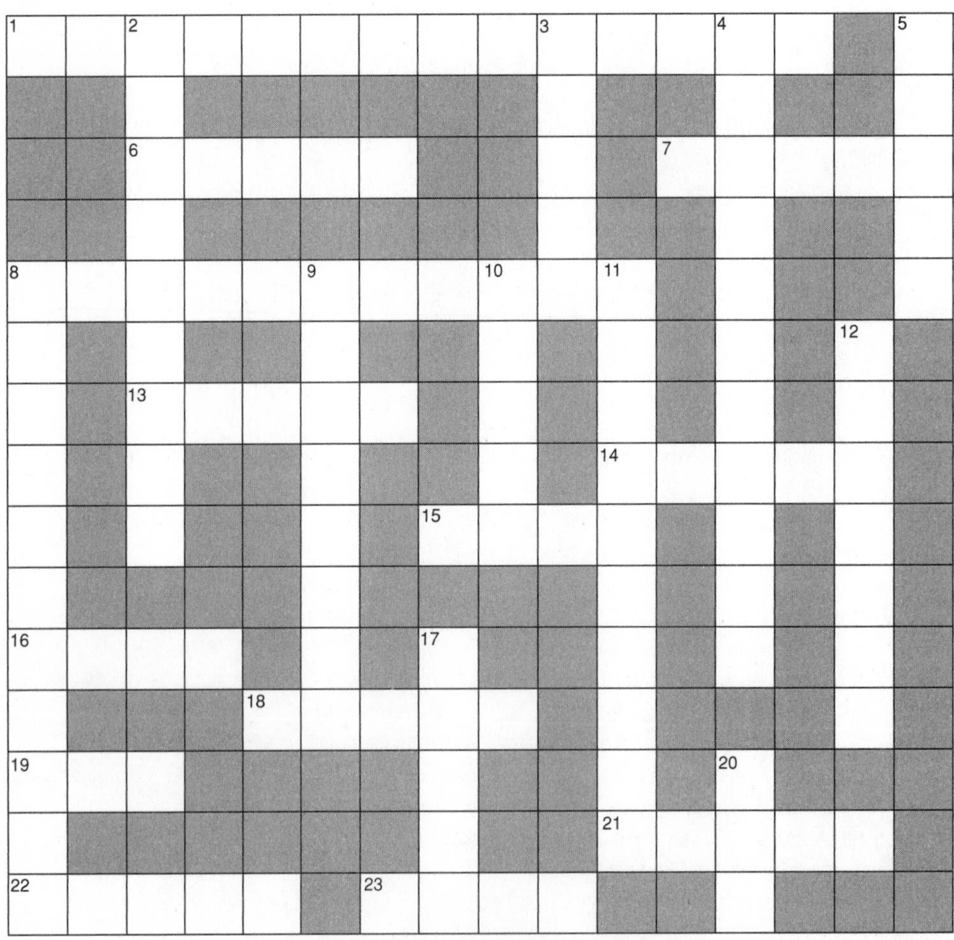

ACROSS

1. The type of interview in which the interviewer uses a list of questions that must be covered
6. Participants can be asked to maintain a journal or ________ that provides rich ongoing data about aspects of ordinary life.
7. Observational data are maintained in ________ notes.
8. The type of observation often undertaken in qualitative studies to "get inside" a social situation is ________ observation.
13. Interviewers may benefit from a ________ guide that specifies the question areas that must be covered.
14. Methodologic ________ document observers' thoughts about their strategies while in the field.
15. A chronology of daily events during field observations is maintained in ________.
16. ________ histories are used to gather personal recollections of events and their perceived causes or consequences.
18. The think ________ method involves having people talk about decisions as they are making them.
19. The ________ can yield rich qualitative data (e.g., through postings in chatrooms) (abbr).
21. A skilled interviewer must learn how to ________ effectively to elicit more detail (backwards).
22. An unstructured interview often begins with a ________ tour question.
23. Observational notes include descriptive and ________ notes (abbr.)

DOWN

2. The person who leads a focus group session
3. Unstructured interviews cons_ _ _ _ _ neither the interviewers nor the participants.
4. Photo ________ is a technique that uses photographs to encourage participant narratives.
5. A record of an observational setting can be made by ________taping it.
8. Observers have to make decisions about ________ themselves so as best to capture the behaviors and events of interest.
9. The technique called ________ incidents focuses on the circumstances surrounding particularly notable incidents.
10. The best method to record unstructured interviews is to ________tape them.
11. Researchers who tape their interviews must then ________ them so that the data can more readily be read, re-read, and analyzed.
12. In a life ________ interview, participants are encouraged to provide a chronologic narration of life experiences.
17. Both semistructured and focus group interviews typically involve use of a topic ________.
20. Participant observers may often have to excuse themselves from a setting to briefly ________ down notes about what is transpiring.

■ B. Study Questions

1. Suppose you were interested in studying the frustrations of patients waiting for treatment in the waiting area of an emergency department. Develop a topic guide for a focused interview on this topic.

2. Below are several research problems. Indicate which type of unstructured approach you might recommend using for each. Defend your response.
   a. By what process do older brothers and sisters of a handicapped child adapt to their sibling's disability?
   b. What is it like to have a persistent wound?
   c. What stresses does the spouse of a terminally ill patient experience?
   d. What type of information does a nurse draw on most heavily in formulating nursing diagnoses?
   e. What are the coping mechanisms and perceived barriers to coping among severely disfigured burn patients?

3. Develop a topic guide that focuses on nursing students' reasons for selecting nursing as a career and their satisfactions and dissatisfactions with their decision. Administer the topic guide to five first-year nursing students in a face-to-face interview situation. Now administer the topic guide in a focus group setting with five nursing students. Compare the kinds of information that the two approaches yielded. What, if anything, did you learn in the group setting that did not emerge in the personal interviews (and *vice versa*)?

4. Would a psychiatric nurse researcher be well suited to undertake a participant observation study of the interactions between psychiatric nurses and their clients? Why or why not?

5. Read one of the following articles, and indicate how, if at all, you would augment the self-report data collected in this study with participant observation:
   - Aldred, H., Gott, M., & Gariballa, S. (2006). Advanced heart failure: Impact on older patients and informed carers. *Journal of Advanced Nursing, 49*(2), 116–124.
   - Bramhagen, A., Axelsson, I., & Hallstrom, I. (2006). Mothers' experiences of feeding situations—An interview study. *Journal of Clinical Nursing, 15*(1), 29–34.
   - Moore, J., & Beckwith, A. (2006). Self-care operations and nursing interventions for children with cancer and their parents. *Nursing Science Quarterly, 19*(2), 147–156.

6. Read the introduction and method sections of one of the following reports. Use the critiquing guidelines in Box 15.3 of the textbook (available as a Word document in the Toolkit ⊗) to critique the data collection aspects of the study:
   - Donnelly, T. (2006). The health-care practices of Vietnamese-Canadian women. *Canadian Journal of Nursing Research, 38*(1), 82–101.
   - Nehring, W., & Faux, S. (2006). Transitional and health issues of adults with neural tube defects. *Journal of Nursing Scholarship, 38*(1), 63–70.

- Sun, F., Long, A., Boore, J., & Tsao, L. (2006). Patients' and nurses' perceptions of ward environmental factors and support systems in the care of suicidal patients. *Journal of Clinical Nursing, 15*(1), 83–92.

■ C. Application Exercises

EXERCISE 1: STUDY IN APPENDIX B

Read the method section of the report by Rew ("Homeless youth") in Appendix B—paying special attention to the procedures subsection. Then answer the following questions:

Questions of Fact

a. Did Rew collect any self-report data? If no, could self-reports have been used? If yes, what concepts were captured by self-report?
b. What specific types of qualitative self-report methods were used?
c. Were examples of questions included in the report?
d. Does the report provide information about how long interviews took, on average?
e. How were the self-report data recorded?
f. Did Rew collect any data through observation? If no, could observation have been used? If yes, what concepts were captured through observation?
g. If there were observations, how were observational data recorded?
h. Who collected the data in this study?

Questions for Discussion

a. Comment on the adequacy of the researcher's description of her data collection methods.
b. Comment on the data collection approaches Rew used. Did she fully capture the concepts of interest in the best possible manner?
c. If examples of specific questions were included in the report, do they appear appropriate for collecting the desired information? If they were not included, does the absence of such examples undermine your ability to fully understand the quality of evidence the study yielded?
d. If the report describes how long the interviews were, do you feel the interviews were sufficiently long to obtain the desired information? If such information was missing, does its absence undermine your ability to fully understand the quality of evidence the study yielded?
e. Comment on the procedures used to collect and record data in this study. Were adequate steps taken to ensure the highest possible quality data?

EXERCISE 2: STUDY IN APPENDIX F

Read the method section of the report by Giddings ("Health disparities") in Appendix F. Then answer the following questions:

Questions of Fact

a. Did Giddings collect any self-report data? If no, could self-reports have been used? If yes, what concepts were captured by self-report?
b. What specific types of qualitative self-report methods were used?
c. Were examples of questions included in the report?
d. Does the report provide information about how long interviews took, on average?
e. How were the self-report data recorded?
f. Did Giddings collect any data through observation? If no, could observation have been used? If yes, what concepts were captured through observation?
g. If there were observations, how were observational data recorded?
h. Who collected the data in this study?

Questions for Discussion

a. Comment on the adequacy of the researcher's description of her data collection methods.
b. Comment on the data collection approaches Giddings used. Did she fully capture the concepts of interest in the best possible manner?
c. If examples of specific questions were included in the report, do they appear appropriate for collecting the desired information? If they were not included, does the absence of such examples undermine your ability to fully understand the quality of evidence the study yielded?
d. If the report describes how long the interviews were, do you feel the interviews were sufficiently long to obtain the desired information? If such information was missing, does its absence undermine your ability to fully understand the quality of evidence the study yielded?
e. Comment on the procedures used to collect and record data in this study. Were adequate steps taken to ensure the highest possible quality data?

■ D. The Toolkit

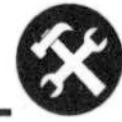

For Chapter 15, the Toolkit on the accompanying CD-ROM contains a Word file with the following:

- Guidelines for Critiquing Unstructured Data Collection Methods (Box 15.3 of the textbook)
- Example of a Topic Guide for a Semistructured Interview
- Example of an Agenda for a Focus Group Session
- Focus Groups Versus In-Depth Personal Interviews: Guide to Selecting a Method
- Example of a Protocol for a Windshield (Community Mapping) Survey
- Examples of Types of Information Relevant in Unstructured Observation (from textbook)
- Example of an Observation Form for Unstructured Observation

CHAPTER 16

Collecting Structured Data

■ A. Crossword Puzzle

Complete the crossword puzzle below, which uses terms and concepts presented in Chapter 16. (Puzzles may be removed for easier viewing.)

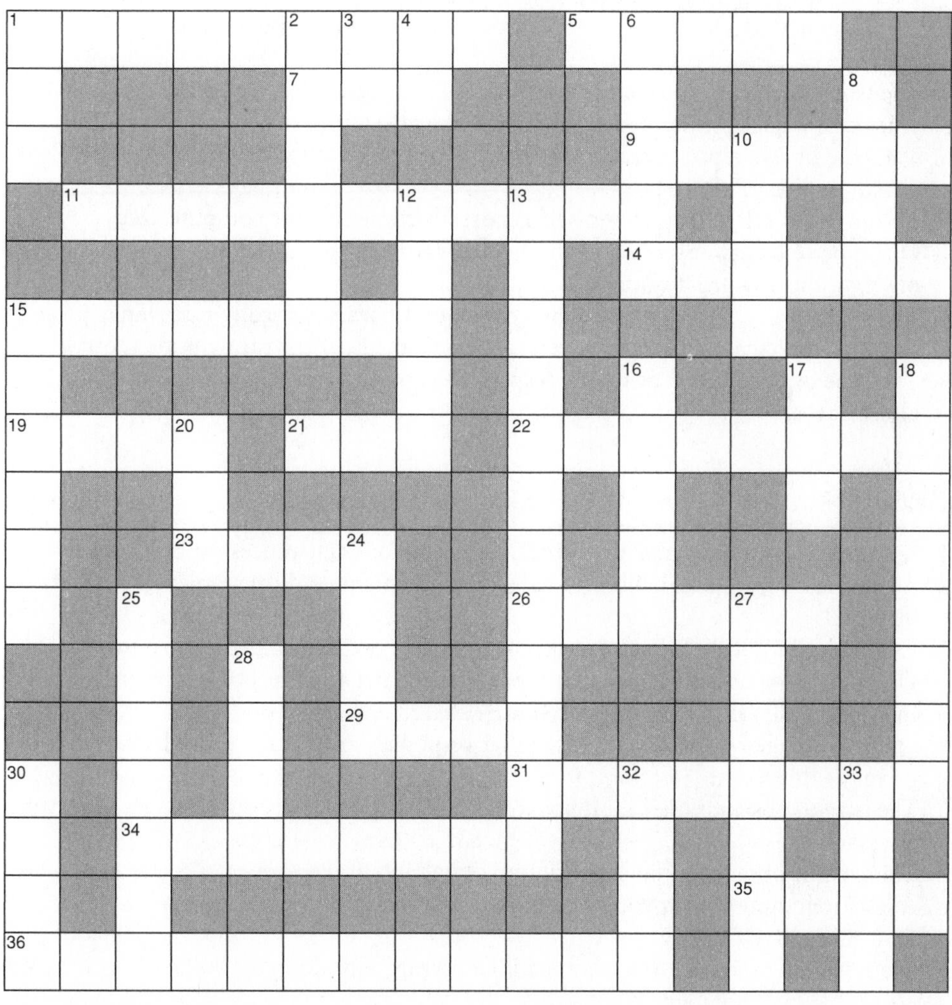

ACROSS

1. In structured observation, a(n) ________ is used with a category system to record the incidence of an observed event.
5. A tool that yields a score placing people on a continuum with regard to an attribute
7. In observation studies, the instruments should be tested by having two or more ________ (abbr.) observers code or rate the event and then comparing results.
9. One method of recording observations is to have observers use ________ scales to provide judgments about the behavioral construct along a continuum.
11. The type of question most prevalent in mailed questionnaires
14. Respondents rate concepts on a series of bipolar rating scales in a ________ differential (abbr.).
15. A description of a situation or person designed to elicit study participants' reactions
19. A ________ card is presented to respondents in interviews when response options are complex or multiple questions have the same options.
21. The tendency to distort self-report information in characteristic ways is a response ________ bias.
22. The two ________ alternatives to "What is your gender?" are "male" and "female."
23. One advantage of using questionnaires is the absence of any interviewer ________.
26. The type of self-report that typically yields better quality data than self-administered questionnaires (abbr.)
29. Acronym for self-administered self-report instruments (not computerized)
31. One type of observation bias is the bias toward central ________, which distorts observations toward a middle ground.
34. The error of ________ occurs when observers characteristically rate things positively.
35. A Likert-type scale may also be referred to as a ________ rating scale (abbr.).
36. The type of question that forces respondents to choose from two competing alternatives.

DOWN

1. A system used to organize observational events or occurrences (abbr.)
2. A summated rating scale used to measure agreement or disagreement with statements
3. Extracting biophysiologic material from people yields ________ vitro measures.
4. On an agreement continuum, the most extreme negative response option (acronym)
6. In Q-sorts, the objects being sorted are ________.
8. One advantage of questionnaires is that responses are ________, which ensures privacy (abbr.).
10. The type of observational sampling approach used to select periods when observations are made
12. The type of observational sampling involving integral episodes
13. A bias stemming from people's wanting to "look good" is called a(n) ________ desirability bias.
15. A questioning method to measure clinical symptoms along a 100-mm continuum is a(n) ________ analogue scale.

16. A self-report approach involving the sorting of statements into different piles along a continuum
17. On a 5-point Likert scale, if SD were scored 5, SA would be scored ________.
18. The error of ________ occurs when observers characteristically rate things too harshly.
20. Self-report instruments can be administered as ________-based surveys over the Internet.
24. Filter questions often involve the use of ________ patterns to route people appropriately through a self-report instrument.
25. A rating scale along the continuum "exhausted" to "energized" is using ________ adjectives.
27. If both positive and negative items were included in a scale, the researcher would need to ________ the scoring of one type or the other.
28. The question "What is it like to be a cancer survivor?" is ________ ended.
30. The most widely used method of data collection by nurse researchers is by ________ report.
32. The number of piles in a Q-sort is typically ________ or eleven.
33. Scales are often called ________ scales because they are a combination of multiple items (abbr.).

■ B. Study Questions

1. Suppose you were interested in studying attitudes toward risky behavior (e.g., unsafe sex, drug use, speeding) among adolescents. Develop the following types of questions designed to measure these attitudes.
   a. Dichotomous item
   b. Multiple choice item
   c. Open-ended item
2. Below are hypothetical responses for Respondent Y and Respondent Z to the statements on the Likert scale presented in Table 16.2 of the textbook. What would the total score for both of these respondents be, using the scoring rules described in Chapter 16?

Item No.	Respondent Y	Respondent Z
1	D	SA
2	A	D
3	SA	D
4	?	A
5	D	SA
6	SA	D

12. Below is a list of five variables. Indicate briefly how you would operationalize each using structured observational procedures.
    a. Fear in hospitalized children
    b. Pain during childbirth
    c. Dependency in psychiatric patients
    d. Empathy in nursing students
    e. Cooperativeness in chemotherapy patients
13. Three nurse researchers were collaborating on a study of the effect of preoperative visits to surgical patients by operating room nurses on the stress levels of those patients just before surgery. One researcher wanted to use the patients' self-reports to measure stress; the second suggested using pulse rate and the Palmer Sweat Index; the third recommended using an observational measure of stress. Which measure do you think would be the most appropriate for this research problem? Can you suggest other possible measures of stress that might be even more appropriate? Justify your response.
14. Read the introduction and method sections of one of the following reports. Use the critiquing guidelines in Box 16.4 of the textbook (available as a Word document in the Toolkit) to critique the data collection aspects of the study:
    - Carter, P. A. (2006). A brief behavioral sleep intervention for family caregivers of persons with cancer. *Cancer Nursing, 29*(2), 95–103.
    - Ramelet, A., Abu-Saad, H., Bulsara, M., Rees, N., & McDonald, S. (2006). Capturing pediatric pain responses in critically ill infants aged 0 to 9 months. *Pediatric Critical Care Medicine,* 7(1), 19–26.
    - Tel, H., & Tel, H. (2006). The effect of individualized education on the transfer anxiety of patients with myocardial infarction and their families. *Heart & Lung, 35*(2), 101–107.

■ C. Application Exercises

EXERCISE 1: STUDY IN APPENDIX C

Read the method section of the report by Wang and Chan ("Culturally tailored diabetes education") in Appendix C. Then answer the following questions:

Questions of Fact

a. Did this study use any self-report measures? What variables were measured by self-report?
b. Were examples of specific questions included in the report?
c. Did the researchers' instruments include both open-ended and closed-ended questions? Did the report mention the use of any specific types of self-reports, such as visual analogue scales, forced-choice questions, event calendar questions, and so on?
d. Were any composite scales used? If yes, were they of the Likert type?
e. Were self-report data gathered by interview or by self-administered questionnaires (or both)?

f. Did the researchers develop their own self-report measures, or did they use instruments or scales that had been developed by others?
g. Did the researchers describe the criteria they used in selecting instruments? Is so, what were they?
h. Did the report mention anything about the readability level of self-report instruments?
i. Did the report describe how long it took, on average, for respondents to complete the self-report instrument?
j. Did the researchers collect any data through observation? If no, could observation have been used to measure key concepts? If yes, what variables were measured through observation?
k. Did the researchers collect any biophysiologic measures? If yes, what variables were measured through biophysiologic methods?
l. Does the report describe the procedures for using biophysiologic measurements? Were procedures standardized?
m. Who gathered the data in this study? How were the data collectors trained?

Questions for Discussion

a. Comment on the adequacy of the researchers' description of their data collection approaches and procedures.
b. Do you think that Wang and Chan operationalized their outcome measures in the best possible manner? Could different or supplementary measures have been used to enhance the quality of the study's evidence?
c. Comment on the procedures used to collect data in this study. Were adequate steps taken to ensure the highest possible quality data?

EXERCISE 2: STUDY IN APPENDIX E

Read the method section of the report by Loeb ("Older men's health") in Appendix E. Then answer the following questions:

Questions of Fact

a. Did Loeb use any self-report measures? What variables were measured by self-report?
b. Were examples of specific questions included in the report?
c. Did the researcher's instruments include both open-ended and closed-ended questions? Did the report mention the use of any specific types of self-reports, such as visual analogue scales, forced-choice questions, event calendar questions, and so on?
d. Were any composite scales used? If yes, were they of the Likert type?
e. Were self-report data gathered by interview or by self-administered questionnaires (or both)?
f. Did Loeb develop her own self-report measures, or did she use instruments or scales that had been developed by others?
g. Did the researcher describe the criteria she used to select instruments? If so, what were they?

h. Did the report mention anything about the readability level of self-report instruments?
i. Did the report describe how long it took, on average, for respondents to complete the self-report instrument?
j. Did Loeb collect any data through observation? If no, could observation have been used to measure key concepts? If yes, what variables were measured through observation?
k. Did Loeb collect any biophysiologic measures? If yes, what variables were measured through biophysiologic methods? If no, should any variables have been operationalized using biophysiologic methods?
l. Who gathered the data in this study? How were the data collectors trained?

Questions for Discussion

a. Comment on the adequacy of the researcher's description of her data collection approaches and procedures.
b. Do you think that Loeb operationalized her variables in the best possible manner? Could different or supplementary measures have been used to enhance the quality of the study's evidence?
c. Comment on the procedures used to collect data in this study. Were adequate steps taken to ensure the highest possible quality data?

■ D. The Toolkit

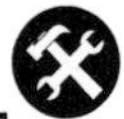

For Chapter 16, the Toolkit on the accompanying CD-ROM contains a Word file with the following:

- Guidelines for Critiquing Structured Data Collection Methods (Box 16.4 of the textbook)
- Example of a Cover Letter for a Mailed Questionnaire (Figure 16.4 of the textbook)
- Example of a Visual Analogue Scale
- Example of a Show Card for a Personal Interview
- Example of a Reminder Postcard for a Mailed Questionnaire
- Example of an Event History Calendar

CHAPTER 17

Assessing Measurement Quality in Quantitative Studies

■ A. Crossword Puzzle

Complete the crossword puzzle below, which uses terms and concepts presented in Chapter 17. (Puzzles may be removed for easier viewing.)

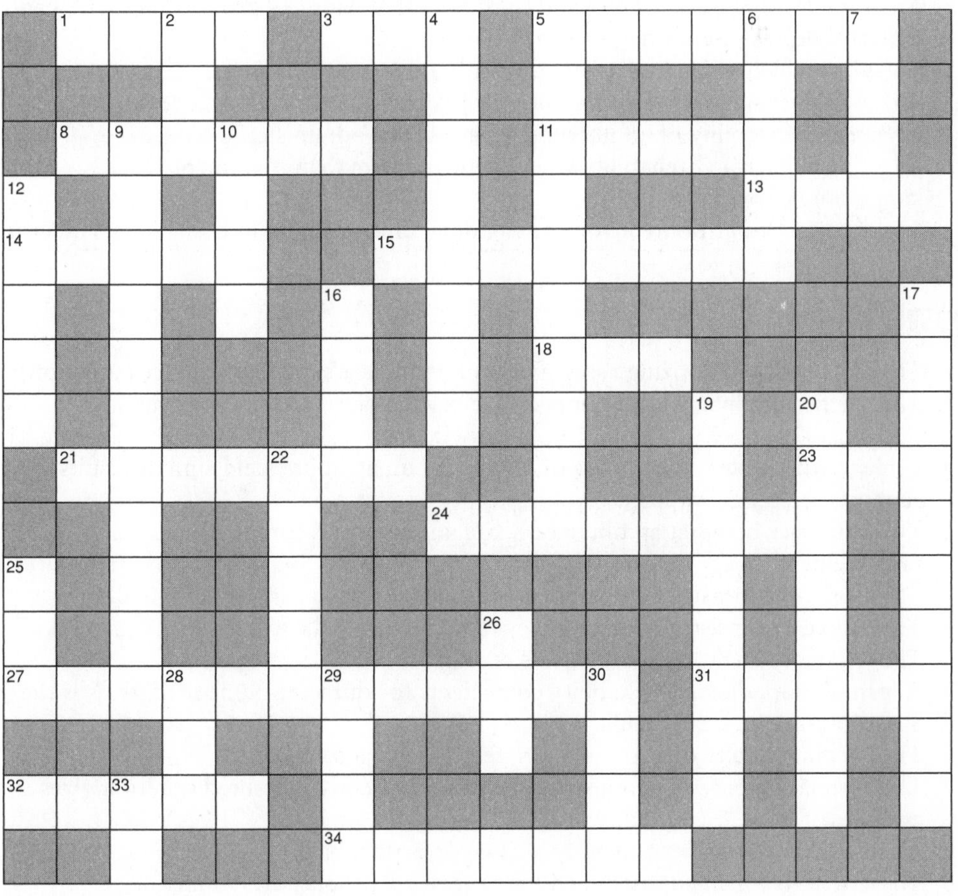

ACROSS

1. The type of validity involving the extent to which a measure "looks" valid
3. Sensitivity is plotted against specificity in a _ _ _ curve (acronym).
5. The type of validity concerned with adequate representation of all aspects of a concept
8. Predictive validity and concurrent validity are aspects of ________-related validity (abbr.).
11. An unreliable instrument could ________ be valid.
13. A receiver ________ curve can be used to determine the best dividing point for cases and noncases in a screening instrument (abbr.).
14. Measurement involves assigning numbers according to established ________.
15. The kappa statistic can be used to estimate inter- ________ reliability.
18. One means of assessing construct validity is through the known ________ technique (acronym).
21. The ability of an instrument to differentiate the construct being measured from other similar concepts (abbr.)
23. An index relating to specificity and sensitivity that captures proportion of area and indicates degree of accuracy (acronym)
24. The most widely evaluated aspect of reliability is a measure's ________ consistency.
27. A thorough evaluation of an instrument involves a(n) ________ assessment.
31. To assess the stability of an instrument, it must be administered ________.
32. To estimate interrater reliability when there are more than two raters, ________-rater kappa can be computed.
33. To ________ an attribute involves assigning numeric values to designate its quantity.

DOWN

2. The indicator summarizing assessments of a measure's content validity (acronym)
4. The coefficient alpha was developed by a psychologist whose last name was ________.
5. Evidence that different methods of measuring an attribute yield similar results supports ________ validity.
6. The difference between an obtained score and the true score is the ________ of measurement.
7. The score on a measure that would be obtained if the measure were infallible
9. The degree of consistency or accuracy of a measure indicates its ________.
10. The reliability method used to assess stability is ________-retest.
12. A formula for adjusting reliability coefficients for different number of items is the Spearman-________ formula.
16. The content validity of items is estimated by this (acronym).
17. The correlation between an instrument and a currently measured criterion gives an estimate of ________ validity.
19. An instrument's ability to identify a case correctly (abbr.)
20. The extent to which an instrument measures what it purports to measure
22. A likelihood ________ summarizes the relationship between specificity and sensitivity in a single number.

25. The proportion of people with a positive result who have the target outcome or disease (backwards acronym)
26. An alternative to classical measurement theory (acronym)
28. In screening instruments, "cases" are separated from "noncases" at the ________off point.
29. A complex technique for exploring construct validity with multiple measures of multiple constructs (acronym)
30. The ________ coefficient is an index used to summarize the magnitude and direction of relationships between variables (abbr.).
33. The ratio of true-positive results to false-positive results is the ___ ___ +.

■ B. Study Questions

1. The reliability of measures of which of the following attributes would *not* be appropriately assessed using a test–retest procedure with 1 month between administrations. Why?
   a. Attitudes toward abortion
   b. Stress
   c. Achievement motivation
   d. Nursing effectiveness
   e. Depression
2. Comment on the meaning and implications of the following statement:

   A researcher found that the internal consistency of her 20-item scale measuring attitudes toward nurse-midwives was .74, using the Cronbach alpha formula.

3. In the following situation, what might be some of the sources of measurement error?

   One hundred nurses who worked in a large metropolitan hospital were asked to complete a 10-item Likert scale designed to measure job satisfaction. The questionnaires were distributed by nursing supervisors at the end of shifts. The staff nurses were asked to complete the forms and return them immediately to their supervisors.

4. Identify what is incorrect about the following statements:
   a. "My scale is highly reliable, so it must be valid."
   b. "My instrument yielded an internal consistency coefficient of .80, so it must be stable."
   c. "The validity coefficient between my scale and a criterion measure was .40; therefore, my scale must be of low validity."
   d. "My scale had a reliability coefficient of .80. Therefore, an obtained score of 20 is indicative of a true score of 16."
   e. "The validation study proved that my measure has construct validity."
   f. "My advisor examined my new measure of dependence in nursing home residents and, based on its content, assured me the measure was valid."

5. Read the introduction and method sections of one of the following reports. Use the critiquing guidelines in Box 17.1 of the textbook (available as a Word document in the Toolkit) to critique the measurement and data quality aspects of the study:
   - Brewer, S., Gleditsch, S., Syblik, D., Tietjens, M., & Vacik, H. (2006). Pediatric anxiety: Child life intervention in day surgery. *Journal of Pediatric Nursing, 21*(1), 13–22.
   - Makabe, R., & Nomizu, T. (2006). Social support and psychological and physical states in Japanese patients with breast cancer and their spouses prior to surgery. *Oncology Nursing Forum, 33*(3), 651–655.
   - Siedliecki, S., & Good, M. (2006). Effect of music on power, depression and disability. *Journal of Advanced Nursing, 54*(5), 553–562.

■ C. Application Exercises

EXERCISE 1: STUDY IN APPENDIX A

Read the method section of the report by Hill and co-researchers ("Chronically ill rural women") in Appendix A—paying special attention to the design and measures subsections. Then answer the following questions:

Questions of Fact

a. Describe what methods (if any) were reported as having been used to assess the reliability of the following instruments—and indicate what the reliability coefficients were in each case:
   - The Personal Resource Questionnaire (PRQ2000)
   - Self-Efficacy Scale
   - Self-Esteem Scale
   - Perceived Stress Scale
   - CES-D Depression Scale
   - UCLA Loneliness Scale

b. Describe what methods (if any) were reported as having been used to assess the validity of the same six instruments.

c. Did Hill and colleagues rely on assessments of quality from other researchers, or did they perform any quality assessments themselves?

d. Was information about the specificity or sensitivity of any of the instruments provided in the report?

Questions for Discussion

a. Describe what some of the sources of measurement error might have been in this study. Did the researchers take adequate steps to minimize measurement error?

b. Comment on the adequacy of information in the report about efforts to select or develop high-quality instruments.

c. Comment on the quality of the measures that Hill and colleagues used in their study. Do you feel confident that instruments yielded adequately reliable and valid indicators of the key constructs?

EXERCISE 2: STUDY IN APPENDIX E

Read the method section of the report by Loeb ("Older men's health") in Appendix E—specifically the subsections on the instruments. Then answer the following questions:

Questions of Fact

a. Describe what methods (if any) were reported as having been used to assess the reliability of the following instruments—and indicate what the reliability coefficients were in each case:
   - The demographics instrument
   - Older Men's Health Program and Screening Inventory
   - Health-Promotion Activities of Older Adults Measure
   - Health Self-Determinism Index

b. Describe what methods (if any) were reported as having been used to assess the validity of the same four instruments.

c. Did Loeb rely on assessments of quality from other researchers, or did she herself perform any quality assessments?

d. Was information about the specificity or sensitivity of any of the instruments provided in the report?

Questions for Discussion

a. Describe what some of the sources of measurement error might have been in this study. Did the researcher take adequate steps to minimize measurement error?

b. Comment on the adequacy of information in the report about efforts to select or develop high-quality instruments.

c. Comment on the quality of the measures that Loeb used in her study. Do you feel confident that they were adequately reliable and valid indicators of the key constructs?

■ D. The Toolkit

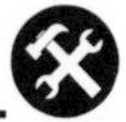

For Chapter 17, the Toolkit on the accompanying CD-ROM contains a Word file with the following:

- Guidelines for Critiquing Data Quality in Quantitative Studies (Box 17.1 of the textbook)
- Suggestions for Enhancing Data Quality and Minimizing Measurement Error in Quantitative Studies

CHAPTER 18

Developing and Testing Self-Report Scales

■ A. Crossword Puzzle

Complete the crossword puzzle below, which uses terms and concepts presented in Chapter 18. (Puzzles may be removed for easier viewing.)

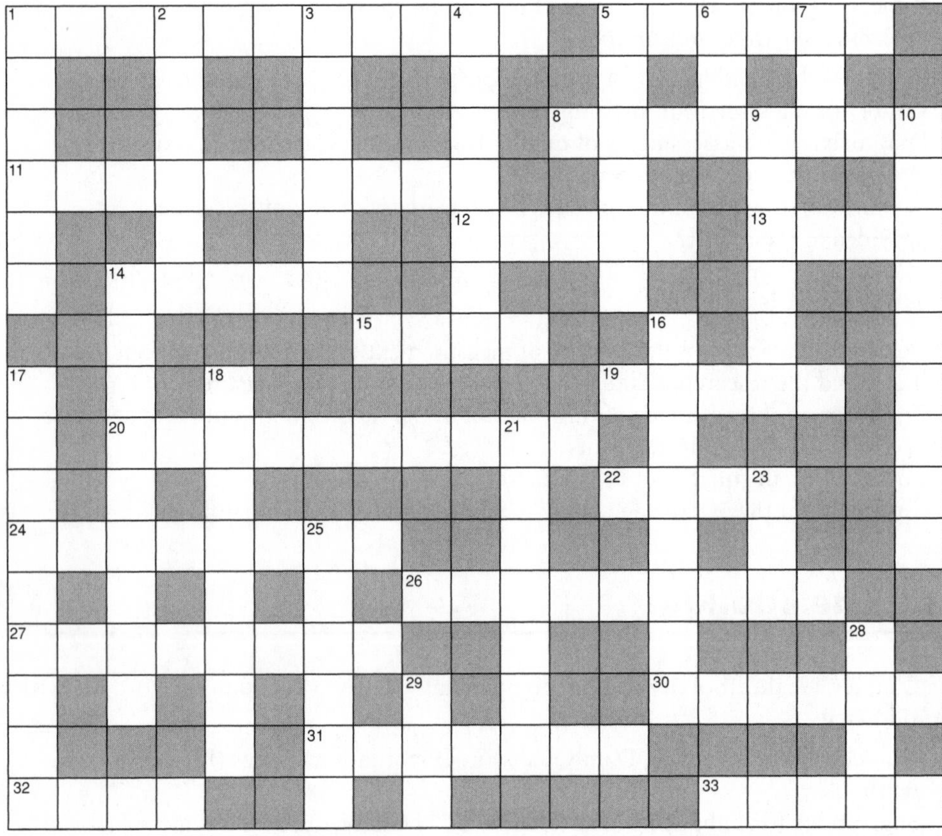

ACROSS

1. The type of factor analysis that stipulates no *a priori* hypotheses about the dimensionality of a set of items
5. ________ analysis is used to shed light on the dimensionality of a set of items.
8. In translations, ________ equivalence concerns the extent to which the meaning of items is the same in the target culture as it was in the original.
11. In principal components analysis, a(n) ________ is equal to the sum of squared weights for a factor.
12. When item difficulty is the only parameter being considered in an IRT analysis, it is said to be a ________ model.
13. Developing a pool of items is often best done as a(n) ________ effort.
14. Initially, it is best to develop 3 to 4 times as many ________ as are believed to be needed for a scale.
15. On a Likert-type scale, each item consists of a declarative ________ and a set of response options.
19. In confirmatory factor analysis, the first phase involves testing of a measurement ________.
20. In EFA, the first phase is called factor ________.
22. One index of readability is the reading ________ score.
24. Most Likert-type scales have five or seven ________ options.
26. The most widely used factor extraction method is ________ components analysis.
27. The purpose of a scale is *not* to place participants into a(n) ________ but rather to array them along a continuum.
30. In scale development, a(n) ________ sampling model is often assumed-random sampling of a set of items from a hypothetical universe of items (backwards).
31. One source of items for a new scale is from a(n) ________ analysis.
32. In item response theory, items with different levels of ________ are sought (abbr.).
33. Development of a high-quality multi-item ________ is a challenging, labor-intensive activity.

DOWN

1. In content validation work, it is necessary to establish a(n) ________ panel to review items.
2. The underlying construct in a scale is sometimes referred to as the ________ variable.
4. If there are negative and positive items on a scale, some have to be ________-scored.
5. The ________-Kincaid grade level is one of several indexes of readability.
6. Factor analysis undertaken to test and confirm hypotheses about items and scales (acronym).
7. One purpose of a panel of content experts is to weed ________ faulty or weak items.
9. Translations are typically done into the ________ tongue of the translator.
10. Translations and back translations typically involve the use of a(n) ________ to arrive at a consensus.
14. For a traditional Likert-type scale, item ________ should be comparable across items.

Questions for Discussion

a. Comment on the adequacy of the scale development process.
b. Comment on the researchers' choice of response options.
c. How effective were the researchers' efforts to establish the content validity of the instrument?
d. Comment on the sampling plan for the psychometric assessment, in terms of both size and sampling method. Overall, how adequate was the sample that was used?
e. How thorough do you think the researchers were in their efforts to determine the psychometric properties of the instrument?
f. How much confidence would you have in the MTQ instrument? Do you feel that the evidence supporting its high quality is persuasive?

■ D. The Toolkit

For Chapter 18, the Toolkit on the accompanying CD-ROM contains a Word file with the following:

- Guidelines for Critiquing Instrument Development and Validation Reports (Box 18.1 of textbook)
- Example of Cognitive Questioning
- Example of a Cover Letter for Expert Content Validity Panel
- Example of a Content Validity Form (Figure 18.1 of textbook)
- Example of a Query Letter for Commercial Publication of an Instrument
- Example of a Table of Contents for an Instrument Manual

PART 5

Analyzing and Interpreting Research Data

CHAPTER 19

Analyzing Qualitative Data

■ A. Crossword Puzzle

Complete the crossword puzzle below, which uses terms and concepts presented in Chapter 19. (Puzzles may be removed for easier viewing.)

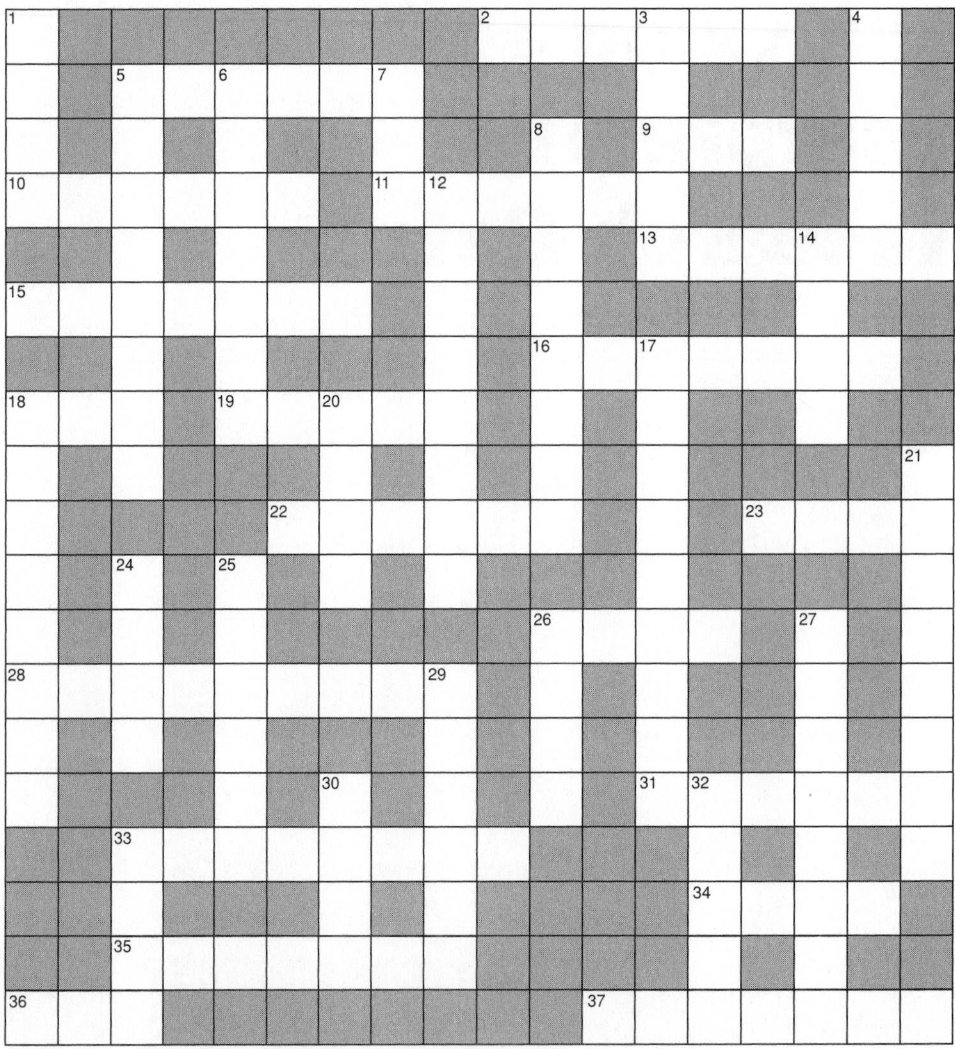

ACROSS

2. Colaizzi's methods involves the use of ________ checks.
5. Phenomenological analysis involves the identification of essential ________.
9. In Glaser and Strauss's method, there are theoretical codes and ________ codes (abbr.).
10. In ethnographies, a broad unit of cultural knowledge
11. *In vivo* codes
13. The hermeneutic ________ involves movement between parts and whole of a text being analyzed.
15. _ _ _ _ _ _ _ i was a prominent analyst and writer in the Duquesne school of phenomenology.
16. In Diekelmann's approach, the discovery of a constitutive ________ forms the highest level of analysis.
18. In grounded theory, the process of identifying characteristics of one piece of data and comparing them with those of another to determine similarity
19. The phenomenologist _ _ _ _ _ i did not espouse validating themes with peers or study participants.
22. The hermeneutic approach developed by ________ includes an analysis of exemplars.
23. Transcribed interviews are usually the main form of ________ in phenomenological analysis.
26. Timelines and ________ charts are devices that can be used to highlight time sequences in qualitative analysis.
28. The most interpretive and subjective qualitative analysis styles
31. After a categorization system is developed, the main task involves ________ the data.
33. A Dutch phenomenologist who encouraged the use of artistic data sources
34. Sometimes qualitative ________ analysis is described as a content analysis.
35. Before analysis can begin, qualitative researchers have to develop a categorization ________.
36. All of a phenomenologist's transcribed interviews would comprise a qualitative data ________.
37. One of the two major schools of phenomenology

DOWN

1. A recurring ________ in a set of interviews can be the basis for an emerging theme.
3. One type of core variable in grounded theory is a ________ social process that evolves over time.
4. A type of coding in Strauss and Corbin's approach wherein the analyst links subcategories
5. A guide for sorting narrative data
6. Grounded theorists and phenomenologists typically use this broad type of qualitative analysis style.
7. In grounded theory, the type of coding focused on the core variable (abbr.)

8. Sometimes used as part of an analytic strategy, especially by interpretive phenomenologists
12. Themes and conceptualizations are viewed as ________ in qualitative analysis.
14. In grounded theory, the ________ category is a central pattern that is relevant to participants.
17. The second level of analysis in Spradley's ethnographic method
18. Glaser proposed 18 ________ of theoretical codes to help grounded theorists conceptualize relationships.
20. The first stage of constant comparison involves ________ coding.
21. ________ cases are strong examples of ways of being in the world.
24. Grounded theorists document an idea in an analytic ________.
25. The nurse researcher who helped develop an alternative approach to grounded theory
26. In manual organization of qualitative data, excerpts are cut up and inserted into a conceptual ________.
27. In Van Manen's ________ approach, the analyst sees the text as a whole and tries to capture its meaning.
29. The field ________ of an ethnographer are an important source of data for analysis.
30. Van ________ was a phenomenologist from the Duquesne school.
32. The point of developing a categorization scheme is to impose ________ on the narrative information.
33. The amount of data collected in a typical qualitative study is ________.

■ B. Study Questions

1. Ask two people to describe their conception of preventive health care and what it means in their daily lives. Pool descriptions with those of other classmates, and develop a coding scheme to organize responses. What major themes emerged?
2. If possible, listen to an audiotaped interview and transcribe a few minutes of it. Compare your transcription with that of another classmate, or with that of the professional transcriber.
3. What is wrong with the following statements?
   a. Hall conducted a grounded theory study about coping with a miscarriage in which she was able to identify four major themes.
   b. Lowe's ethnographic analysis of Haitian clinics involved gleaning related thematic material from French poetry.
   c. Allen's phenomenological study of the lived experience of Parkinson's disease focused on the domain of fatigue.
   d. Dodd's grounded theory study of widowhood yielded a taxonomy of coping strategies.
   e. In her ethnographic study of the culture of a nursing home, MacLean used a rural nursing home as a paradigm case.

4. In her study of homeless youth (Appendix B), Rew presented a list of study participants and some of their demographic and identifying characteristics (Table 1). Instead of using a table, Rew could have described the sample in paragraph form. Try your hand at writing a short paragraph describing a segment of the sample (e.g., the males or the females, the minorities or the Whites, etc.).

5. A category scheme for coding interviews with recently divorced women follows:

CODING SCHEME FOR STUDY OF ADJUSTMENT TO DIVORCE

1. Divorce-related issues
   a. Adjustment to divorce
   b. Divorce-induced problems
   c. Advantages of divorce
2. General psychological state
   a. Before divorce
   b. During divorce
   c. Current
3. Physical health
   a. Before divorce
   b. During divorce
   c. Current
4. Relationship with children
   a. General quality
   b. Communication
   c. Shared activities
   d. Structure of relationship
5. Parenting
   a. Discipline and child-rearing
   b. Feelings about parenthood
   c. Feelings about single-parenthood
6. Friendship/social participation
   a. Dating and marriage
   b. Friendships
   c. Social groups, leisure
   d. Social support
7. Employment/education
   a. Employment experiences
   b. Educational experiences
   c. Job and career goals
   d. Educational goals
8. Workload
   a. Coping with workload
   b. Schedule
   c. Child care arrangements
9. Finances

Read the following excerpt, taken from a real interview. Use the coding scheme to code the topics discussed in this excerpt.

> I think raising the children is so much easier without the father around. There isn't two people conflicting back and forth. You know, like . . . like you discipline them during the day. They do something wrong, you're not saying, "When daddy gets home, you're going to get a spanking." You know, you do that. The kid gets a spanking right then and there. But when two people live together, they have their ways of raising and you have your ways of raising the children and it's so hard for two people to raise children. It's so much easier for one person. The only reason a male would be around is financial-wise. But me and the kids are happier now, and we get along with each other better, cause like, there isn't this competitive thing. My husband always wanted all the attention around here.

6. Read the method and results sections of one of the following reports. Use the critiquing guidelines in Box 19.3 of the textbook (available as a Word document in the Toolkit ⊗) to critique the data analysis aspects of the study:
   - DeSanto-Madeya, S. (2006). The meaning of living with spinal cord injury 5 to 10 years after the injury. *Western Journal of Nursing Research, 28*(3), 265–289.
   - Johnston, B., & Smith, L. (2006). Nurses' and patients' perceptions of expert palliative nursing care. *Journal of Advanced Nursing, 54*(6), 700–709.
   - Kearney, A. (2006). Increasing our understanding of breast self-examination: Women talk about cancer, the health care system, and being women. *Qualitative Health Research, 16*(6), 802–820.

■ C. Application Exercises

EXERCISE 1: STUDY IN APPENDIX B

Read the data analysis and results sections of the report by Rew ("Homeless youth") in Appendix B. Then answer the following questions:

Questions of Fact

a. How many pages of transcribed interview data did the study yield? How many pages of field notes were there?
b. Was constant comparison used in analyzing the data?
c. Did Rew create conceptual files?
d. Was a computer used to analyze the data? If yes, what software was used?
e. Did Rew calculate any quasi-statistics?
f. Which grounded theory analytic approach was adopted in this study?
g. Did Rew prepare any analytic memos?
h. Did Rew describe the open coding process? If so, what did she say?
i. Did Rew describe axial coding? If so, what did she say?

j. How many categories initially emerged in Rew's analysis?
k. How many major categories were ultimately developed and refined? What were they?
l. What was the BSP? What does the BSP entail?

Questions for Discussion

a. Discuss the thoroughness of Rew's description of her data analysis efforts. Did the report present adequate information about the coding of the data and the steps taken to analyze the data?
b. Was there any evidence of "method slurring"—that is, did Rew apply any analytic procedures that are inappropriate for a grounded theory approach?
c. Discuss the effectiveness of Rew's presentation of results. Does the analysis seem sensible, thoughtful, and thorough? Was sufficient evidence provided to support the findings? Were data presented in a manner that allows you to be confident about Rew's conclusions?
d. Did the model in Figure 1 effectively display the grounded theory? Did it adequately communicate the core variable?

EXERCISE 2: STUDY IN APPENDIX D

Read the data analysis and results sections of the report by Beck ("Post-traumatic stress disorder") in Appendix D. Then answer the following questions:

Questions of Fact

a. Did Beck organize her data manually or with the assistance of computer software? If the latter, what software was used?
b. Did Beck calculate any quasi-statistics?
c. Which phenomenological analytic approach was adopted in this study?
d. Did Beck prepare any analytic memos?
e. Did Beck describe the coding process? If so, what did she say?
f. How many themes emerged in Beck's analysis? What were they?
g. Did Beck provide supporting evidence for her themes, in the form of excerpts from the data?

Questions for Discussion

a. Discuss the thoroughness of Beck's description of her data analysis efforts. Did the report present adequate information about the steps taken to analyze the data?
b. Was there any evidence of "method slurring"—that is, did Beck apply any analytic procedures that are inappropriate for a phenomenological approach?
c. Discuss the effectiveness of Beck's presentation of results. Does the analysis seem sensible, thoughtful, and thorough? Was sufficient evidence provided to support the findings? Were data presented in a manner that allows you to be confident about Beck's conclusions?

■ D. The Toolkit

For Chapter 19, the Toolkit on the CD-ROM provided with this Resource Manual contains the following:

- Guidelines for Critiquing Qualitative Data Analyses (Box 19.3 of the textbook)
- Example of a Memo From Beck's (2002) Study on Mothering Multiples
- Example of a Codebook from Beck's (2005) Study of the Benefits of Participating in Internet Interviews
- Example of Coding Hierarchy from Beck's (2002) Study on Mothering Multiples
- Example of a Simple Meta-Matrix (Adapted from Happ et al., 2006)

CHAPTER 20

Enhancing Quality and Integrity in Qualitative Research

■ A. Crossword Puzzle

Complete the crossword puzzle below, which uses terms and concepts presented in Chapter 20. (Puzzles may be removed for easier viewing.)

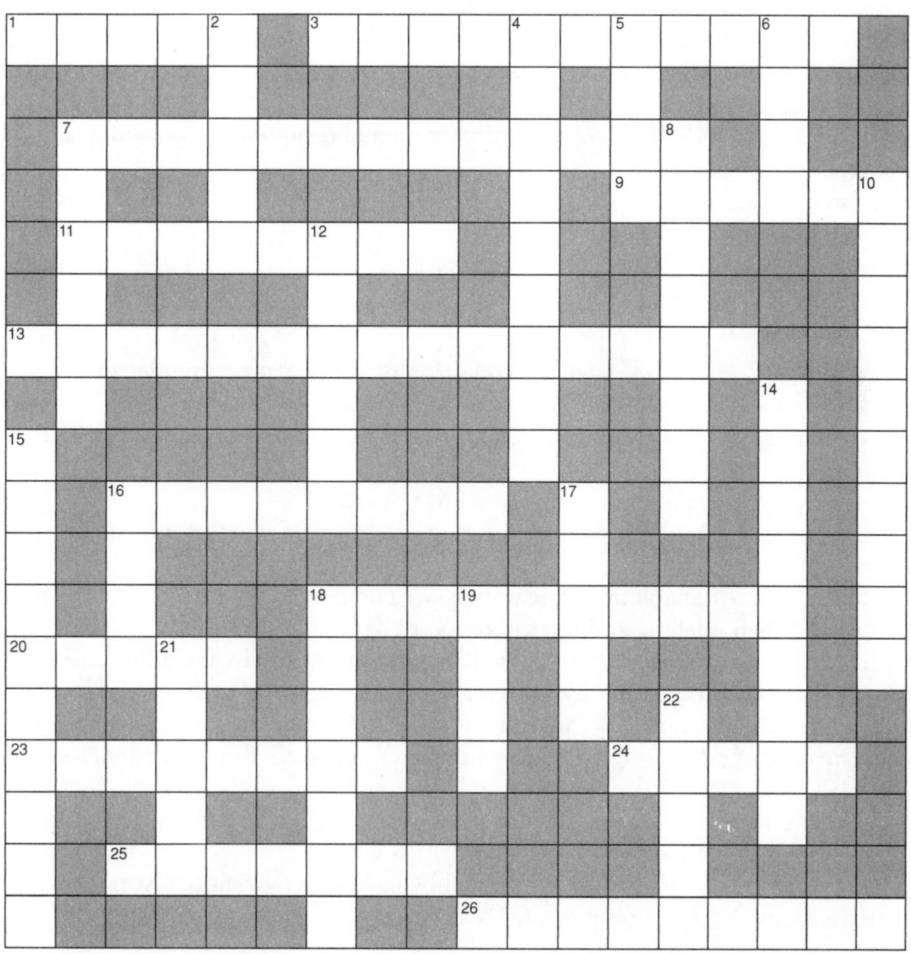

ACROSS

1. Confirmability can be addressed through a scrutiny of documents and procedures in an inquiry ________.
3. A key criterion for assessing quality in qualitative studies, in both frameworks described in the textbook
7. Use of multiple means of converging on the truth
9. The stability of data over time and conditions, analogous to reliability (abbr.)
11. A secondary criterion in the Whittemore et al. framework, referring to the ability to follow researchers' decisions and interpretations (abbr.)
13. Extent to which qualitative findings can be applied to other settings
16. Auditability can be enhanced by a(n) ________ trail that documents judgments and choices.
18. A secondary criterion in the Whittemore et al. framework, referring to interconnectedness
20. Collecting data in multiple sites is a form of ________ triangulation.
23. Credibility in qualitative inquiry has been described as analogous to ________ validity in quantitative inquiry.
24. ________ness involves the presentation of rich, artful descriptions that highlight salient themes in the data.
25. A(n) ________ audit involves a scrutiny of data and supporting documents by an external reviewer.
26. Persistent ________ refers to a focus on the aspects of a situation that are relevant to the phenomena being studied (abbr.)

DOWN

2. An audit ________ is a systematic collection of materials for an independent auditor
4. A word used by some as an overarching goal for qualitative inquiry, in lieu of validity
5. A music player (brand name—unrelated to research!)
6. ________ triangulation involves collecting data about a phenomenon at different points.
7. With ________triangulation, researchers use competing hypotheses or conceptualizations in their analysis and interpretation of data.
8. A process by which researchers revise their interpretations by including cases that appear to disconfirm earlier hypotheses is a ________ case analysis.
10. Credibility can be enhanced through a thorough search for ________ing evidence.
12. One method of addressing credibility involves going back to participants to do member ________.
14. A quality criterion indicating the extent to which the researchers fairly and faithfully show a range of different realities (abbr.)
15. The type of triangulation that is achieved by having two or more researchers make key decisions and interpretations (abbr.)

16. Interviewing patients *and* family members about a phenomenon is an example of ________ source triangulation.
17. Qualitative researchers strive for the ________worthiness of their data and their methods.
18. A secondary criterion in the Whittemore et al. framework, reflecting challenges to traditional ways of thinking (abbr.)
19. Lincoln and ________ proposed criteria for evaluating the trustworthiness of qualitative inquiries.
21. Researchers typically "________" transcribed data by comparing transcriptions to recordings and making necessary corrections.
22. A term that is hotly debated in terms of appropriateness for evaluating quality in qualitative inquiry

■ B. Study Questions

1. Suppose you were conducting a grounded theory study of couples' coming to terms with infertility. What might you do to incorporate various types of triangulation into your study?

2. In the previous chapter, one of the study questions involved a class exercise to elicit descriptions of people's conceptions of preventive health care and what it means in their daily lives (Study Question 1 in Chapter 19, p. 110). Describe efforts you could take to enhance the integrity of this inquiry.

3. What is your opinion about the value of member checking as a strategy to enhance credibility? Defend your position.

4. Read a research report in a recent issue of the journal *Qualitative Health Research*. Identify several examples of "thick description." Also, identify areas of the report in which you feel additional thick description would have enhanced the inquiry.

5. Read one of the following reports. Use the critiquing guidelines in Box 20.1 of the textbook (available as a Word document in the Toolkit ⊗) to evaluate the integrity and quality of the study—augmented, as appropriate, by questions in Table 20.1 of the textbook:
   - Edvardsson, D., Sandman, P., & Rasmussen, B. (2006). Caring or uncaring: Meanings of being in an oncology environment. *Journal of Advanced Nursing, 55*(2), 188–197.
   - Gudmundsdottir, M., & Chesla, C. (2006). Building a new world: Habits and practices of healing following the death of a child. *Journal of Family Nursing, 12*(2), 143–164.
   - Houldin, A., & Lewis, F. (2006). Salvaging their normal lives: A qualitative study of patients with recently diagnosed advanced colorectal cancer. *Oncology Nursing Forum, 33*(4), 719–725.

▪ C. Application Exercises

EXERCISE 1: STUDY IN APPENDIX B

Read the report by Rew ("Homeless youth") in Appendix B. Then answer the following questions:

Questions of Fact

a. What types of triangulation, if any, were used in Rew's study?
b. Were any of the following methods used to enhance the credibility of the study and its data?
    - Prolonged engagement and/or persistent observation
    - Peer debriefing
    - Member checks
    - Search for disconfirming evidence
    - Researcher credibility
    - Other methods

c. Describe what methods (if any) were used to enhance the following aspects of the study:
    - Dependability; confirmability/auditability
    - Transferability
    - Authenticity
    - Explicitness

Questions for Discussion

a. Discuss the thoroughness with which Rew described her efforts to enhance and evaluate the quality and integrity of her study.
b. Discuss the extent to which Rew made efforts to enhance the transferability of her study findings.
c. How would you characterize the integrity and trustworthiness of this study, based on Rew's documentation?

EXERCISE 2: STUDY IN APPENDIX F

Read the report by Giddings ("Health disparities") in Appendix F. Then answer the following questions:

Questions of Fact

a. What types of triangulation, if any, were used in Giddings's study?
b. Were any of the following methods used to enhance the credibility of the study and its data?
    - Prolonged engagement and/or persistent observation
    - Peer debriefing

- Member checks
- Search for disconfirming evidence
- Researcher credibility

c. Describe what methods (if any) were used to enhance the following aspects of the study:
   - Dependability
   - Confirmability/auditability
   - Transferability
   - Authenticity
   - Explicitness
   - Sensitivity

Questions for Discussion

a. Discuss the thoroughness with which Giddings described her efforts to enhance and evaluate the quality and integrity of her study.
b. Discuss the extent to which Giddings made efforts to enhance the transferability of her study findings.
c. How would you characterize the integrity and trustworthiness of this study, based on Giddings's documentation?

■ D. The Toolkit

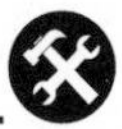

For Chapter 20, the Toolkit on the accompanying CD-ROM contains a Word file with the following:

- Guidelines for Evaluating Quality and Integrity in Qualitative Studies (Box 20.1 of the textbook)
- Questions for Self-Scrutiny During a Study: Whittemore et al.'s Primary Qualitative Validity Criteria (based on Table 20.1 of the textbook)
- Questions for Self-Scrutiny During a Study: Whittemore et al.'s Secondary Qualitative Validity Criteria (based on Table 20.1 of the textbook)
- Questions for *Post Hoc* Assessments of a Study: Whittemore et al.'s Primary Qualitative Validity Criteria (based on Table 20.1 of the textbook)
- Questions for *Post Hoc* Assessments of a Study: Whittemore et al.'s Secondary Qualitative Validity Criteria (based on Table 20.1 of the textbook)

CHAPTER 21

Describing Data Through Statistics

■ A. Crossword Puzzle

Complete the crossword puzzle below, which uses terms and concepts presented in Chapter 21. (Puzzles may be removed for easier viewing.)

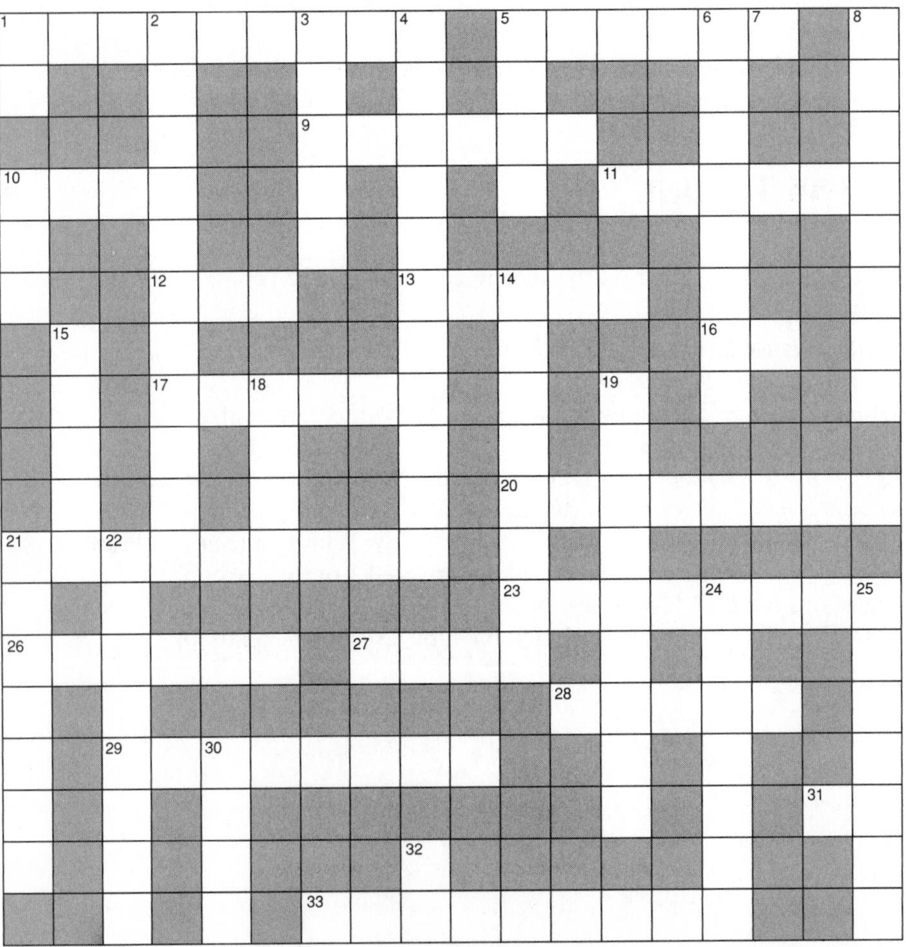

ACROSS

1. Frequency distributions that have a peak in the center and each half mirrors the other
5. Intercorrelations among key variables are frequently displayed in a correlation ________.
9. A unimodal, symmetric distribution that is not too peaked or too flat
10. The ratio of two probabilities (the probability of an event occurring to the probability that it will not occur
11. Distributions whose peaks are "off center"
12. A correlation index for ordinal-level data
13. Each variable can be described in terms of its ________ of measurement, which affects appropriate mathematic operations.
16. A common risk index—the simple proportion of people who experienced an undesirable outcome (acronym)
17. The most common correlation index: the Pearson product ________ coefficient
20. Interval measures provide no information about ________ magnitude.
21. A way to display a bivariate distribution is in a ________ table (abbr.).
23. Another name for a bivariate display (see 21 Across)
26. In nominal measurement, the ________ used to code a variable has no inherent quantitative meaning.
27. A measure of central tendency indicating the most "popular" value
28. The number needed to ________ is an estimate of how many people would need to receive an intervention to prevent an undesirable outcome.
29. When the tail of a frequency distribution points to the left, the skew is ________.
31. An index of central tendency that indicates the midpoint of a distribution (abbr.)
33. An index of a sample is a statistic; an index of a population is a(n) ________.

DOWN

1. The most frequently used index of variability or dispersion (acronym)
2. There are four levels of ________ for research variables.
3. A crude index of variability—the highest value minus the lowest
4. Relationships between two variables can be described through ________ procedures.
5. The sum of all data values, divided by the number of cases
6. The level of measurement in which distances between values is equal, but there is no rational zero
7. A bar over this is used as a symbol for the mean.
8. The mean is the most commonly used index of central ________.
14. The standard deviation squared
15. The highest level of measurement
18. In lay terms, the *average*
19. One type of graphic display of frequency distribution data
21. A distribution of data can be described by its shape, ________ tendency, and variability.

22. The variable *gender* is measured on this level.
24. Bivariate relationships can be graphed on a ________ plot.
25. A distribution that has two peaks
30. Another name for a bell-shaped curve is a ________ distribution (abbr.).
32. The most commonly reported risk index in nursing journals (acronym).

■ B. Study Questions

1. For each of the following variables, specify the *highest* possible level of measurement that you think a researcher could attain.
   a. Attitudes toward the mentally handicapped
   b. Birth order
   c. Length of time in labor
   d. White blood cell count
   e. Blood type
   f. Tidal volume
   g. Degrees Celsius
   h. Unit assignment for nursing staff
   i. Scores on a fear of death scale
   j. Amount of sputum
2. Prepare a frequency distribution and histogram for the following set of data values, which represent the ages of 30 women receiving estrogen replacement therapy:

   47 50 51 50 48 51 50 51 49 51

   54 49 49 53 51 52 51 52 50 53

   49 51 52 51 50 55 48 54 53 52

   Describe the resulting distribution in terms of its symmetry and modality.
3. Calculate the mean, median, and mode for the following pulse rates:

   78 84 69 98 102 72 87 75 79 84 88 84 83 71 73
4. Study the contingency table from an SPSS printout on the next page. The table presents data from a study of sexually active teenagers in which both males and females were asked how old they were when they first had sexual intercourse. Each row in the table indicates the ages specified by the respondents. The last row contains the code for respondents who could not remember how old they were, coded 88. Answer the following questions about this contingency table:
   a. How many males were included in the study?
   b. How many females first had sexual intercourse at age 14?
   c. What percentage of respondents were 16 years of age when they first had sexual intercourse?
   d. What percentage of males did not know at what age they first had sexual intercourse?

e. Of those respondents who were 13 years of age when they first had sexual intercourse, what percentage was female?

			GENDER		
			Male	**Female**	**Total**
AGE	13	Count	1	2	3
		% within AGE	33.3%	66.7%	100.0%
		% within GENDER	2.2%	4.4%	3.3%
		% of Total	1.1%	2.2%	3.3%
	14	Count	6	3	9
		% within AGE	66.7%	33.3%	100.0%
		% within GENDER	13.3%	6.7%	10.0%
		% of Total	6.7%	3.3%	10.0%
	15	Count	9	6	15
		% within AGE	60.0%	40.0%	100.0%
		% within GENDER	20.0%	13.3%	16.7%
		% of Total	10.0%	6.7%	16.7%
	16	Count	15	10	25
		% within AGE	60.0%	40.0%	100.0%
		% within GENDER	33.3%	22.2%	27.8%
		% of Total	16.7%	11.1%	27.8%
	17	Count	11	14	25
		% within AGE	44.0%	56.0%	100.0%
		% within GENDER	24.4%	31.1%	27.8%
		% of Total	12.2%	15.6%	27.8%
	18	Count	2	8	10
		% within AGE	20.0%	80.0%	100.0%
		% within GENDER	4.4%	17.8%	11.1%
		% of Total	2.2%	8.9%	11.1%
	88 Don't Remember	Count	1	2	3
		% within AGE	33.3%	66.7%	100.0%
		% within GENDER	2.2%	4.4%	3.3%
		% of Total	1.1%	2.2%	3.3%
Total		Count	45	45	90
		% within AGE	50.0%	50.0%	100.0%
		% within GENDER	100.0%	100.0%	100.0%
		% of Total	50.0%	50.0%	100.0%

5. Suppose a researcher has conducted a study concerning lactose intolerance in children. The data reveal that 12 boys and 16 girls have lactose intolerance, out of a sample of 60 children of each gender. Construct a contingency table and calculate the row, column, and total percentages for each cell in the table. Discuss the meaning of these statistics.

- On what day(s) did some people in the intervention group get *no* massage?
- Did everyone in the sample get pain control from medication? Was there ever a day when a person got *no* medication?

c. Referring to Table 3 and the accompanying text, answer the following questions:
- Does this table present information about study outcomes (dependent variables)?
- What descriptive statistical indexes are presented in this table?
- Which group had more difficulty washing their back, members of the intervention or control group?
- Which group was more variable with regard to the difficulty they reported in removing something from their back pocket?
- Which of the four tasks in the table did the intervention group have most difficulty with at the first follow up? Was the same task reported as most difficult for those in the control group?

Questions for Discussion

a. Discuss the effectiveness of the presentation of information in the tables. What, if anything, could be done to make the tables more informative, more comprehensible, or more efficient? Should there have been other tables?

d. Did Forchuk and colleagues use the appropriate statistics to describe their data? For example, did the statistics correspond to the levels of measurement of the variables? Could additional descriptive statistics have been used to more fully describe the data?

■ D. The Toolkit

For Chapter 21, the Toolkit on the accompanying CD-ROM contains a Word file with the following:

- Guidelines for Critiquing Descriptive Statistics (Box 21.1 of the textbook)
- Table Templates for Presenting Selected Descriptive Analyses
  - Table Template 1: Sample Description Table
  - Table Template 2: Contingency Table
  - Table Template 3: Correlation Matrix

CHAPTER 22

Using Inferential Statistics to Test Hypotheses

■ A. Crossword Puzzle

Complete the crossword puzzle below, which uses terms and concepts presented in Chapter 22. (Puzzles may be removed for easier viewing.)

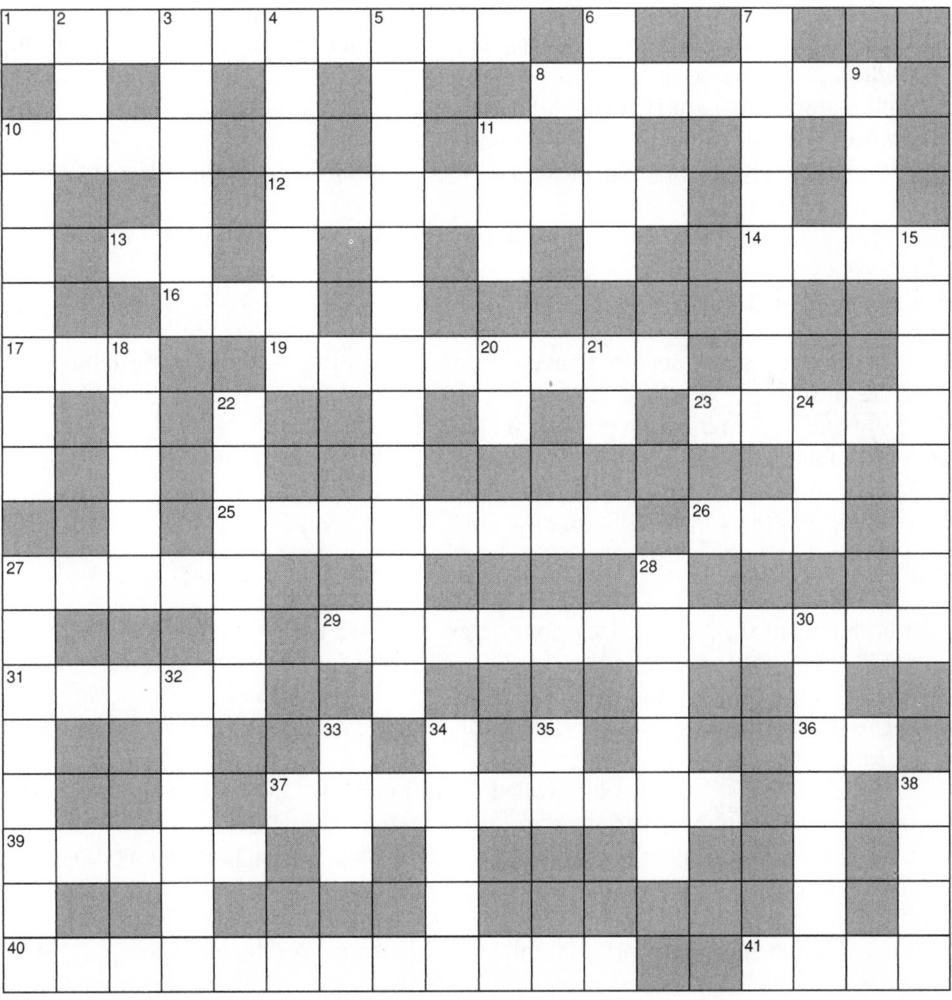

ACROSS

1. A(n)________ interval indicates degree of precision in parameter estimation.
8. One of the two broad approaches in statistical inference is hypothesis ________.
10. The probability of committing a Type II error
12. Data from a design in which there are multiple measurements of the outcome variable can be analyzed using a(n) ________-measures ANOVA.
13. In statistical testing, the error that reflects a false negative is a Type ________ error.
14. A nonparametric analog to a *t*-test is the ________ Whitney *U* test.
16. A test comparing the means of three groups is a ________-way analysis of variance.
17. An ES index in an ANOVA situation is ________ squared.
19. The ________ error of the mean is the SD of a theoretical distribution of means.
23. A Bonferroni correction involves a correction to ________ to reflect multiple tests with the same data.
25. The ________ region of a theoretical distribution indicates whether the null hypothesis is *improbable.*
26. The test most often used when a hypothesis concerns differences in proportions is ________ square.
27. When sample sizes are very small, Fisher's ________ test should be used to test differences in proportions.
29. In statistical testing, an alpha of .05 is, by convention, the minimum level of ________.
31. A(n)________ analysis can be used during the planning of a study to estimate sample size needs.
36. If the computer indicated a $p = .15$, this would indicate the relationship being tested was ________ (abbr.).
37. Even though researchers often have directional hypotheses, they most often report the results of _____-______ tests.
39. In statistical testing, a false positive is a(n) ________ error.
40. A sampling ________ is theoretical, not based on actual data values.
41. Most statistical _ _ _ _yses involve inferential statistics.

DOWN

2. If both tails of the sampling distribution are not used to test the null hypothesis, the test is called ________ tailed.
3. The statistic computed in analysis of variance
4. Each statistical analysis is associated with certain ________ of freedom that usually reflect sample size.
5. The class of statistics that is also called distribution-free and that has less restrictive assumptions about how variables are distributed
6. An alpha of .01 is a more stringent ________ of significance than one of .05.
7. For dichotomous variables, the sampling distribution is called a(n) ________ distribution.
9. The overall mean for an entire sample, with all groups combined, is the _ _ _ _d mean.

10. An independent groups statistical test is used for ________-subjects designs.
11. With ordinal data, one correlation index is Kendall's ________.
15. When the null hypothesis is not rejected, results are sometimes described as ________.
18. The analysis used to compare three or more group means (acronym)
20. The number of observations free to vary about a parameter (acronym)
21. If pretest and posttest means were compared for two groups, one analytic approach would be _ _-ANOVA (acronym).
22. In a repeated measures analysis, the within-subjects analysis effect involves a time ________.
24. An index describing the relationship between two dichotomous variables
27. In an analysis of contingency table data, observed frequencies are contrasted with ________ frequencies.
28. The nonparametric analogue of a paired *t*-test is the Wilcoxon ________ rank test.
30. A ________ result indicates that the null hypothesis cannot be rejected (abbr.).
32. Cohen's *d* is an index used to estimate ________ size in a two-group mean difference situation.
33. The simplest type of multifactor ANOVA is a ________-way ANOVA.
34. Two group means can be compared using a(n) ___-_____.
35. The following might be the information for a 95% ________: (−1.25, .78)
38. In hypothesis testing, researchers typically seek to reject the ________ hypothesis.

■ B. Study Questions

1. A nurse researcher measured the amount of time (in minutes) spent in recreational activities by a sample of 200 hospitalized paraplegic patients. She compared male and female patients, as well as those 50 years of age and younger versus those older than 50 years. The four group means were as follows:

	Male	Female
≤ 50	98.2 (n = 50)	70.1 (n = 50)
> 50	50.8 (n = 50)	68.3 (n = 50)

A two-way ANOVA yielded the following results:

	F	*df*	*p*
Gender	3.61	1196	>.05
Age group	5.87	1196	<.05
Gender × age group	6.96	1196	<.01

Discuss the meaning of these results.

2. The correlation between the number of days absent per year and annual salary in a sample of 100 employees of an insurance company was found to be −.23 (p = .02). Discuss this result in terms of significance levels and meaning.

3. Indicate which statistical test(s) you would use to analyze data for the following variables:
   a. Variable 1 is psychiatric patients' gender; variable 2 is whether or not the patient has attempted suicide in the past 12 months.
   b. Variable 1 is the participation versus nonparticipation of patients with a pulmonary embolus in a special intervention group; variable 2 is the pH of the patients' arterial blood gases.
   c. Variable 1 is serum creatinine concentration levels; variable 2 is daily urine output.
   d. Variable 1 is patients' marital status—married versus single (never married) versus divorced or widowed; variable 2 is the patients' degrees of self-reported depression on a 30-item depression scale.

4. On the next page is a correlation matrix produced by an SPSS run, based on real data from a study of low-income mothers. The variables in this matrix are as follows:

   Scores on a scale measuring stressful life events
   Total household income in the prior month
   Scores on the CES-D depression scale
   Scores on the physical health subscale of the SF-12
   Scores on the mental health subscale of the SF-12

   Answer the following questions with respect to this matrix:
   a. How many respondents completed the stressful life event scale?
   b. What is the correlation between total household income and scores on the physical health subscale?
   c. Is the correlation between physical health and mental health subscale scores significant at conventional levels?
   d. What is the probability that the correlation between depression scores and total household income in this sample is simply a function of chance?
   e. With which variable(s) is stressful life event scale scores significantly related at conventional levels?
   f. Explain what is meant by the correlation between the depression and mental health scale scores.

5. Below is a list of variables. Assume that you have data from 500 nurses on these variables. Develop two or three hypotheses regarding the relationships among these variables, and indicate what statistical tests you would use to test your hypotheses.

   Number of years of nursing experience
   Type of employment setting (hospital, nursing school, public school system, industry)
   Salary
   Marital status
   Job satisfaction ("dissatisfied," "neither dissatisfied nor satisfied," or "satisfied")
   Number of children younger than 18 years

Correlation

		Stressful Life Event Score	Total Household Income	CES-D Score (Range 0 to 60)	SF12: Physical Health Component Score	SF12: Mental Health Component Score
Stressful Life Event Score	Pearson Correlation	1.000	−.024	.275**	−.136	−.265**
	Sig. (2-tailed)		.485	.000	.000	.000
	N	958	887	950	907	907
Total Household Income	Pearson Correlation	−.024	1.000	−.105**	.113**	.055
	Sig. (2-tailed)	.485		.002	.001	.113
	N	887	935	893	843	843
CES-D Score (Range 0 to 60)	Pearson Correlation	.275**	−.105**	1.000	−.181	−.643**
	Sig. (2-tailed)	.000	.002		.000	.000
	N	950	893	963	903	903
SF12: Physical Health Component Score	Pearson Correlation	−1.36**	.113	−181**	1.000	.078*
	Sig. (2-tailed)	.000	.001	.000		.019
	N	907	843	903	909	909
SF12: Mental Health Component Score	Pearson Correlation	−.265**	.055	−.643**	.078*	1.000
	Sig. (2-tailed)	.000	.113	.000	.019	
	N	907	843	903	909	909

**Correlation is significiant at the 0.01 level (2-tailed).
* Correlation is significiant at the 0.05 level (2-tailed).

Gender
Type of nursing preparation (diploma, Associate's, Bachelor's)

6. Estimate the required total sample sizes for the following situations:
   a. Comparison of two group means: $\alpha = .01$; power = .90; ES = .35.
   b. Correlation of two variables: $\alpha = .01$; power = .80; $\rho = .27$.

7. Read one of the following research reports and use the critiquing guidelines in Box 22.1 of the textbook (available as a Word document in the Toolkit for this chapter) to critique the researchers' analyses, ignoring at this point discussions of multivariate statistics such as multiple regression:
   - Artinian, N., Washington, O., Flack, J., Hockman, E., & Jen, K. (2006). Depression, stress, and blood pressure in urban African-American women. *Progress in Cardiovascular Nursing, 21*(2), 68–75.
   - Sveinsdottir, H., & Olafsson, R. (2006). Women's attitudes to hormone replacement therapy in the aftermath. *Journal of Advanced Nursing, 54*(5), 572–584.
   - Voyer, P., Cole, M., McCusker, J., & Belzile, E. (2006). Prevalence and symptoms of delirium superimposed on dementia. *Clinical Nursing Research, 15*(1), 46–66.

■ C. Application Exercises

EXERCISE 1: STUDY IN APPENDIX A

Read the results section of the report by Hill and colleagues ("Chronically ill rural women") in Appendix A. Then answer the following questions:

Questions of Fact

a. Which bivariate statistical tests discussed in Chapter 22 did Hill and colleagues use?
b. Did Hill and colleagues present information about hypothesis tests? about parameter estimation? about effect sizes?
c. Referring to Table 3, answer the following questions:
   - What was the correlation between the women's Depression and Self-Efficacy scores?
   - Which variables were negatively correlated with Loneliness scores?
   - Scores on the Stress scale were significantly correlated with which other variables?
   - What is the strongest correlation in this matrix?
   - What is the weakest correlation in this matrix?
   - How many correlations were statistically significant at or beyond the .05 level? How many were *not* statistically significant?
   - What is the name of the test statistic presented in this table?

d. Referring to Table 5 and the accompanying text, answer the following questions:
   - What is the independent variable in the analyses presented in this table?
   - Are the analyses between-subjects or within-subjects tests?
   - Explain what the results for the Empowerment scale scores mean.
   - Explain what the results for the Self-Efficacy scores mean.
   - For how many dependent variables were differences in experimental–control group changes significant at the .05 level?
   - For how many dependent variables were there significant changes over time for the sample as a whole at the .05 level?
   - What statistical test was used in the analyses presented in this table?

e. Did the report indicate that a power analysis was done while planning the study to estimate sample size needs?

Questions for Discussion

a. Discuss the effectiveness of the presentation of information in the tables. What, if anything, could be done to make the tables more informative, more comprehensible, or more efficient? Should there have been other tables?
b. Did Hill and colleagues use the appropriate statistical tests to analyze their data? If not, what tests should have been performed?
c. Did the researchers present a sufficient amount of information about their statistical tests? What additional information would have been helpful?

EXERCISE 2: STUDY IN APPENDIX E

Read the results section of the report by Loeb ("Older men's health") in Appendix E. Then answer the following questions:

Questions of Fact

a. Which bivariate statistical tests discussed in Chapter 22 did Loeb use?
b. Did Loeb present information about hypothesis tests? about parameter estimation? about effect sizes?
c. Referring to Table 1, answer the following questions:
   - What was the correlation between the men's Healthiness of Lifestyle scores and Health-promoting behaviors (HPAOAM) scores?
   - What variables were negatively correlated with the variable "Total screenings"?
   - Scores on the HSDI (Health motivation) were significantly correlated with which other variables?
   - What is the strongest correlation in this matrix? What is the probability level associated with it?
   - What is the weakest correlation in this matrix? What is the probability associated with it?
   - What is the name of the test statistic presented in this table?
   - Are any of the variables in this table nominal-level measures?
   - According to this table, were men who attended more health-promoting programs significantly more likely than other men to participate in appropriate health screenings?
d. Referring to Table 3 and the accompanying text, answer the following questions:
   - What is the independent variable in the analyses presented in this table?
   - What statistical test was used in the analyses presented in this table?
   - Which group had higher average scores on the HSDI? Was the group difference statistically significant? What does this mean?
   - For which dependent variables were the groups significantly different?
e. Referring to Table 4 and the accompanying text, answer the following questions:
   - What is the independent variable in the analyses presented in this table?
   - The title of Table 4 is incorrect. What should it be?
   - What statistical test was used in the analyses presented in this table?
   - Which group had higher average scores on the HPAOAM? Was the group difference statistically significant?
   - For which dependent variables were the groups significantly different?
f. Did the report indicate that a power analysis was done while planning the study to estimate sample size needs?

Questions for Discussion

a. Discuss the effectiveness of the presentation of information in the tables. What, if anything, could be done to make the tables more informative, more comprehensible, or more efficient? Should there have been other tables?

b. Did Loeb use the appropriate statistical tests to analyze her data? If not, what tests should have been performed?
c. Did Loeb present a sufficient amount of information about the statistical tests? What additional information would have been helpful?

■ D. The Toolkit

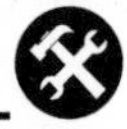

For Chapter 22, the Toolkit on the accompanying CD-ROM contains a Word file with the following:

- Guidelines for Critiquing Bivariate Inferential Analyses (Box 22.1 of the textbook)
- Table Templates for Presenting Selected Bivariate Analyses
  - Table Template 1A: Independent *t*-Tests
  - Table Template 1B: Independent *t*-Tests (Alternative Format)
  - Table Template 2: Paired *t*-Tests
  - Table Template 3: One-Way ANOVA
  - Table Template 4: RM-ANOVA
  - Table Template 5A: Chi-Square Tests (For Two-Group Comparisons)
  - Table Template 5B: Chi-Square Tests (For Two or More Group Comparisons)

CHAPTER 23

Using Multivariate Statistics to Analyze Complex Relationships

■ A. Crossword Puzzle

Complete the crossword puzzle below, which uses terms and concepts presented in Chapter 23. (Puzzles may be removed for easier viewing.)

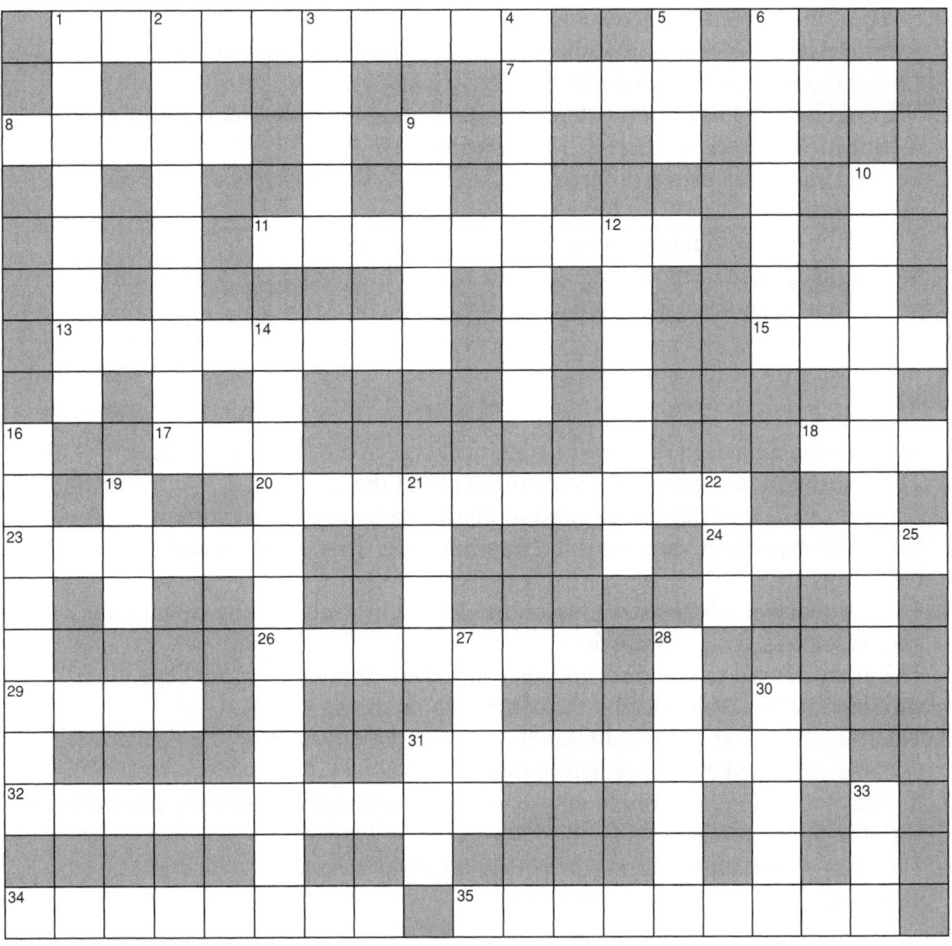

c. A researcher wants to test the effects of (a) two drug treatments and (b) two dosages of each drug on (a) blood pressure and (b) the pH and PO_2 levels of arterial blood gases.
d. A researcher wants to predict hospital staff absentee rates based on month of the year, staff rank, shift, number of years with the hospital, and marital status.

3. Below is a list of variables that a nurse researcher might be interested in predicting. For each, suggest at least three independent variables that could be used in a multiple regression analysis.
   a. Amount of time spent exercising weekly among teenagers
   b. Nurses' frequency of administering pain medication
   c. Body mass index (a common measure of obesity)
   d. Patients' level of fatigue
   e. Anxiety levels of prostatectomy patients
4. Wang, Redeker, Moreyra, and Diamond, in their 2001 study (*Clinical Nursing Research, 10*, 29–38), used a series of *t*-tests and chi-square tests to compare two groups of patients who underwent cardiac catheterization with regard to measures of safety, comfort, and satisfaction: those with 4 hours versus those with 6 hours of bed rest. Identify two or three multivariate procedures that could have been used to analyze the data, being as specific as possible (e.g., if you suggest ANCOVA, identify appropriate covariates).
5. Read one of the following studies and use the critiquing guidelines in Box 22.1 of the textbook (available as a Word document in the Toolkit for the previous chapter) to evaluate the multivariate statistical analyses:
   - Amar, A. (2006). College women's experience of stalking: Mental health symptoms and changes in routine. *Archives of Psychiatric Nursing, 20*(3), 108–116.
   - Jones, L., Courneya, K., Vallance, J., Ladha, A., Mant, M., Belch, A., & Reiman, T. (2006). Understanding the determinants of exercise intentions in multiple myeloma cancer survivors: An application of the Theory of Planned Behavior. *Cancer Nursing, 29*(3), 167–175.
   - Kosteniuk, J., D'Arcy, C., Stewart, N., & Smith, B. (2006). Central and peripheral information source use among rural and remote Registered Nurses. *Journal of Advanced Nursing, 55*(1), 100–114.

■ C. Application Exercises

EXERCISE 1: STUDIES IN APPENDICES A, C, AND G

Skim the method and results sections of the reports in Appendices A, C, and G. Then answer the following questions:

Questions of Fact

a. Did any of these studies use multiple regression analysis? If yes, what were the dependent variables and what were the predictors?

b. Did any of these studies use ANCOVA? If yes, what groups were being compared? What were the dependent variables and what were the covariates?
c. Did any of these studies use other types of multivariate analyses discussed in this chapter? If yes, which ones?

Questions for Discussion

a. Could any of these studies that did *not* use ANCOVA or multiple regression have potentially benefited from a multivariate approach?
b. If you recommend a multivariate rather than a bivariate analysis for any of these studies, what variables would you want to control statistically?

EXERCISE 2: STUDY IN APPENDIX E

Read the results section of the report by Loeb ("Older men's health") in Appendix E. Then answer the following questions:

Questions of Fact

a. What approach to entering variables into the multiple regression equation was used in this study?
b. Referring to Table 2 and the accompanying text, answer the following questions:
    - What was the dependent variable in the multiple regression analysis?
    - What predictor variable was most strongly correlated with the dependent variable?
    - What was the value of R^2 after the first variable entered the regression equation?
    - How many predictor variables in total were used in the final regression equation, as shown in the table?
    - Were there other variables that Loeb tried to include in the regression analysis? Why were these variables not used? Were any of these variables statistically significant at the bivariate level?
    - What was the final value of R^2?
c. Did the authors assess the risk for multicollinearity for their regression analysis? If yes, what did they conclude?

Questions for Discussion

a. Comment on Loeb's strategy for entering variables into the regression equation. Would you recommend an alternative approach?
b. Were there other multivariate analyses that Loeb could have used but did not? Would you recommend the use of such analyses? Why or why not?

■ D. The Toolkit

For Chapter 23, the Toolkit on the CD-ROM provided with this Resource Manual contains the following:

- Table Templates for Presenting Selected Multivariate Statistics
  - Table Template 1: Simultaneous Multiple Regression
  - Table Template 2: Hierarchical Multiple Regression
  - Table Template 3: ANCOVA
  - Table Template 4: Logistic Regression

CHAPTER 24

Designing a Quantitative Analysis Strategy: From Data Collection to Interpretation

■ A. Crossword Puzzle

Complete the crossword puzzle below, which uses terms and concepts presented in Chapter 24. (Puzzles may be removed for easier viewing.)

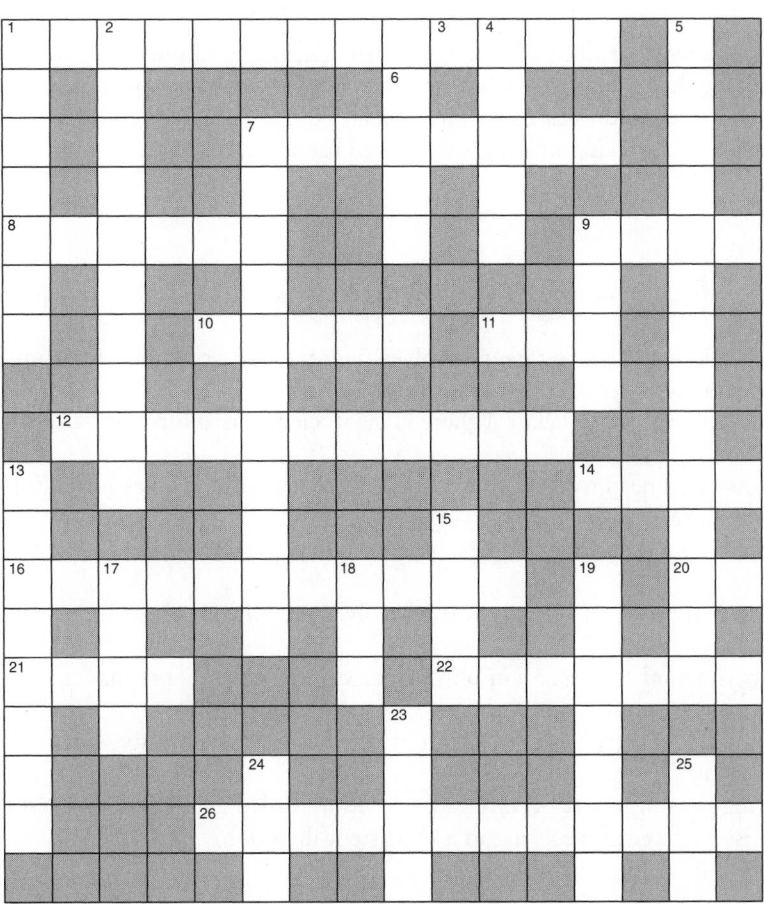

ACROSS

1. The removal of cases with missing data on an analysis-by-analysis basis
3. To better understand the meaning of results, it is useful to compute ________ sizes.
7. Coding decisions are documented in a ________.
8. When sample ________ extends over a long period of time, tests for cohort effects are advisable.
9. When there are missing items on a scale, ________ substitution involves using the mean item score for that person on other items on the scale.
10. When some hypotheses are upheld and others are not, results are said to be ________.
11. An important issue in deciding a missing values strategy is whether the data are ________ (acronym).
12. Data cleaning includes ________ checks, which examine whether there are any contradictions in the data within individual cases.
14. Before the principal analyses are undertaken, researchers should make assessments for various types of ________.
16. To test for the robustness of results, researchers sometimes undertake ________ analyses.
20. Each case in a data set should be assigned a(n) ________ number.
21. A coded value that is impossible within the coding scheme is a(n) ________ code.
22. Refusals and skipped questions require special ________ values codes.
26. One strategy for resolving missing values is to use mean ________.

DOWN

1. When there are multiple sites, it is useful to test for whether ________ across sites is appropriate.
2. One broad missing values strategy involves the ________ of values to estimate those that are missing.
4. A(n) ________ effect can occur if there is insufficient possibility for variation in low scores.
5. Researchers often need to do a data ________ to get coded values into a form appropriate for analysis.
6. After determining that their findings are credible, researchers need to interpret what they ________.
7. The first step in doing an interpretation involves establishing the ________ of the findings.
9. In nonexperimental studies, an important maxim to remember is that ________ does not prove causation (abbr.).
13. When entire cases are removed from a data set because of extensive missing values, the deletion is ________.
15. In preparing to compute scale values, a procedure called ________ reversal is sometimes necessary to ensure scoring in a consistent direction.

17. It is difficult to use traditional hypothesis testing to test a hypothesis that is actually the ________ (absence of a relationship).
18. Sometimes a transformation involves creating a dummy ________ for multivariate analysis (abbr.).
19. The findings of a study are also called the ________.
23. Researchers strive for a rectangular ________ for key variables in their data set (abbr.).
24. An extreme value outside the normal range is called a(n) _ _ _ lier.
25. A type of transformation that can render skewed data more normal (abbr.)

■ B. Study Questions

1. Read the following study and (a) indicate which steps in the process shown in Figure 24.1 of the textbook were described in the report and (b) comment on whether the absence of other information affected the quality of the research evidence.
   - Smith, S., & Michel, Y. (2006). A pilot study on the effects of aquatic exercises on discomforts in pregnancy. *Journal of Obstetric, Gynecologic, & Neonatal Nursing, 35*(3), 315–323.
2. Read the following study, which involved some data transformations. Comment on the researchers' decision to use transformations and the results that were achieved.
   - Fernandes, C., Worster, A., Eva, K., Hill, S., & McCallum, C. (2006). Pneumatic tube delivery system for blood samples reduces turnaround times without affecting sample quality. *Journal of Emergency Nursing, 32*(2), 139–143.
3. Read one of the following studies and evaluate the extent to which the researchers assessed possible biases—can you think of analyses that could have been performed to strengthen the credibility of the results?
   - Doorenbos, A., Given, B., Given, C., & Verbitsky, N. (2006). Physical functioning: Effect of a behavioral intervention for symptoms among individuals with cancer. *Nursing Research, 55*(3), 161–171.
   - Mantler, J., Armstrong-Stassen, M., Horsburgh, M., & Cameron, S. (2006). Reactions of hospital staff nurses to recruitment incentives. *Western Journal of Nursing Research, 28*(1), 70–84.
4. In the following research article, a team of researchers reported that they obtained nonsignificant results that were not consistent with expectations. Review and critique the researchers' interpretation of the findings and suggest some possible alternatives.
   - Holzemer, W., Bakken, S., Portillo, C., Grimes, R., Welch, J., Wantland, D., & Mullan, J. (2006). Testing a nurse-tailored HIV medication adherence intervention. *Nursing Research, 55*(3), 189–197.

C. Application Exercises

EXERCISE 1: STUDY IN APPENDIX A

Read the method, results, and discussion sections of the report by Hill and colleagues ("Chronically ill rural women") in Appendix A. Then answer the following questions:

Questions of Fact

a. Did the report provide information about how missing data were handled?
b. Did the researchers indicate that tests were performed to assess the degree to which their data met assumptions for parametric tests such as RM-ANOVA?
c. Did the researchers provide evidence about the success of randomization—i.e., whether experimentals and controls were equivalent at the outset and, thus, selection biases were absent?
d. Did any study participants withdraw from the study? What was the rate of attrition in the two groups? Did the researchers report an analysis of attrition biases?
e. Was the analysis an intention-to-treat analysis?
f. With regard to Aim #1 (intercorrelations among psychosocial variables), were hypotheses supported, nonsupported, or mixed?
g. With regard to Aim #2 (experimental-control group differences on psychosocial variables), were hypotheses supported, nonsupported, or mixed?
h. Did the report provide information about the precision of results through confidence intervals?
i. Did the report provide information about magnitude of effects through calculation of effect sizes?
j. In the Discussion section, was there any explicit discussion about the study's internal validity?
k. In the Discussion section, was there any explicit discussion about the study's external validity?
l. In the Discussion section, was there any explicit discussion about the study's statistical conclusion validity?
m. Did the Discussion section link study findings to findings from prior research—i.e., did the authors place their findings into a broader context?
n. Did the Discussion section explicitly mention any study limitations?

Questions for Discussion

a. Discuss the thoroughness of the researchers' description about their analytic and data management strategy.
b. Critique the analysis of biases in this report and possible resulting effects on the interpretation of the findings.
c. Do you agree with the researchers' interpretations of their results? Why or why not?
d. Discuss the extent to which the Discussion included all important results.
e. Compare your assessment about the external validity of the study with that of the researchers.

f. To what extent do you think the researchers adequately described the study's limitations and strengths?
g. Discuss the extent to which the results as described in this report would facilitate an EBP-type assessment of the evidence.

EXERCISE 2: STUDY IN APPENDIX C

Read the methods, results, and discussion sections of the report by Wang and Chan ("Culturally tailored diabetes education") in Appendix C. Then answer the following questions:

Questions of Fact

a. Did the report provide information about how missing data were handled?
b. Did the report indicate that tests were performed to assess the degree to which their data met assumptions for parametric tests such as *t*-tests?
c. Did all study participants fully complete the intervention? What was the rate of attrition? Did all participants provide follow-up data? Did the researchers report an analysis of attrition biases?
d. One of the stated purposes of this study was to "evaluate the preliminary efficacy of the interventions." Were inferential statistics used in this evaluation? If yes, were results reported?
e. Did the report provide information about the precision of results through confidence intervals?
f. Did the report provide information about magnitude of effects through calculation of effect sizes?
g. Did the Discussion section link study findings to findings from prior research?
h. Did the Discussion section explicitly mention any "lessons learned" in this pilot study?
i. Did the Discussion section explicitly mention any study limitations?

Questions for Discussion

a. Discuss the thoroughness of the researchers' description about their analytic and data management strategy.
b. Do you agree with the researchers' interpretations of their results? Why or why not?
c. Discuss the extent to which the Discussion included all important results.
d. To what extent do you think the researchers adequately described the study's limitations and strengths?

■ D. The Toolkit

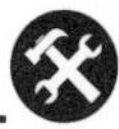

For Chapter 24, the Toolkit on the accompanying CD-ROM contains a Word file with the following:

- Guidelines for Critiquing Interpretations in a Quantitative Research Report (Box 24.1 of the textbook)

PART 6

Building an Evidence Base for Nursing Practice

CHAPTER 25

Integrating Research Evidence: Meta-Analysis and Metasynthesis

■ A. Crossword Puzzle

Complete the crossword puzzle below, which uses terms and concepts presented in Chapter 25. (Puzzles may be removed for easier viewing.)

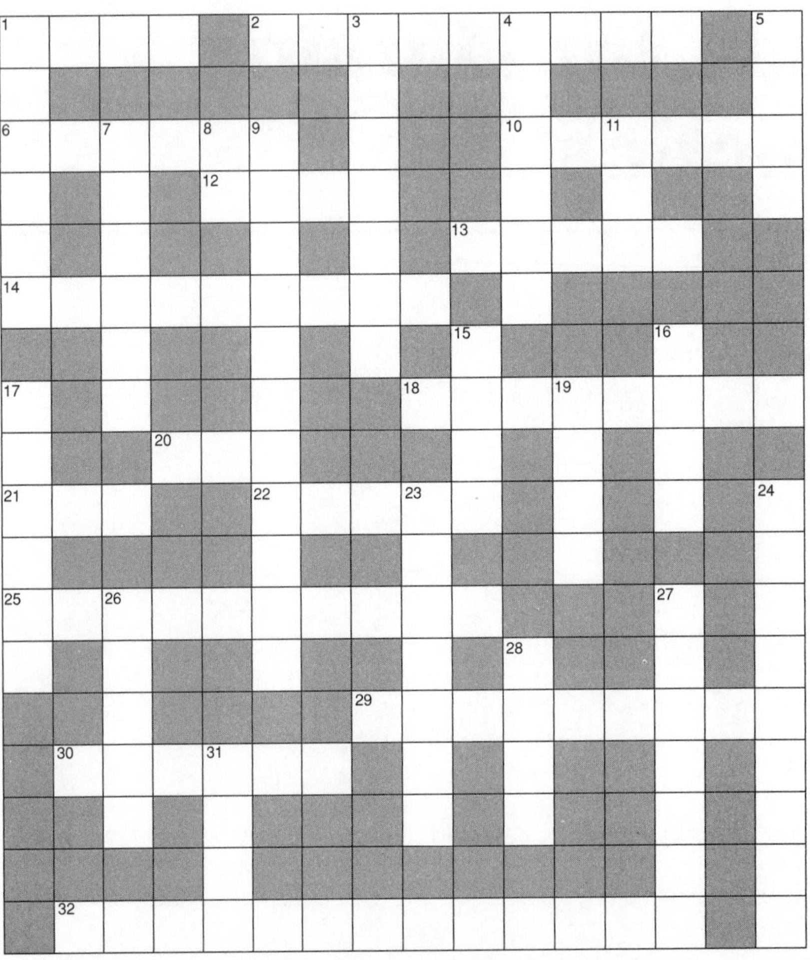

ACROSS

1. A(n) ________ safe number estimates the number of studies with nonsignificant results that would be needed to reverse the conclusion of a significant effect.
2. A(n) ________ effect size is the ratio of reports with a particular thematic finding, divided by all reports relating to a phenomenon.
6. The type of model used in meta-analysis that takes both within-study and between-studies variability into account is called ________ effects.
10. One theory-building integration approach is ________ grounded theory.
12. A method of analyzing the effect of clinical and method factors on variation in effect size is meta-________ (abbr.).
13. Study quality can be examined in relation to effect size using either a component or ________ approach.
14. The ________ level ($5k + 10$) is the number against which a fail-safe number is compared.
18. A(n) ________ analysis involves examining the extent to which effects differ for different types of studies or types of people.
20. The numerator for computing a weighted average effect is the ________ of each primary study's ES times the weight for each study.
21. A common test of the null hypothesis for heterogeneity is the ________ squared test.
22. Analysts must choose a ________ for the meta-analysis that addresses the issue of heterogeneity.
25. Another name for the effect index d is: standardized mean ________.
29. A concern in a systematic review is the ________ bias that stems from identifying only studies in journals and books (abbr.).
30. One way to address primary study quality is to do a(n) ________ analysis that includes and then excludes studies of low quality (abbr.).
32. A meta-analyst must make decisions about how to address the inevitable ________ of effects across studies.

DOWN

1. A(n)________ plot is a graphic display of the effect size (including CIs around them) of each primary study.
3. A preanalysis task in systematic reviews is to ________ information about study and sample characteristics from each primary study.
4. Each primary study in a meta-analysis must yield a quantitative estimate of the ________ of the independent variable on the dependent variable.
5. A problem in quality appraisal is that there is no ________ standard for determining study rigor.
7. One of the originators of a widely used approach to metasynthesis/metaethnography.
8. One of several effect indicators for dichotomous outcomes (acronym)
9. A(n) ________, which involves calculating manifest effect sizes, can lay the foundation for a metasynthesis.

11. The RR is an effect index of ________, rather than absolute, risk (abbr.).
15. There is evidence of a bias against the ________ hypothesis in published studies.
16. An early question in a systematic review is whether it is justifiable to ________ results across studies statistically.
17. In a meta-analysis, after extracting information from primary studies, it is necessary to ________ it so that it can be included in the analysis.
19. The body of unpublished studies is sometimes referred to as ________ literature.
23. In a meta-analysis, researchers often decide to ________ primary studies written in a language other than English.
24. A(n) ________ effect size is the ratio of the number of themes represented in one report, divided by all relevant themes relating to a phenomenon across all reports.
26. In a(n) ________ effects model, it is assumed that one true effect size underlies all study results.
27. ________appraisal is undertaken in most meta-analyses, although approaches to using the information vary.
28. A funnel ________ is often used to detect publication biases.
31. The index *d* provides an estimate of effect ________ for comparing means.

■ B. Study Questions

1. Read one of the following meta-analysis reports:
   - Conn, V., Valentine, J., & Cooper, H. (2002). Interventions to increase physical activity among aging adults: A meta-analysis. *Annals of Behavioral Medicine, 24,* 190–200.
   - Floyd, J., Medler, S., Ager, J., & Janisse, J. (2000). Age-related changes in initiation and maintenance of sleep: A meta-analysis. *Research in Nursing & Health, 23,* 106–117.
   - Peters, R. (1999). The effectiveness of therapeutic touch: A meta-analytic review. *Nursing Science Quarterly, 12*(1), 52–61.

Then, search the literature for related quantitative primary studies published *after* this meta-analysis. Are new study results consistent with the conclusions drawn in the meta-analytic report? Are there enough new studies to warrant a new meta-analysis?

2. Read one of the following metasynthesis reports:
   - Burke, S., Kauffmann, E., Costello, E., Wiskin, N., & Harrison, M. (1998). Stressors in families with a child with a chronic illness: An analysis of qualitative studies and a framework. *Canadian Journal of Nursing Research, 30,* 71–95.
   - Russell, C., Bunting, S., & Gregory, S. (1997). Protective care-receiving: The active role of care recipients. *Journal of Advanced Nursing, 25,* 532–540.
   - Sherwood, G. (1997). Meta-synthesis of qualitative analysis of caring: Defining a therapeutic model of nursing. *Advanced Practice Nursing Quarterly, 3,* 32–42.

Then, search the literature for related qualitative primary studies published *after* this metasynthesis. Are new study results consistent with the conclusions drawn in the metasynthesis report? Are there enough new studies to warrant a new metasynthesis?

3. Read the following report, which involved a systematic review without a meta-analysis. Did the authors adequately justify their decision not to conduct a meta-analysis?
   - McGillion, M., Watt-Watson, J., Kim, J., & Yamada, J. (2004). A systematic review of psychoeducational intervention trials for the management of stable angina. *Journal of Nursing Management, 12*(3), 174–182.
4. Read one of the following reports, and use the critiquing guidelines in Box 25.1 (available as a Word document in the accompanying Toolkit ⊗) to evaluate the integration.
   - Carroll, S. (2004). Nonvocal ventilated patients' perceptions of being understood. *Western Journal of Nursing Research, 26*(1), 85–103.
   - Hsieh, H., & Lee, F. (2005). Graduated compression stockings as prophylaxis for flight-related venous thrombosis: Systematic literature review. *Journal of Advanced Nursing, 51*(1), 83–98.
   - Lefler, L., & Bondy, L. (2004). Women's delay in seeking treatment with myocardial infarction: A meta-synthesis. *Journal of Cardiovascular Nursing, 19*(4), 251–268.
   - Mahon, N., Yarcheski, A, Yarcheski, T., Cannella, B., & Hanks, M. (2006). A meta-analytic study of predictors for loneliness during adolescence. *Nursing Research, 55*(5), 308–315.
   - Nelson, A. (2003). Transition to motherhood. *Journal of Obstetric, Gynecologic, & Neonatal Nursing, 43*(4), 465–477.

■ C. Application Exercises

EXERCISE 1: STUDY IN APPENDIX J

Read the report on the meta-analysis by Taylor-Piliae and Froelicher ("Effectiveness of Tai Chi") in Appendix J. Then answer the following questions:

Questions of Fact

a. What was the stated purpose of this review?
b. How many bibliographic databases were searched? Was there an effort to identify and locate "grey literature"?
c. How many initial citations were obtained? How many citations were reviewed in-depth? How many primary studies were included in the analysis?
d. If a primary study was an RCT that examined the effect of Tai Chi on blood pressure, would it have been included in the review?

e. How many of the studies included in this meta-analysis used an experimental or quasi-experimental design? How many were nonexperimental?
f. Did the researchers develop quality assessment scores for each study in the data set? If yes, how many study elements were appraised? What was the highest possible quality score? What was the average quality score for the studies used in the meta-analysis? How many people scored the studies for quality? Was interrater agreement assessed?
g. Did the researchers set a threshold for study quality as part of their inclusion criteria? If yes, what was it? Were any studies excluded because of a low quality rating?
h. What effect size measure was used in the analysis? What were the effect sizes weighted by?
i. How many subjects were there in total, in all studies combined?
j. Answer the following questions regarding information in Table 1:
    - What are the citations for the studies that used a true experimental design?
    - What were the control conditions in the four studies in Table 1?
    - In which study (and for which group) was the effect size the largest? Was this effect size statistically significant?
    - In which study (and for which group) was the effect size the smallest? Was this effect size statistically significant?
k. Answer the following questions regarding information in Table 2:
    - In which study was the average age of subjects in the Tai Chi group most different from subjects in the comparison group? What type of threat to internal validity does this suggest?
    - For which group of subjects, in which study, was aerobic capacity the greatest, on average?
    - In which study (and for which group) was the effect size the largest? Was this effect size statistically significant?
l. Did the researchers perform any tests for heterogeneity?
m. Was a fixed effects model or random effects model used?
n. Answer the following questions about the results presented in Figures 1 and 2:
    - What is the name for this type of figure?
    - Across all seven studies, did any of the effects favor controls? If yes, which ones?
    - What was the average effect size for the experimental studies? Is this statistically significant? What was the average effect size for the nonexperimental studies? Was this statistically significant?
    - Looking at these two figures, how would you characterize heterogeneity across studies?
o. Were any subgroup analyses performed? If yes, were the subgroups based on methodologic features? Subject characteristics? Intervention characteristics?
p. Was the average effect size higher for the classical Yang style of Tai Chi or for other types? Among men or women?
q. Was a meta-regression performed?
r. Did the researchers do any sensitivity analyses based on study quality or sample size?
s. Did this meta-analysis address the issue of publication bias?

Questions for Discussion

a. Was the size of the sample (studies and subjects) sufficiently large to draw conclusions about the overall effect of Tai Chi and about subgroup effects?
b. What other subgroups might have been interesting to examine (assuming there was sufficient information in the original studies)?
c. Did the researchers draw reasonable conclusions about the quality, quantity, and consistency of evidence?
d. Discuss the implications of the discrepant findings for the experimental and nonexperimental studies.
e. How would you assess the overall rigor of this meta-analysis? What would you recommend to improve the quality of this systematic review?

EXERCISE 2: STUDY IN APPENDIX K

Read the report on the metasynthesis by Swartz ("Parenting preterm infants") in Appendix K. Then answer the following questions:

Questions of Fact

a. What was the stated purpose of this integration?
b. How many bibliographic databases were searched? Was there an effort to identify and locate "grey literature"?
c. How many initial citations were obtained? How many primary studies were included in the integration?
d. What was Swartz's position in the controversy regarding integration across research traditions?
e. Were primary studies appraised for quality? Were any studies excluded because of poor quality?
f. Were the data in the primary studies derived from interviews, observations, or both?
g. Did both mothers and fathers provide data for the analysis? Did any other type of parent figures provide data?
h. What approach was used to conduct this metasynthesis?
i. Was a meta-summary performed?
j. How many study participants were there in all of the studies combined?
k. How many shared themes were identified in this meta-synthesis? What were those themes?
l. Was Swartz's analysis supported through the inclusion of raw data from the primary studies?
m. Did the report mention any limitations of this metasynthesis?

Questions for Discussion

a. Was the size of the sample (studies and subjects) sufficiently large to conduct a meaningful metasynthesis? Did the diversity of the sample (in terms of participant characteristics, timing of data collection, or research tradition) enhance the study or weaken it?

b. Did the analysis and integration appear reasonable and thorough?
c. Were primary studies adequately described?
d. How would you assess the overall rigor of this metasynthesis? What would you recommend to improve its quality?

■ D. The Toolkit

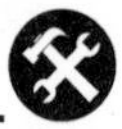

For Chapter 25, the Toolkit on the accompanying CD-ROM contains a Word file with the following:

- Guidelines for Critiquing Systematic Reviews and Metasyntheses (Box 25.1 of the textbook)
- Example of a Data Extraction Form for a Meta-Analysis
- Selected Formulas for Calculating a Standardized Mean Difference Effect Size (*d*)
- Template for a Table Summarizing Characteristics of Studies Included in a Meta-Analysis or Systematic Review
- Template for a Summary Table for a Metasynthesis
- Template for a Table Summarizing Meta-Findings in a Meta-Summary

CHAPTER 26

Disseminating Evidence: Reporting Research Findings

■ A. Crossword Puzzle

Complete the crossword puzzle below, which uses terms and concepts presented in Chapter 26. (Puzzles may be removed for easier viewing.)

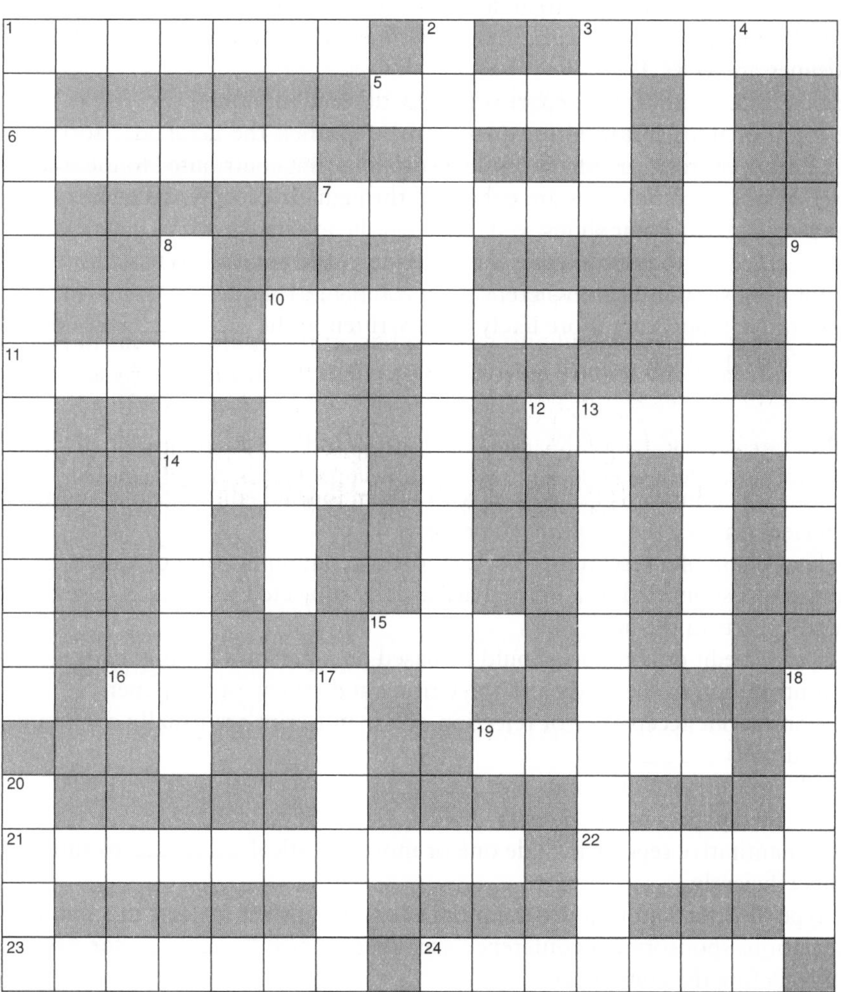

■ C. Application Exercises

STUDIES IN APPENDICES A–K

Answer the following questions with regard to the 11 research reports (Appendices A–K) included in appendices in this Resource Manual:

Questions of Fact

a. Which articles in the appendices were published in journals that had an impact factor greater than 1.00 in 2005? Which articles were published in journals with an impact factor between .70 and .99?
b. Which, if any, of the reports in the appendices deviated from a traditional IMRAD format?
c. In reports that were multiply authored, were the authors listed alphabetically?
d. Which, if any, of the reports used first-person narratives to describe aspects of the study methods or results?

Questions for Discussion

a. Comment on the extent to which the abstracts for the studies in the appendices adequately captured key concepts and the population of interest.
b. Which report title had the greatest appeal to you—that is, which one most intrigued you and made you want to read the study?
c. Select one or two reports and comment on how effectively the authors used figures and tables to enhance or streamline communication.

■ D. The Toolkit

For Chapter 26, the Toolkit on the CD-ROM provided with this Resource Manual contains the following:

- Guidelines for Critiquing the Presentation of a Research Report (Box 26.2 of the textbook)
- CONSORT Checklist of Items to Include When Reporting a Randomized Trial
- The CONSORT Flow Chart

CHAPTER 27

Writing Proposals to Generate Evidence

■ A. Crossword Puzzle

Complete the crossword puzzle below, which uses terms and concepts presented in Chapter 27. (Puzzles may be removed for easier viewing.)

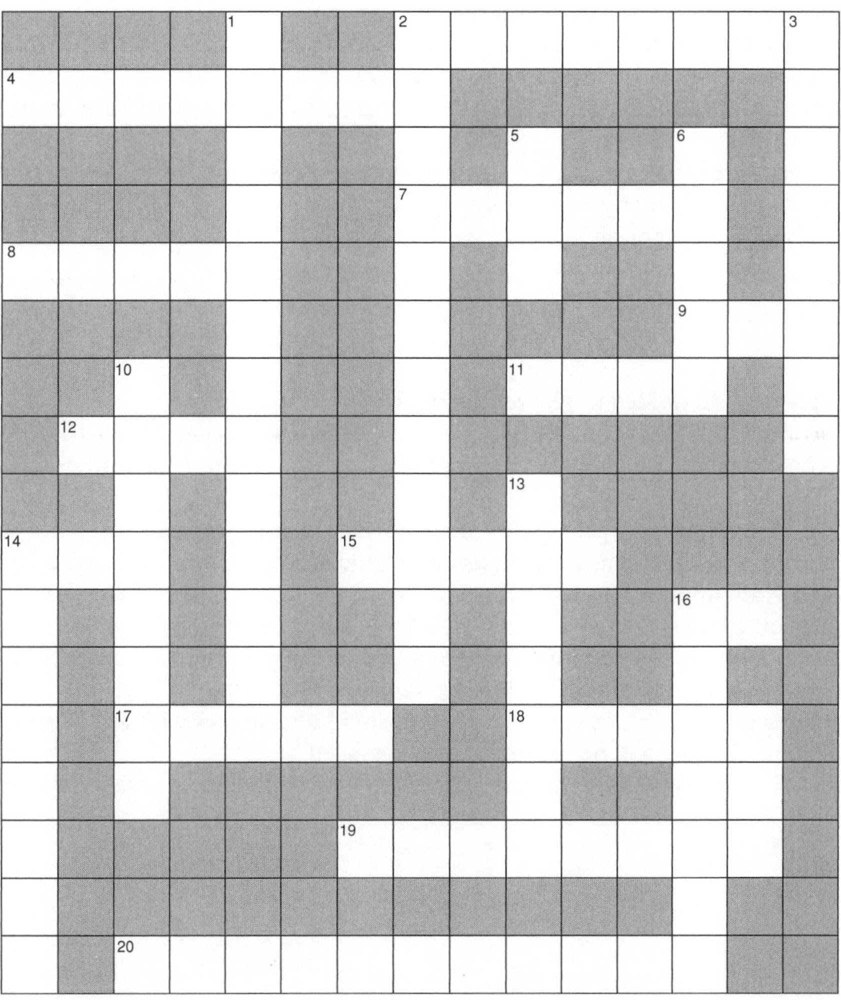

ACROSS

2. In applications to NIH, the study purpose is described in the section called ________ Aims.
4. The costs of a project over and above specific project-related costs
7. Specific project-related costs
8. The funding mechanism that gives researchers considerable discretion in what to study and how best to study it
9. A mechanism for soliciting grant application using broad guidelines about the type of projects of interest (acronym)
11. In the United States and most countries, the entity that funds most research (abbr.)
12. A type of NIH award for institutions that have not historically received much NIH funding is an R15 or ________ grant (acronym).
14. Applications to NIH typically go through ________ rounds of review.
15. A frequent criticism of grant applications to NIH is insufficient ________ work.
16. The form used for NIH grant submissions is the __ __ 424.
17. It is prudent to consider whether there is a current "hot ________" that will make a grant application more appealing to reviewers.
18. The R03, or ________ Grant Program, is mainly for pilot or feasibility studies (backwards).
19. Indirect costs, or ________, are institutional costs associated with doing research (e.g., for space, administrators, etc.).
20. In an NIH grant application, pilot work is described in the section called ________ Studies.

DOWN

1. The set of skills needed to secure funding for a research project
2. The informal name for an NIH peer review group (two words)
3. The funding mechanism for a specific study that a government or entity wants to have done
5. The formal name for a peer review panel for NIH (acronym)
6. Writing proposals is time-consuming, so a good strategy is to ________ early!
10. Scored grant applications to NIH are given a(n) ________ score that reflects average ratings of merit.
13. ________ budgets, paid in blocks of $25,000, are appropriate for most NIH applications requesting $250,000 or less per year of direct costs.
14. Including a(n) ________ with a proposal provides reviewers with an understanding of how the project will be organized and managed.
16. Each applicant to NIH is sent a(n) ________ sheet that includes reviewers' comments.

■ B. Study Questions

1. Chapter 27 of the textbook describes four major sections of U.S. Public Health Service grant applications (Specific Aims, Background and Significance, Preliminary Studies, and Research Design and Methods). In which section would the following statements ordinarily be found?
   a. Study participants, who will include young adults who have been treated for a drug overdose, will initially be recruited through the emergency department of a local hospital. Network sampling will then be used to contact a broader population of those with an overdose experience.
   b. It is hypothesized that paraplegics who receive pool therapy will perform better on tests of muscle strength than those who receive other types of exercise.
   c. Two members of the research team have recently completed an in-depth longitudinal study of the coping mechanisms of parents with a Down syndrome infant.
   d. The major threat to the internal validity of the proposed study is selection bias, which will be dealt with through the careful selection of comparison subjects and through statistical adjustment of preexisting differences.
   e. Prior studies have found that people undergoing cancer treatment experience a complex array of disease- and treatment-related symptoms.
   f. The proposed research will have the potential of restructuring the delivery of health care in rural areas.

2. Go to the CRISP database (*http://crisp.cit.nih.gov/*) and find an NINR-funded grant nearing completion, on a topic that interests you. Write to the Principal Investigator (PI) to inquire about any conference presentations or published papers that have resulted from the grant.

■ C. Application Exercises

EXERCISE 1: APPENDIX L

Appendix L contains a successful grant application, "Older adults' response to health care practitioner pain communication." This application was submitted by Dr. Deborah Dillon McDonald to NINR for funding under a program announcement PA-03-152, "Biobehavioral Pain Research." Before reviewing Dr. McDonald's grant application and the associated materials in Appendix L, scan the program announcement (available at *http://grants.nih.gov/grants/guide/pa-files/pa-03-152.html*) and answer the following questions:

a. Did this PA fund projects through the R01 mechanism only?
b. When did this program announcement expire for R01 applications?
c. How many institutes within NIH, besides NINR, participated in this program announcement?

d. Would this funding mechanism be appropriate for funding research on the effectiveness of pain treatments and interventions?
e. Would this funding mechanism be appropriate for funding basic research on affective responses to pain?
f. The four major sections of a grant application (Specific Aims Through Research Design and Methods) are usually required to be no more than 25 pages. For this PA, what were the page restrictions?

EXERCISE 2: APPENDIX L

Read through the grant application forms and research proposal submitted by Dr. McDonald in Appendix L. (Note that this application was submitted on form PHS398, the form that was used before the SF424 electronic filing form became mandated.) Then answer the following questions:

Questions of Fact

a. What were the total *direct* costs requested for the entire research project for all project years? What are the *total* requested funds, for both direct and indirect costs?
b. What were the proposed timeframes for the study?
c. How many people were listed as key personnel for the proposed study? How much of the PI's time was proposed for this project?
d. Did the research plan section of the grant application conform to the page restrictions for this PA?
e. In what section of the application did McDonald present her hypothesis? Is this placement consistent with guidelines?
f. In what section did McDonald describe her own prior research relating to pain communication? How many relevant prior studies had she undertaken?
g. McDonald divided her "Research Design and Methods" section into several subsections. What were they?
h. What type of research design did McDonald propose?
i. What sample size did McDonald propose? Was the proposed sample size based on a power analysis?
j. According to the proposal, who would be blinded in this study?
k. Did the application stipulate that a stipend would be given to subjects? If yes, what incentive would be offered?
l. In the analysis plan, were any multivariate analyses proposed? If so, what type of analysis would be undertaken?

Questions for Discussion

a. Before reading any of the reviewers' comments, critique McDonald's proposed design, sampling plan, data collection, and data analysis strategies. Then compare your comments with the reviewers' comments about the proposed methods.
b. What do you think the weakest aspect of the proposed project is?

EXERCISE 3: APPENDIX L

Appendix L also includes the summary sheet for McDonald's grant application, together with McDonald's response to reviewers' concerns. Read through these materials and then answer the following questions.

a. The application number indicates the NIH funding mechanism for the proposed project. What was the funding mechanism?
b. Which study section reviewed the grant application? On what date did the study section meet?
c. What was this grant application's priority score?
d. What was the primary concern of the study section—that is, what part was deemed "unacceptable" and required McDonald to elaborate on proposed methods?

■ D. The Toolkit

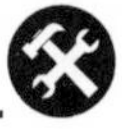

For Chapter 27, the Toolkit on the accompanying CD-ROM contains a Word file with the following:

- Checklist for a Quantitative Grant Application
- Example of a Grant-Writing Timeline (Figure 27.1 of the textbook)
- NIH Grant Application Forms (Not Fillable—for Review Purposes Only)

APPENDIX A

INFLUENCE OF A COMPUTER INTERVENTION ON THE PSYCHOLOGICAL STATUS OF CHRONICALLY ILL RURAL WOMEN

Preliminary Results

Wade Hill • Clarann Weinert • Shirley Cudney

- **Background:** Adaptation to chronic illness is a lifelong process presenting numerous psychological challenges. It has been shown to be influenced by participating in support groups. Rural women with chronic illness face additional burdens as access to information, healthcare resources, and sources of support are often limited. Developing virtual support groups and testing the effects on psychosocial indicators associated with adaptation to chronic illness may help remove barriers to adaptation.
- **Objective:** To examine the effects of a computer-delivered intervention on measures of psychosocial health in chronically ill rural women including social support, self-esteem, empowerment, self-efficacy, depression, loneliness, and stress.
- **Methods:** An experimental design was used to test a computer-delivered intervention and examine differences in psychosocial health between women who participated in the intervention ($n = 44$) and women in a control group ($n = 56$).
- **Results:** Differences between women who participated in the intervention and controls were found for self-esteem, $F(1,98) = 5.97$, $p = .016$; social support, $F(1,98) = 4.43$, $p = .038$; and empowerment, $F(1,98) = 6.06$, $p = .016$. A comparison of means for depression, loneliness, self-efficacy, and stress suggests that differences for other psychosocial variables are possible.
- **Discussion:** The computer-based intervention tested appears to result in improved self-esteem, social support, and empowerment among rural women with chronic illness. Descriptive but nonsignificant differences were found for other psychosocial variables (depression, loneliness, self-efficacy, and stress); women who participated in the intervention appeared to improve more than women in the control group.

- **Key Words:** chronic illness · computer-based intervention · psychosocial outcomes · rural

Adaptation to chronic disease is a lifelong challenge to persons with long-term health problems. Being diagnosed with a chronic illness, unlike an acute illness, is a profound and life-altering event that can result in alterations in physical functioning, loss of control over life circumstances, and subsequently emotional strain (Emery, 2003). The psychological task imposed on these individuals is that of maintaining an acceptable quality of life while living with the changes in lifestyle that long-term illness imposes. For chronically ill, middle-aged, rural women who live where there are relatively few healthcare resources and limited access to those that do exist, it is particularly difficult to maintain a semblance of normalcy and balance in their lives. They often must struggle in isolation to meet the psychological challenges of adapting to their chronic illnesses.

Emotional distress often accompanies these challenges, yet not all experience significant emotional problems (Earll, Johnson, & Mitchell, 1993), particularly if they have adequate social support and access to quality health information. Social support has been demonstrated to be a constructive influence on the experience of dealing with illness (Finfgeld-Connett, 2005; Hegyvary, 2004) and positively affects psychosocial adjustment, enhances quality of life, and reduces the incidence of depression. Those with intact psychosocial health can live healthier lives and better manage living with long-term illness (Stuifbergen, Seraphine, & Roberts, 2000). Historically, traditional support groups where participants interact in person are known to influence psychosocial health (Hunter & Hall, 1989; Lin, Simeone, Ensel, & Kuo, 1979; Williams, 1990), although little is known about the effects of virtual support groups.

■ Background

Social support, based on the work of Weiss (1969), includes the provision of attachment or intimacy, facilitation of social integration, opportunity for nurturant behavior, reassurance of self-worth, and availability of informational and material assistance. Social support can buffer the negative effects of life events on health (Paykel, 1994; Pollachek, 2001; Thomas, 1995) and positively influence psychosocial adjustment and self-management of the chronic illness experience (Gallant, 2003; Symister & Friend, 2003). Inadequate social support can contribute to increased levels of depression and stress (Connell, Davis, Gallant, & Sharpe, 1994; Gray & Cason, 2002). Not all persons with chronic illness suffer from significant emotional problems (Earll et al., 1993), particularly if they have adequate social support and access to quality health information that enable them to live healthy and productive lives while successfully adapting to and managing the many challenges of chronic illness. Social support resources may buffer the consequences of a chronic disease by enhancing recovery, increasing adherence to treatment recommendations, and promoting overall psychological adaptation (Wallston, Alagna, DeVellis, & DeVellis, 1983; Wortman & Conway, 1985). An effective and efficient means of providing support and facilitating the mobilization of support is through self-help groups (Schaefer, 1995). For those who live in geographically isolated areas, distance, travel time, weather, and road conditions often prohibit contact with others like themselves who are attempting to maintain psychosocial health (Sullivan, Weinert, & Cudney, 2003).

Computer-based support systems can be one solution to the problem of isolation. It has been shown that ill individuals using a computer-based health support system had better health outcomes, exerted greater efforts to improve functioning, and demonstrated greater resistance to psychological dysfunction (Gustafson et al., 1999).

The diagnosis of a chronic illness sets in motion a complex process of adaptation that requires balancing the demands of the situation and the individual's ability to respond (Pollock, Christian, & Sands, 1990). Adaptation has been a major theoretical concept guiding nursing practice over the past 20 years as delineated in the Roy Adaptation Model (RAM; Roy & Andrews, 1999). Pollock et al. (Pollock, 1986, 1993; Pollock et al., 1990) used the RAM as the theoretical framework for integrating the major variables of chronicity, stress, hardiness, and adaptive behavior. Their investigation identified and measured selected intervening variables that influenced adaptation. These variables included the ability to tolerate stress, presence of the hardiness characteristic, demographic characteristics, involvement in health promotion activities, and participation in health education programs (which enhance optimal self-management). The end result or level of adaptation was the individual's functioning as measured in the psychological and physiologic domains (Pollock, 1986). Chen (2005) tested the fit of the RAM as a framework for studying the nutritional health of community-dwelling elders using a conceptual–theoretical–empirical approach for examining factors that influence adaptation level. Stuifbergen et al. (2000) developed a model of health promotion and quality of life (QOL) in chronic disabling conditions that has implications for associating optimal self-management with QOL. The central concept for management of chronic illness throughout the literature has been psychosocial health and represents the key component of interest in this study.

One example of a computer-based intervention designed to support adaptation for chronically ill rural women was the Women to Women Project (WTW; Cudney & Weinert, 2000; Cudney, Winters, Weinert, & Anderson, 2005; Weinert, 2000; Weinert, Cudney, & Winters, 2005). The WTW was an online self-help support group designed to enhance social support and teach women the computer literacy skills necessary to find and evaluate health information available on the World Wide Web (WWW). Indicators of the potential for adaptation used in this project were social support, self-esteem, empowerment, self-efficacy, stress, depression, and loneliness. The purposes of this article are: to (a) examine the relationships among the psychosocial indicators and (b) determine the effect of the intervention on social support, self-esteem, empowerment, self-efficacy, stress, depression, and loneliness.

▪ Method

DESIGN

This research was approved and monitored through the university's institutional review board for protection of human subjects. Women for this study were recruited (N = 125) from the Intermountain West using a variety of techniques including mass media, agency and service organization newsletters, and word of mouth (see Figure 1). After eliminating the names of five women who lived in urbanized areas, 120 women were randomized into intervention and control groups (intervention = 61; control = 59). At the completion of the intervention, 17 women from the intervention group dropped out due to declining health, inadequate time for participation, or moving to urban areas. Only two women from the control group dropped from the study due to failing to return the questionnaires. Data analyzed here are based on 43 women that completed the intervention and 57 women in the control group. One woman from the intervention group was dropped due to missing data.

To determine the impact of the intervention on the women's psychological status, measures were administered via a mail questionnaire composed of psychosocial health indicators: social support, self-esteem, empowerment, self-efficacy, stress, depression, and loneliness. *Illustrative comments from the women's online conversations were added to* illuminate the data related to emotional and informational support. A detailed description of the intervention is provided elsewhere (Weinert et al., 2005); thus, only a limited description of WTW will be repeated here.

The intervention included 22 weeks of participation in an online, asynchronous, peer-led support group and health teaching units. The WebCT (2005) platform was used to deliver the intervention and was available 24 hours a day, 7 days a week, thus allowing women to participate at any convenient time. Women in the intervention group had access to "Koffee Klatch," an asynchronous chat room in which they exchanged feelings, expressed concerns, provided support, and shared life experiences. The e-mail function ("Mailbox") gave the women private access to each other and to the research team. Women also engaged in health teaching unit activities independently, which included accessing health information on the WWW and participating in expert-facilitated chat room ("Health Roundtable") discussions related to the health teaching unit activities.

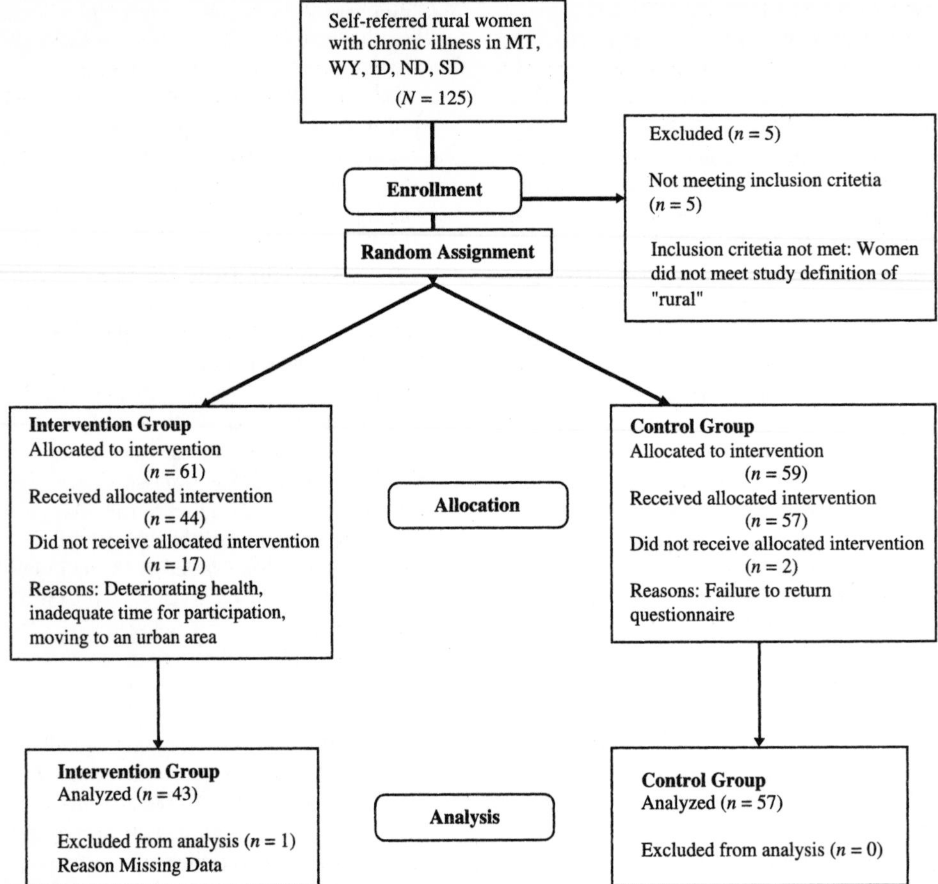

Figure 1. Participant progression.

SAMPLE

The sample consisted of 100 chronically ill rural women. Participants were required to be 35–65 years of age and have a chronic illness such as diabetes, rheumatoid condition, heart disease, cancer, or multiple sclerosis. They lived at least 25 miles outside an urbanized area (a city of 12,500 or more) on a ranch, farm, or small town in Montana, Idaho, North Dakota, South Dakota, or Wyoming. On average, women in the sample traveled almost 57 (*SD* = 74.2) miles one-way for routine healthcare. The women were primarily older than 40 years of age (92%), were married or living with someone (80%), and had 13 or more years of education (77%). A majority of the sample were not employed outside of the home (64%) and household income varied from less than $15,000 (21%) to $55,000 or greater (16%). The length of chronic illness (time since diagnosis) was 1–51 years with a mean of 13.0 years (*SD* = 11.1). Additional demographic details are presented in Table 1.

MEASURES

Disease may coexist with health in the same person at any point in the life span; thus, health maintenance is an important part of the quality of life equation for people with chronic illness. Promoting health, even in the

Table 1. Sample Characteristics

	Participants (N = 100)	Sample (%)
Age		
30–39	8	8
40–49	27	27
50–59	50	50
60–69	15	15
Ethnicity		
White	93	93
Hispanic or Latina	1	1
American Indian or Alaskan	3	3
Native		
Other	3	3
Marital status		
Married	79	79
Divorced	13	13
Separated	1	1
Widowed/Never married	15	15
Living together	1	1
Education (years of school completed)		
12 or less	23	23
13–15	47	47
16–18	29	29
19 or greater	1	1
Income		
Less than $15,000	21	21
$15,000–24,999	14	14
$25,000–34,999	16	16
$35,000–44,999	16	16
$45,000–54,999	17	17
$55,000–64,999	8	8
$65,000–74,999	4	4
$75,000–84,999	4	4
Employment (outside home)		
Yes	36	36
No	64	64

presence of chronic illness, includes activities that educate, guide, and motivate the individual to take personal actions which improve the likelihood of sustained good health (Fries, 1997). Factors considered to influence the success of these activities in promoting good health are social support, self-esteem, empowerment, self-efficacy, stress, depression, and loneliness. These factors can be conceptualized as psychosocial health indicators of the individual's potential to adapt to and manage chronic illness. The instruments used to measure the psychosocial concepts were selected based on the strength of their psychometric properties, prior use in research with chronic illness, conceptual fit, use by the research team, and because there is evidence in earlier work and the literature that they are amenable to change, based on a support and health education intervention. For all instruments used, higher scores indicate higher levels of the measured construct (e.g., higher depression scores indicate more depression symptomatology; higher social support scores indicate a greater degree of social support). See Table 2 for published information on reliability and validity for each instrument along with the alphas obtained in the current study.

Social Support. Social support can be conceptualized as the provision of intimacy, facilitation of social integration, opportunity for nurturant behavior, reassurance of self-worth, and the availability of assistance (Weiss, 1969), and it can buffer the negative effects of life events on health (Pollachek, 2001). Social support can positively influence psychosocial adjustment and management of the chronic illness (Symister & Friend, 2003) and inadequate support can increase depression and stress (Gray & Cason, 2002). Interventions designed to enhance social support can facilitate coping and problem solving (Spiegel, 1993) and encourage the reciprocal aspects of providing comfort and support to others, which is critical to many women's sense of worth and well-being. The Personal Resource Questionnaire (PRQ) was developed to measure situational support and perceived support (Brandt & Weinert, 1981) and has systematically and consistently undergone psychometric evaluation over the past 20 years resulting in the current 15-item version, the PRQ2000 (Weinert, 2003).

Table 2. Psychological Concepts, Indicators, Items, Reliability, Validity

Concepts	Indicators	No. of Items	Reported α	Study α	Validity
Self-efficacy	Self-Efficacy Scale (Sherer et al., 1982)	23	.71–.86	.88	Construct criterion
Self-esteem	Self-Esteem Scale (Rosenberg, 1965)	10	.77–.88	.87	Convergent discriminant
Empowerment	Diabetes Empowerment Scale (Anderson et al., 2000)	10	.91	.96	Concurrent
Social support	PRQ2000 (Weinert, 2003)	15	.87–.92	.90	Construct divergent
Stress	Perceived Stress Scale (Cohen et al., 1983)	14	.84–.86	.90	Convergent discriminant
Depression	CES-D (Devine & Orme, 1985)	20	.84–.90	.90	Convergent discriminant
Loneliness	UCLA Loneliness Scale (Rosenberg, 1965)	20	.94	.94	Convergent discriminant

Self-Esteem. Self-esteem is the extent to which people value, approve, or like themselves (Baumeister, Campbell, Krueger, & Vohs, 2003). Self-esteem is considered an indicator, among others, of psychological well-being and can be thought of as one dimension of the potential to manage chronic illness. People who have a positive sense of self-worth, believe in their own control, and are optimistic about the future may be more likely to exhibit better health behaviors (Taylor, Kemeny, Reed, Bower, & Gruenewald, 2000). The Rosenberg Self-Esteem Scale (SES) was designed originally to measure global feelings of self-worth or self-acceptance for ease of administration, economy of time, and unidimensionality. The 10 items are a self-report of feelings about the self (Robinson, Shaver, & Wrightsman, 1991).

Empowerment. In its most general sense, empowerment refers to the ability of people to gain understanding and control over personal, social, economic, and political forces to take action to improve their life situations. Control over destiny emerges as a disease risk factor and a strategy for health promotion (Wallerstein, 2002); lack of control of destiny enhances susceptibility to illness. These deficits can be overcome through the use of computer-based support systems that have been shown to be extremely valuable in helping participants understand their illness and as a result became a source of empowerment (Gustafson et al., 1993). For this study, the Diabetes Empowerment Scale (Anderson, Funnell, Fitzgerald, & Marrero, 2000) was modified with the permission of the author of the tool. The 10-item Setting and Achieving Goals subscale was used after changing the word "diabetes" in the stem to "chronic illness."

Self-Efficacy. Self-efficacy is the belief that by personal behavior one may be able to affect health or other futures and is an essential key to subsequent changes in health risk behavior (Fries, Koop, Sokolov, Beadle, & Wright, 1998). One hallmark of a successful information and support program is its power to develop individuals' skills and confidence in their ability to take responsibility for managing their healthcare and provide access to social support to foster self-efficacy (Gustafson et al., 1999). The Self-Efficacy Scale

(Sherer et al., 1982) was designed to measure generalized self-efficacy expectations dependent on past experiences and on tendencies to attribute success to skill as opposed to chance. The items were written to measure general self-efficacy expectancies in areas such as social skills or vocational competence (17 items) and social self-efficacy (6 items).

Stress. Chronic illness and stress are closely aligned. The diagnosis and treatment of a chronic illness affects an individual's physical, psychological, and social self, and it affects sense of stress and well-being (Pollachek, 2001). Developing the capacity to manage stress is often helpful in managing the additional problems of a chronic illness (Cagle, 2004). The Perceived Stress Scale (PSS; Cohen, Kamarck, & Mermelstein, 1983) measures the degree to which situations in one's life are perceived as stressful. The PSS is based on the argument that the causal event is the cognitively mediated response to the objective event, not the objective event itself.

Depression. Depression is very common among people who have chronic illness and can impair their ability to cope with their diseases and detract from their quality of life (Davis & Gershtein, 2003). Chronic physical conditions affect depression directly and indirectly by affecting domestic relationships, reducing occupational performance, imposing economic strains, and undermining personal resources (e.g., self-esteem and empowerment; Vilhjalmsson, 1998). The Center for Epidemiological Studies Depression Scale (CES-D) is a 20-item self-report measure of depressive symptomatology that was initially developed for use in epidemiology surveys of depression within the general population (Devine & Orme, 1985). The CES-D assesses the frequency and duration of cognitive, affective, behavioral, and somatic symptoms associated with depression in the preceding week. Positive affect is also assessed by the instrument.

Loneliness. Loneliness can be defined as a deficit in human intimacy and negative feelings about being alone (Hall & Havens, 1999). The significance of loneliness is that it often results in human suffering, whereas freedom from loneliness contributes to a feeling of well-being and a positive mental health outlook (Perlman, Gerson, & Spinner, 1977). For chronically ill rural women, the risk for loneliness is compounded by their geographic isolation. The UCLA Loneliness Scale (Version 3), a widely used measure of loneliness, was used in this study (Robinson et al., 1991). It is a Likert-type measure focusing on the quality of a respondent's relationships with others. Advantages of the scale are that the word "loneliness" does not appear in any of the items, which helps reduce response bias, and loneliness is conceptualized as a unidimensional affective state.

■ Results

For the first aim, bivariate correlations were produced to examine the relationships among the psychosocial variables of interest from data collected at baseline. On Table 3, the correlations among self-efficacy, self-esteem, empowerment, social support, stress, depression, and loneliness are shown. All correlations were statistically significant ($p = .01$, two-tailed) and in the anticipated direction. For example, self-esteem is positively associated with social support ($r = .414$), empowerment ($r = .354$), and self-efficacy ($r = .566$). Alternatively, psychosocial outcomes such as stress, loneliness, and depression were negatively associated with positive outcomes such as self-esteem, social support, empowerment, and self-efficacy. The highest absolute correlations are found between loneliness and stress ($r = .716$), depression and stress ($r = .708$), depression and loneliness ($r = .701$), and social support and loneliness ($r = -.646$).

For the second aim, repeated-measures analysis of variance was conducted to evaluate the effects of the computerized intervention on changes in the seven psychosocial outcomes of interest. The models tested included the dependent variable of scale scores for the SES (self-esteem), the PRQ (social support), Chronic

Table 3. Correlations Among Psychosocial Measures

	Self-esteem	Social Support	Empowerment	Self-efficacy	Depression	Loneliness
Social support	.414					
Empowerment	.354	.488				
Self-efficacy	.566	.546	.564			
Depression	−.599	−.447	−.487	−.586		
Loneliness	−.686	−.646	−.390	−.549	.701	
Stress	−.600	−.413	−.380	−.454	.708	.716

Note. Correlation is significant at the .01 level (two-tailed).

Illness Empowerment Scale (CIES; empowerment), Self-Efficacy Scale (Sherer et al., 1982), CES-D (depression), University of California, Los Angeles (UCLA) Loneliness Scale (version 3), and PSS (stress) (Cohen et al.) scales, one within-subjects factor of time (i.e., baseline measurement to the 3-month measurement, at the conclusion of the computer intervention) and one between-subjects factor of membership in the intervention or control groups. The means and standard deviations for all scale scores found for both time periods are presented in Table 4.

Table 4. Baseline and 3-month Means for Psychosocial Measures ($N = 100$)

	Baseline Mean (*SD*)	3-Month Mean (*SD*)
Self-esteem		
Intervention	29.57 (5.83)	30.83 (5.17)
Control	31.82 (4.82)	31.21 (5.32)
Social support		
Intervention	79.05 (13.40)	83.46 (12.42)
Control	79.91 (14.86)	78.96 (17.15)
Empowerment		
Intervention	36.79 (7.15)	40.30 (4.83)
Control	35.73 (7.24)	36.14 (6.48)
Self-efficacy		
Intervention	110.33 (21.08)	111.26 (18.86)
Control	109.61 (17.32)	106.09 (19.82)
Depression		
Intervention	18.52 (11.64)	15.50 (11.90)
Control	18.13 (10.34)	16.91 (11.82)
Loneliness		
Intervention	45.73 (9.99)	43.15 (8.69)
Control	43.97 (10.53)	43.11 (10.94)
Stress		
Intervention	28.49 (7.51)	26.15 (7.83)
Control	28.46 (7.32)	27.28 (8.80)

Table 5. ANOVA Results for Effect of Intervention on Psychosocial Measures

	Sum of Squares	*df*	Mean Square	*F*	*p*
Self-esteem					
Time	5.15	1	5.15	0.733	.394
Time × Treatment	41.92	1	41.92	5.973	.016
Social support					
Time	142.38	1	142.38	1.855	.176
Time × Treatment	340.15	1	340.15	4.432	.038
Empowerment					
Time	187.10	1	187.10	9.699	.002
Time × Treatment	116.94	1	116.94	6.062	.016
Self-efficacy					
Time	81.43	1	81.43	0.90	.346
Time × Treatment	240.62	1	240.62	2.65	.107
Depression					
Time	215.54	1	215.54	5.00	.028
Time × Treatment	39.29	1	39.29	0.91	.342
Loneliness					
Time	141.94	1	141.94	6.51	.012
Time × Treatment	35.29	1	35.29	1.62	.206
Stress					
Time	144.931	1	144.93	8.44	.005
Time × Treatment	15.58	1	15.58	0.91	.343

After assurance that ANOVA assumptions were met (e.g., normality, homogeneity of variance), the results for the ANOVAs indicate that significant Time × Treatment interactions exist for self-esteem, $F(1,98) = 5.97$, $p = .016$, social support, $F(1,98) = 4.43$, $p = .038$, and empowerment, $F(1,98) = 6.06$, $p = .016$, thereby suggesting that the group's scores changed differently across time. An examination of the means and standard deviations in Table 4 shows that for all three psychosocial outcomes the intervention group improved across time; for example, social support increased from 79.05 at baseline to 83.46 at 3 months, whereas the control groups either improved very little or decreased. These results suggest that the intervention had an appreciable effect on self-esteem, social support, and empowerment within the sample.

The results for the other psychosocial outcomes of interest are less clear (see Table 5). ANOVA results for depression, loneliness, and stress show that significant main effects for time only are evident, suggesting that the groups together changed significantly across time, but did not differ statistically. For depression, $F(1,98) = 5.00$, $p = .028$, results of the ANOVA and descriptive statistics indicate that both groups became less depressed over time, although subjects in the treatment group showed a much greater change (i.e., treatment group declined by 3.02; control declined by 1.22). Likewise, both loneliness, $F(1,98) = 6.51$, $p = .012$, and stress, $F(1,98) = 8.44$, $p = .005$, yield main effects for time, but do not indicate statistical differences between groups despite greater improvements made among the participants of the intervention when examining descriptive statistics. These findings suggest that cautious optimism is warranted in conclusions that the computer intervention had effects on depression, loneliness, and stress.

■ Discussion

The purpose of this study was to examine the impact of a computer-delivered intervention on measures of psychosocial health (social support, self-esteem, empowerment, self-efficacy, depression, loneliness, and stress) in chronically ill rural women. Although statistically significant differences between intervention and control groups were found only for social support, self-esteem, and empowerment, all psychosocial indicators improved in the intervention group and declined or remained stable among controls.

SOCIAL SUPPORT

Although the nature and function of social support on various states of health is debated, agreement exists that social support and social networks have important causal influences on health (Finfgeld-Connett, 2005). As expected, the intervention had appreciable effects on social support because women in the intervention group were provided access to others with similar conditions and the means, via computers, to access an asynchronous support environment. Essentially, women created new social networks and provided and received support at will, without regard to time of day or distance between participants.

Self-esteem is thought to mediate the relationships between social support and variables such as depression that have been used to define psychological adjustment to chronic illness (Druley & Townsend, 1998). Although it is unknown whether manipulating self-esteem regulates the relationship between social support and psychological adjustment, or alternatively if persons with high or low self-esteem receive differential support or perceive support differently, recent research supports the idea that social support operates through self-esteem and can influence both optimism and depression (Symister & Friend, 2003). Bivariate relationships from previous studies compare favorably with the findings here, providing further evidence about the connectedness of self-esteem, social support, and depression. Symister and Friend (2003) used a sample of 86 people with end-stage renal disease to study psychosocial response to chronic illness and found correlations of .47 ($p < .001$) between social support and self-esteem, −.51 ($p < .001$) between social support and depression, and −.62 ($p < .001$) between self-esteem and depression. Our findings for the relationships between social support and self-esteem, social support and depression, and self-esteem and depression were .41 ($p < .01$), −.45 ($p < .01$), and −.60 ($p < .01$), respectively. Our ability to demonstrate positive effects on self-esteem and social support suggests that Web-based interventions may be an effective tool to assist persons with adjusting to chronic illness.

Paterson (2001) noted that discussions about patient participation in healthcare decisions and self-care are based on a model of empowerment. Findings from the current study suggest that women participating in the intervention improved in their ratings of empowerment more significantly than women in the control group. Professional dominance may delegitimize knowledge and experience of people with chronic illness (Paterson, 2001) and understanding where power resides becomes central to the idea of empowerment (Wallerstein, 2002). In this study, we suggest that the mechanism for empowering women who participated in the intervention includes learning and practicing with a new set of skills that guide them in the use of the WWW to find information and subsequently evaluate that information for credibility and usefulness. As rural residents, many of these women relied solely on healthcare providers and informal networks for health information. By having access to the WWW and the experience provided through participation in the intervention (Hill & Weinert, 2004), the women had a new and valuable source of information with which to make self-care decisions or lessen the maldistribution of power between themselves and their health-care providers.

LIMITATIONS

Despite favorable initial findings from this ongoing study, several limitations are important to note. First, the total anticipated sample was not available for analysis and this decreased our statistical power and may have led to nonsignificant findings for changes in self-efficacy, depression, loneliness, and stress. Further analysis of these data will be necessary in the future as sample size increases and the program continues to evolve. Second, it is unknown whether effects resulting from the intervention will be sustained over time. The posttest measurements on which the analysis was based were performed immediately after participants concluded the intervention when anticipated effects were thought to be greatest. Because psychosocial adjustment to chronic illness is thought to be a dynamic process where individuals must respond to daily challenges, it will be important to examine effects over time to determine whether this intervention provides lasting benefits. Third, because this intervention was tested with rural chronically ill women who were predominantly white, generalization to urban dwellers, men, and communities of color is not possible. Fourth, statistically significant results presented here indicate apparently small differences between the groups on self-esteem and empowerment and moderate differences in social support. For individual psychosocial factors, caution is warranted in interpreting these findings as clinically significant. However, taken together, small changes in many of the psychosocial factors representing adaptation may have a compounding effect on the ability of women to adapt to their chronic illnesses. Future research should examine the effects of similar interventions among more heterogeneous populations.

STRENGTHS

Despite these limitations, this study has a number of strengths. Much of the previous research on adaptation to chronic illness generally uses homogenous samples where single illnesses are selected (Stuifbergen, Seraphine, Harrison, & Adachi, 2005; Symister & Friend, 2003). A particular strength of this study is that psychosocial benefits of participation in a Web-based intervention were tested among women with a variety of chronic illnesses. Thus, external validity is somewhat improved. Second, rural populations that have limited access to health information and resources were targeted. An efficient way to meet the needs of geographically isolated populations was demonstrated through the efficacy of this intervention.

As technology becomes increasingly available among rural populations, strategies for using computers and the WWW to improve health need to be developed and tested. The success of the WTW project in making a difference in women's psychosocial outcomes provides impetus to researchers and clinicians interested in harnessing technology to assist people in adapting to chronic illness.

Wade Hill, *PhD, RN, is Assistant Professor;* ***Clarann Weinert***, *SC, PhD, RN, FAAN, is Professor; and* ***Shirley Cudney***, *MA, RN, GNP, is Retired Associate Professor, College of Nursing, Montana State University.*

Accepted for publication August 7, 2005.
Funded by The NIH/National Institute of Nursing Research (1RO1NR07908-01), SC Ministry Foundation, Arthritis Foundation.
Correspondence: Wade Hill, PhD, RN, College of Nursing, Montana State University, MT 59717 (e-mail: whill@montana.edu).

REFERENCES

Anderson, R. M., Funnell, M. M., Fitzgerald, J. T., & Marrero, D. G. (2000). The Diabetes Empowerment Scale: A measure of psychosocial self-efficacy. *Diabetes Care, 23*(6), 739–743.

Baumeister, R. F., Campbell, J. D., Krueger, J. I., & Vohs, K. D. (2003). Does high self-esteem cause better performance, interpersonal success, happiness, or healthier lifestyles? *Psychological Science in the Public Interest, 4*(1), 1–44.

Brandt, P. A., & Weinert, C. (1981). The PRQ—A social support measure. *Nursing Research, 30*(5), 277–280.

Cagle, C. S. (2004). 3 themes described how self care management was learned and experienced by patients with chronic illness. *Evidence-Based Nursing, 7*(3), 94.

Chen, C. C. (2005). A framework for studying the nutritional health of community-dwelling elders. *Nursing Research, 54*(1), 13–21.

Cohen, S., Kamarck, T., & Mermclstein, R. (1983). A global measure of perceived stress. *Journal of Health and Social Behavior, 24*(4), 385–396.

Connell, C. M., Davis, W. K., Gallant, M. P., & Sharpe, P. A. (1994). Impact of social support, social cognitive variables, and perceived threat on depression among adults with diabetes. *Health Psychology, 13*(3), 263–273.

Cudney, S., Winters, C., Weinert, C., & Anderson, K. (2005). Social support in cyberspace: Lessons learned. *Rehabilitation Nursing, 30*(1), 25–29.

Cudney, S. A., & Weinert, C. (2000). Computer-based support groups. Nursing in cyberspace. *Computers in Nursing, 18*(1), 35–43.

Davis, J. M., & Gershtein, C. M. (2003). Screening for depression in patients with chronic illness: Why and how? *Disease Management & Health Outcomes, 11*(6), 375–378.

Devine, G., & Orme, C. (1985). Center for epidemiologic studies depression scale. In D. J. Keyser & R. C. Sweetland (Eds.), *Test critiques* (Vol. I, pp. 144–160).

Druley, J. A., & Townsend, A. L. (1998). Self-esteem as a mediator between spousal support and depressive symptoms: A comparison of healthy individuals and individuals coping with arthritis. *Health Psychology, 17*(3), 255–261.

Earll, L., Johnson, M., & Mitchell, E. (1993). Coping with motor neuron disease—An analysis using self-regulation theory. *Palliative Medicine*, 7(4 Suppl.), 21–30.

Emery, C. (2003). Women living with chronic illness experienced transition that involved stages of distress and a quest for ordinariness. *Evidence-Based Nursing*, 6(2), 63.

Finfgeld-Connett, D. (2005). Clarification of social support. *Journal of Nursing Scholarship*, *37*(1), 4–9.

Fries, J. F. (1997). Reducing the need and demand for medical care: Implications for quality management and outcome improvement. *Quality Management in Health Care*, 6(1), 34–44.

Fries, J. F., Koop, C. E., Sokolov, J., Beadle, C. E., & Wright, D. (1998). Beyond health promotion: Reducing need and demand for medical care. *Health Affairs*, *17*(2), 70–84.

Gallant, M. P. (2003). The influence of social support on chronic illness self-management: A review and directions for research. *Health Education & Behavior*. *30*(2), 170–195.

Gray, J., & Cason, C. L. (2002). Mastery over stress among women with HIV/AIDS. *Journal of the Association of Nurses in AIDS Care*, *13*(4), 43–51.

Gustafson, D., Wise, M., McTavish, F., Taylor, J. O., Wolberg, W., Stewart, J., et al. (1993). Development and pilot evaluation of a computer based support system for women with breast cancer. *Journal of Psychosocial Oncology*, *11*(4), 69–93.

Gustafson, D. H., McTavish, F. M., Boberg, E., Owens, B. H., Sherbeck, C., Wise, M., et al. (1999). Empowering patients using computer based health support systems. *Quality in Health Care*, *8*(1), 49–56.

Hall, M., & Havens, B. (1999). *The effects of social isolation and loneliness on the health of older women*. Winnipeg, Manitoba: Prairie Women's Health Center of Excellence.

Hegyvary, S. T. (2004). Clarifying social support. *Journal of Nursing Scholarship*, *36*(4), 287.

Hill, W., & Weinert, C. (2004). An evaluation of an online intervention to provide social support and health education. *CIN: Computers, Informatics, Nursing*, *22*(5), 282–288.

Hunter, S. M., & Hall, S. S. (1989). The effect of an educational support program on dyspnea and the emotional status of COPD clients. *Rehabilitation Nursing*, *14*(4), 200–202.

Israel, B. A., Checkoway, B., Schulz, A., & Zimmerman, M. (1994). Health education and community empowerment: Conceptualizing and measuring perceptions of individual, organizational, and community control. *Health Education Quarterly*, *21*(2), 149–170.

Lin, N., Simeone, R. S., Ensel, W. M., & Kuo, W. (1979). Social support, stressful life events, and illness: A model and an empirical test. *Journal of Health and Social Behavior*, *20*(2), 108–119.

Paterson, B. (2001). Myth of empowerment in chronic illness. *Journal of Advanced Nursing*, *34*(5), 574–581.

Paykel, E. S. (1994). Life events, social support and depression. *Acta Psychiatrica Scandinavica Supplementum*, 377, 50–58.

Perlman, D., Gerson, A., & Spinner, B. (1977). Loneliness among senior citizens: A report. *Essence*, 6, 3–17.

Pollachek, J. B. (2001). *The relationship of hardiness, social support, and health promoting behaviors to well-being in chronic illness*. Newark, NJ: Rutgers, The State University of New Jersey.

Pollock, S. E. (1986). Human responses to chronic illness: Physiologic and psychosocial adaptation. *Nursing Research*, *35*(2), 90–95.

Pollock, S. E. (1993). Adaptation to chronic illness: A program of research for testing nursing theory. *Nursing Science Quarterly, 6*(2), 86–92.

Pollock, S. E., Christian, B. J., & Sands, D. (1990). Responses to chronic illness: Analysis of psychological and physiological adaptation. *Nursing Research, 39*(5), 300–304.

Robinson, J., Shaver, P., & Wrightsman, L. (1991). *Measures of personality and social psychological attitudes.* New York: Academic Press.

Rosenberg, M. (1965). *Society and the adolescent self image.* Princeton, NJ: University Press.

Roy, C., & Andrews, H. A. (1999). *The Roy Adaptation Model* (2nd ed.). Stamford, CT: Appleton & Lange.

Schaefer, K. M. (1995). Women living in paradox: Loss and discovery in chronic illness. *Holistic Nursing Practice, 9*(3), 63–74.

Sherer, M., Maddix, J., Mercandante, B., Prentice-Dunn, S., Jacobs, B., & Rogers, R. (1982). The Self-Efficacy Scale: Construction and validation. *Psychological Reports, 51*, 663–671.

Spiegel, D. (1993). Psychosocial intervention in cancer. *Journal of the National Cancer Institute, 85*(15), 1198–1205.

Stuifbergen, A. K., Seraphine, A., Harrison, T., & Adachi, E. (2005). An explanatory model of health promotion and quality of life for persons with post-polio syndrome. *Social Science and Medicine, 60*(2), 383–393.

Stuifbergen, A. K., Seraphine, A., & Roberts, G. (2000). An explanatory model of health promotion and quality of life in chronic disabling conditions. *Nursing Research, 49*(3), 122–129.

Sullivan, T., Weinert, C., & Cudney, S. (2003). Management of chronic illness: Voices of rural women. *Journal of Advanced Nursing, 44*(6), 566–574.

Symister, P., & Friend, R. (2003). The influence of social support and problematic support on optimism and depression in chronic illness: A prospective study evaluating self-esteem as a mediator. *Health Psychology, 22*(2), 123–129.

Taylor, S. E., Kemeny, M. E., Reed, G. M., Bower, J. E., & Gruenewald, T. L. (2000). Psychological resources, positive illusions, and health. *American Psychologist, 55*(1), 99–109.

Thomas, S. P. (1995). Psychosocial correlates of women's health in middle adulthood. *Issues in Mental Health Nursing, 16*(4), 285–314.

Vilhjalmsson, R. (1998). Direct and indirect effects of chronic physical conditions on depression: A preliminary investigation. *Social Science and Medicine, 47*(5), 603–611.

Wallerstein, N. (2002). Empowerment to reduce health disparities. *Scandinavian Journal of Public Health Supplement, 59*, 72–77.

Wallston, B. S., Alagna, S. W., DeVellis, B. M., & DeVellis, R. F. (1983). Social support and physical health. *Health Psychology, 2*, 367–391.

WebCT campus edition. (2005). Retrieved July 5, 2005, from http://www.webct.com/software/viewpage?name=software_campus_edition.

Weinert, C. (2000). Social support in cyberspace for women with chronic illness. *Rehabilitation Nursing, 25*(4), 129–135.

Weinert, C. (2003). Measuring social support: PRQ2000. In O. Strickland & C. Dilorio (Eds.), *Measurement of nursing outcomes: Self care and coping* (Vol. 3, pp. 161–172). New York: Springer.

Weinert, C., Cudney, S., & Winters, C. (2005). Social support in cyberspace: The next generation. *CIN: Computers, Informatics, Nursing, 23*(1), 7–15.

Weiss, R. (1969). The fund of sociability. *Transaction, 6*, 36–43.

Williams, M. H. (1990). The self-help movement in head injury. *Rehabilitation Nursing, 15*(6), 311–315.

Wortman, C. B., & Conway, T. L. (1985). The role of social support in adaptation and recovery from physical illness. In S. Cohen & S. L. Syme (Eds.), *Social support and health* (pp. 281–302). Orlando, FL: Academic Press.

APPENDIX B

A Theory of Taking Care of Oneself Grounded in Experiences of Homeless Youth

Lynn Rew

- ▶ ***Background:*** Homeless adolescents are vulnerable to poor health outcomes owing to the dangerous and stressful environments in which they live. Despite their vulnerability, many of them are motivated to engage in self-care behaviors.
- ▶ ***Objective:*** The specific aim of this study was to explore self-care attitudes and behaviors of homeless adolescents.
- ▶ ***Method:*** Individual interviews were conducted with 15 homeless adolescents. Interviews were audiotaped, transcribed verbatim, and analyzed using the constant comparative method of grounded theory.
- ▶ ***Results:*** Findings revealed a basic social process of taking care of oneself in a high-risk environment. This basic social process was supported by three categories: Becoming Aware of Oneself, Staying Alive With Limited Resources, and Handling One's Own Health, each including two processes.
- ▶ ***Discussion:*** Findings support Orem's conceptualizations of self-care and self-care agency and suggest the need for programs to support further healthy growth and development among homeless adolescents.

- ▶ ***Key Words:*** adolescence · grounded theory · homelessness

Homeless adolescents in the United States (US) comprise a population vulnerable to myriad health risks and adverse health outcomes. Numbering nearly two million, these youths include individuals who have run away from home, been removed from their homes by child protective authorities, or who have been thrown out of their homes by their parents (Shane, 1996). Living in the streets, abandoned buildings, cars, trucks, and public parks, these youths encounter environmental conditions that are both stressful and hazardous to their health (van der Ploeg & Scholte, 1997). Despite their early childhood experiences and high-risk lifestyles, many homeless youths are characterized as resilient (Rew, Taylor-Seehafer, Thomas, & Yockey, 2001). Several studies have focused on the health-risk behaviors of homeless adolescents (Rew, Taylor-Seehafer, & Fitzgerald, 2001; Rotheram-Borus, Mahler, Koopman, & Langabeer, 1996; Sullivan, 1996; Yoder, Hoyt, & Whitbeck 1998), yet there is little known about the attitudes and behaviors that reflect their self-care and health-promoting behaviors. The purpose of this study was to develop a descriptive theory of self-care attitudes and practices grounded in the experiences of older youths who are homeless.

SELF-CARE PHILOSOPHY AND THEORY

The history of a self-care philosophy of health in the US can be traced back to the early to mid-1800s when Americans espoused their beliefs in personal responsibility for health and in having control over their own destiny (Steiger & Lipson, 1985). The concept of self-care in nursing is generally attributed to Orem (1971; 2001), but it can be traced to Nightingale's (1859/1946) work a century earlier. Orem conceptualized self-care as "the personal care that human beings required each day and that may be modified by health state, environmental conditions, the effects of medical care, and other factors" (1985, p. 19). Her conceptualizations led to the development of the theory of self-care deficits. Orem (1991) noted that self-care involved taking actions to regulate one's own functioning and development. She identified persons as self-care agents (2001) who (a) determined requirements for healthy functioning; (b) decided what needs must be met and how to meet them; (c) performed the needed actions; and (d) identified the outcomes of such actions. Conditioning factors (e.g., age, sociocultural orientation, patterns of living) affect a person's ability to engage in self-care (Orem, 2001).

Numerous studies of self-care have been done with children (McNabb, Quinn, Murphy, Thorp, & Cook, 1994; Moore, 1995; Rew, 1987), adolescents (Canty-Mitchell, 2001; Christian, D'Auria, & Fox, 1999; McCaleb & Cull, 2000; Shilling, Grey, & Knafl, 2002), and adults (Leenerts & Magilvy, 2000). However, few have explored this phenomenon in high-risk homeless adolescents.

HEALTH IN HOMELESS YOUTH

Homelessness is a highly stressful situation for most people (Craft-Rosenberg, Powell, Culp, & Iowa Homeless Research Team, 2000). By definition, homeless youths live in temporary quarters such as abandoned cars or buildings and have limited access to nutritional meals and healthcare services (Rew, 1996). Alcohol and other drugs are readily available among street people and this is a major health threat for adolescents who run away or are thrown out of their homes (Bailey, Camlin, & Ennett, 1998; Greene, Ennett, & Ringwalt, 1997; Koopman, Rosario, & Rotheram-Borus, 1994; Rew, Taylor-Seehafer, & Fitzgerald, 2001). Rew, Chambers, and Kulkarni (2002) conducted focus groups with homeless adolescents and found that these youths encountered numerous barriers in seeking healthcare services for symptoms of disease. These barriers included lack of available and/or accessible services, not knowing where to go, mistrust of healthcare providers, and inability to pay for care.

McCormack and MacIntosh (2001) conducted a grounded theory study of 11 homeless persons living in shelters and found that in spite of their homelessness, these persons were actively involved in promoting their health. The resulting theory focused on the concepts of person (who directs action), and health (the outcome of action that becomes the stimulus for further action). These researchers noted that pathways to health followed by this population began with accepting responsibility for self-care. Rew (2000) interviewed homeless youths and found that they used numerous strategies (e.g., making friends and keeping pets) to cope with the stress and loneliness that was part of their lifestyle.

Montgomery (1994) interviewed homeless women and identified a number of strengths among the participants, which included "stubborn pride," a positive orientation to life, moral structure, stoic determination, and creation of self. It was argued that the social meaning of homelessness has a negative connotation but nurses should recognize the many strengths of these individuals and advocate for social change that does not blame and further marginalize them.

It is well documented that homeless adolescents are vulnerable to poor health outcomes owing to the dangerous and stressful environments in which they live. Recent studies of homeless persons, including adolescents, suggest that despite the vulnerability associated with homelessness, many individuals display strengths that reflect their ability to engage in self-care behaviors. The purpose of this research was to explore self-care attitudes and behaviors of homeless youth.

■ Method

DESIGN

A grounded theory design (Strauss & Corbin, 1994) was selected because of its potential to address the patterns of behaviors within and between members of a particular social group (Strauss & Corbin, 1998). Data were collected by individual interviews that were audiotaped and through observations of the participants recorded in field notes.

■ Participants

Theoretical sampling of homeless youths living temporarily in an urban area was used to insure a wide range of self-care experiences. Potential participants were recruited from youths seeking health and social services from a street outreach program (i.e., a clinic set up in a church basement) in central Texas. Criteria for inclusion were (a) 16–20 years of age, (b) ability to understand and speak English, (c) willingness to volunteer for an interview. This age group represented the majority of youths seeking services from this program. Fifteen youths (7 males, 6 females, and 2 transgendered) who were an average of 18.8 years of age volunteered to participate. Saturation (sufficient or adequate data had been collected to meet the goal of the study) was reached at the end of 12 interviews; three additional participants were recruited to verify the findings (Morse, 1998). These participants had been homeless for an average of 4.0 years. In the past year, the majority (n = 13) had lived in "squats," which are temporary campsites claimed by youths and other homeless persons. Demographic data and personal characteristics of these participants were summarized and pseudonyms were used to protect the identity of all participants (Table 1).

PROCEDURE

Prior to data collection, the investigator wrote down inital preconceptions, values, and beliefs about the population based on previous experiences with them and from a review of the literature. These initial ideas were held in abeyance until all data were collected and initial coding was done. The study protocol and consent forms were approved by the university Institutional Review Board for the protection of human subjects. The setting for the study was a street outreach program housed in the basement of a church. Potential participants were told about the study by program personnel. Upon agreeing to participate, the youths were referred to the investigator who described the purpose of the study in greater detail and obtained written consent. Demographic data were collected by self-report, using a paper-pencil information form. Interviews were conducted either in a private area in the basement of the church or outside in a quiet courtyard area.

All interviews were tape-recorded with permission from the participants. Interviews lasted an average of 30 minutes and were guided by two main tour questions: (a) What helps you remain healthy living as you do? and (b) What would you like to tell me about how you take care of yourself? Upon completion of the interview, each participant received compensation of $10, a snack bar, and a beverage. The investigator also recorded field notes that detailed the youths' physical appearance and gestures during the interviews. Following each interview, the investigator's personal impressions of the participant and the participant's responses were written in a journal. This formed a portion of the audit trail, which was continued throughout the analyses as the conceptual development of the theory was documented (Morse, 1998).

DATA ANALYSIS

All interviews were transcribed verbatim by a professional transcriptionist. Confidentiality was maintained as (i.e., no names were used) during the interviews. The transcriptions yielded 193 pages of narrative data. Each transcribed interview was read and analyzed along with the accompanying field notes and

Table 1. Participants in a Theory of Self-Care Grounded in Experiences of Homeless Youth

Pseudonym	Age	Sex	Ethnicity	Identifying Characteristics
Bev	18	F	White	Traveler; dropped out of school, has GED
Brett	20	M/T	Mulatto	Mother abandoned at age 14
Judi	19	F	White	Mother died when she was 16
Dawn	19	F	White	Traveler; smoking with family at age 11
Hal	18	M	White	Thrown out by family at age 16
Roy	20	M	Mixed	Abused by stepfather; disabled
Gene	20	M	White	Ran out of money in college; on his own
Cody	16	M	White	Used alcohol and marijuana at age 11 with father and brother; parents divorced
Chad	19	M	Latino	Wants to show parents he can be on his own
Liz	20	F	Mixed	Grew up in poverty; boyfriend committed suicide
Amber	18	F	Maltese	Wants to go to school for artists
Clarice	19	F	White	Traveler; looking for inspiration
Lee	19	M/T	White	Sexually abused by father; in foster care 8–18
Skip	19	M	Latino	Arrested at age 14 for stealing (not guilty)
Jerry	18	M	Native American	Emotionally and physically abused by parents

Note. F = female; M = male; M/T = male/transgendered.

journal entry prior to the next interview. The constant comparative method was used to develop open coding, analytic memos, and categories (Strauss & Corbin, 1994). To increase rigor in the initial coding process, the NUD*IST Q5 software program was used (Richards & Richards, 1998) to analyze the first eight interviews and verify initial codings. Coding from the software program was identical to the hands-on method used for the remainder of the study. To validate the interpretations of the data, member checks were conducted with three participants who agreed that the interpretations were accurate.

Each of the 15 interviews was analyzed line-by-line during (a) open coding, (b) the process of examining, (c) comparing, (d) conceptualizing, and (e) categorizing the data (Strauss & Corbin, 1994, p. 61). These initial codes used the language of the participants. Each interview was analyzed by comparing it to all previous interviews for preliminary conceptualizations. These early conceptualizations were recorded in analytic memos that were used in an iterative process of rereading and recoding. Axial coding produced categories in terms of causes, dimensions, and context. Twelve categories emerged and were diagrammed to indicate relationships between them. This resulted in the identification of some subcategories that were later clarified as processes of the three major categories. Continued refinement, including rereading the transcripts, rediagramming the concepts and categories, and returning to the literature, completed the process of analysis. Pseudonyms for the participants were used in analysis and presentation of findings.

■ Results

BASIC SOCIAL PROCESS

The basic social process, Taking Care of Oneself in a High-Risk Environment, linked the three categories together to form a descriptive theory of self-care for homeless/ street youth. The three categories were: Becoming Aware of Oneself, Staying Alive with Limited Resources, and Handling One's Own Health. Each category contains two processes and several strategies (Figure 1). Taking care of oneself, self-care for homeless/ street youths, is a process of deciding and acting in ways that enhance basic self-respect (caring about oneself) and that promote health. For the majority of street youths in this sample, this process begins with an awareness that life at home was intolerable and unhealthy and that they would have a better chance for survival and happiness if they were not living with parents or guardians. Many have had poor role models at home and learned to distrust "the system," represented by parents and institutions (e.g., schools, medical care agencies, child protective agencies). Most are more willing to listen to other youths from similar backgrounds (who they will find on the streets) than adults because in the past important adults in their lives have violated their trust.

Street life respresents freedom and a pathway to health and happiness for some youth. Given that many adolescents who live on the streets have made a conscious decision to leave an abusive or dysfunctional family, this avenue may be perceived as freedom from the oppression and unhappiness they experienced at home. Brett said, "This is a learning experience. The streets are a stepping stone." This metaphor is supported by various experiences that youths have trying to figure out where they are going in life.

CATEGORY: BECOMING AWARE OF ONESELF

Self-awareness is a perception of oneself borne out of interactions with other people. Processes for attaining self-awareness are

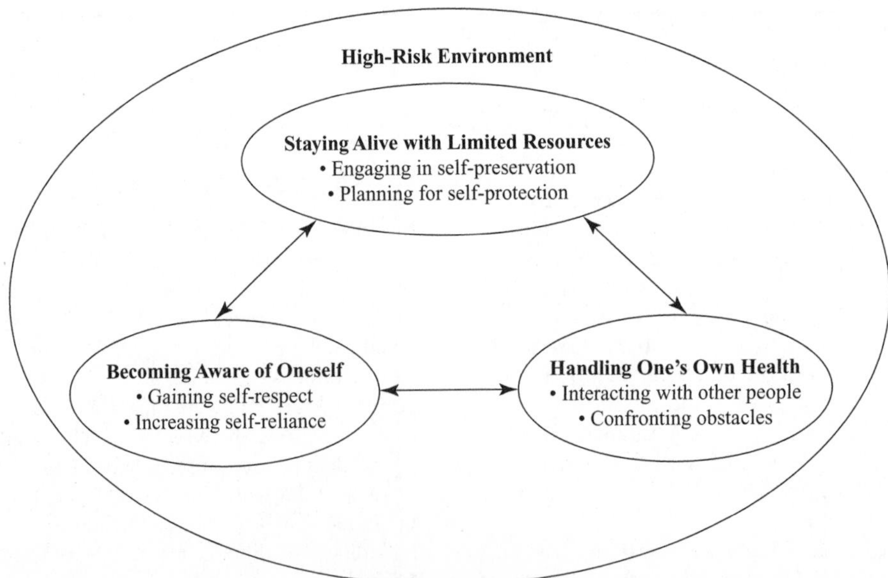

Figure 1. Taking care of oneself in a high-risk environment.

gaining self-respect and increasing self-reliance. Becoming aware of oneself begins with the adolescent's interactions with biologic and/or foster parents. Most of the youths in this sample described growing up in an environment that did not support healthy growth and development of children. Liz grew up in extreme poverty on an Indian reservation. "I didn't even really have shoes that fit, you know, I didn't really even have clothes. I'd be lucky if I got fed. My parents' idea of babysitting was to stick me in a closet with my brother and lock the closet until they come back." Lee, a 19-year-old transgendered youth, was sexually abused by his father who was also violent toward other family members. After his father locked Lee and his sister in a car, child protective services removed the children from their home and placed them in foster care. Lee ran away from this home because of conflict with the foster family about his sexual orientation. He spent some time in a shelter before entering the streets.

Brett was sexually molested by his grandfather, enjoyed wearing his grandmother's clothing as a child, and was taken to a gay bar by his mother when he was 13. By the time he was 14, his mother had moved out of their apartment, abandoning him to take care of himself. His school grades plummeted and he had repeated psychiatric hospitalizations after faking suicide attempts, which he said were "for attention." He subsequently ran away from a hospital and remained on the street.

Out of such home-life situations, these adolescents grappled with a developing sense of self. Lee said, "I already knew who I was. I am in the wrong body—I am *so* in the wrong body." Amber also acknowledged her growing self-awareness when she said, in reference to a Mardi Gras party, "I'm like, no, you know, that's not me. Why would I want to do that [expose her breasts in public]?" Judi expressed her developing self-awareness related to interactions with her father: "Frankly, I'm more mature than him in a lot of ways . . . like in understanding human relations."

Developing a sense of self within families where the youth's sexual orientation led to conflict or where parents failed to provide mature care and guidance to the child led many of these youths to conclude that they were more capable of caring for and about themselves than their natural parents or those they encountered in foster homes. As Clarice put it, "I made my decision not to be around them [family]. I had to learn to build my self-confidence." Lee added, "I knew I could probably take care of myself pretty well."

Process: Gaining Self-Respect. After coming to the streets, these youths developed additional self-awareness through two processes: (a) gaining self-respect, and (b) increasing self-reliance. Gaining self-respect was reflected in the attitudes they expressed towards themselves and the strategies they used to stay alive and healthy on the streets. Brett philosophized, "I'm never truly going to be happy or find anybody if I have no respect for myself." Amber spoke of her practice of avoiding casual sexual encounters with other street kids: "I respect myself more . . . I think it's [exhibitionism] so degrading." Lee spoke of defending his sexual orientation: "I'm not scared of no one [sic] . . . to an extent I'm very proud of myself because I've come a long way. I need to learn to respect myself and care for myself." This process of gaining self-respect contributed to a sense of healing from the brutal experiences of childhood.

Process: Increasing Self-Reliance. Increasing self-reliance was expressed as the tendency to trust one's own judgment and actions taken on one's own behalf above the judgment and caring actions of others. This process was expressed by all 15 of the participants. Many of these youths believed they could deal with any health problems encountered on the street with very little help from professional sources. Brett said, "I'm taking care of myself now better than I ever have in my life." Dawn, who knows she has anemia, said, "I, like, know what I have and how I'm supposed to deal with it." She, like several others, did not care to use prescribed medications (partly because the cost was prohibitive) or to pursue a more conventional lifestyle. Bev, who has asthma, added that she would not seek healthcare services for this chronic health problem unless it was very serious. She said, "If it's not life-threatening or anything, you're just going to be miserable . . . for a day or two . . . I mean, I don't want it [healthcare]." Roy and Judi described themselves as stubborn, saying, "I'm too stubborn to get treated for it" (Judi, speaking of her depression); and "I'm an independent person so I do it myself. I'm stubborn like that" (Roy).

Increasing self-reliance meant that these street youths such as Cody did not "wait for somebody to come do something for you." Strategies that increased their self-reliance included (a) taking care of a dog, (b) obtaining essentials without asking for help, (c) using natural remedies to treat cuts and upset stomachs, (d) improvising places to sleep and ways to travel, and (e) staying aware of their surroundings.

Despite their early experiences in homes that did not promote healthy growth and development, these street youths were becoming aware of themselves as agents of change. Most of the participants recognized unhealthy environments at home or in foster homes and relied on their abilities to protect themselves. By gaining self-respect and self-reliance through new experiences (e.g., taking care of themselves and their pets on the streets, traveling with friends, improvising to maintain their health), they were changing old patterns of feeling devalued and victimized into new patterns of feeling worthy and capable.

CATEGORY: STAYING ALIVE WITH LIMITED RESOURCES

Becoming more self-aware through gaining self-respect and increasing self-reliance led these participants to engage in daily self-care practices to promote and maintain their health. Living on the streets for these participants meant staying alive even though they had few resources such as regular meals, clean clothing, and a consistent place to sleep that would contribute to optimal growth and healthy development. However, these youths persevered toward their goal of finding a better way to live by meeting their own survival needs and protecting themselves from harm.

Process: Engaging in Self-Preservation. Engaging in self-preservation included strategies such as holding part-time jobs and panhandling ("flying a sign") to get food and getting into fights to preserve one's dignity. Engaging in self-preservation was examplified in many commonsense self-care behaviors (e.g., eating fruits and vegetables instead of sweets or junk food, drinking plenty of water, getting lots of exercise [mostly walking], and staying clean). Most participants learned to care for their feet knowing that "boot rot" (tinnea pedis) would cause immobility. These youths also knew that sleeping restfully and staying out of inclement weather (rain and cold) were important strategies in staying alive and healthy, As Chad said, "This [living on the streets] really does take some work."

Process: Planning for Self-Protection. Aware that this environment was dangerous, youths described (a) having a dog for protection, (b) carrying weapons (usually a knife or chain), (c) staying with familiar people, (d) avoiding dark places and drug addicts, and (e) remaining cautious about the surroundings. Others were very specific about protecting themselves from sexually transmitted diseases by using condoms and getting immunizations for hepatitis B. Females, in particular, expressed an interest in learning more about self-defense. Clarice said, "I'm pretty good with self-defense and protecting myself—not making myself a potential victim."

There were diverse opinions about the topic of carrying weapons. Gene noted, "Several kids carry weapons. Some kids broadcast the fact they have these knives and these other types of weapons on them and I mean, that makes you actually afraid of what if these people do get drunk one of these nights?" Jerry added, "Nah [carry a knife?], some of my friends carry knives, but I figure I'd just get hurt more if I do that. I just stay away from dangerous situations." In describing how she protects herself on the streets, Liz said, "I've got my big huge dog and I know how to fight and I carry weapons [knife]." Bev also said, "Try not to go down dark places . . . if I'm by myself, show my knife. Yeah, I had a really big dog for a very long time—that was kind of my knife, I guess you could say. Nobody ever messed with me with him, you know."

By engaging in self-preservation activities and protecting themselves, participants showed how they persevered with limited resources. They were (a) highly motivated to survive, (b) knowledgeable of health and hygiene, and (c) resourceful in protecting their health and their lives.

CATEGORY: HANDLING ONE'S OWN HEALTH

Participants identified two major processes in handling their own health. These were interacting with other people and overcoming obstacles. Learning to handle one's own health was experienced through other people at home, at school, and in healthcare facilities as they were growing up. As independents, they become more aware of their knowledge about healthy behaviors and their lack of trust of authority figures and institutions. Judi claimed, "I'm very wary of Western medicine."

Process: Interacting With Other People. Participants were aware of healthcare resources available at the street outreach center where this study was conducted. Other people they met while on the streets or while obtaining services from the outreach center helped them to survive by giving them food and shelter. Traveling companions provided a safety net, a shield against loneliness. Clarice said, "I'm constantly around people so it's not so lonely." Interacting with peers as well as professionals became part of handling their own health.

Process: Confronting Obstacles. They identified a number of obstacles to taking care of themselves on the street. Many identified inconveniences in trying to find regular meals and a comfortable place to sleep. For example, Dawn said that although the street outreach program gave her cans of food, she could not cook: "It's hard enough to find a can opener." Clarice voiced her concern about adequate sleep: "Sometimes we sleep on real hard concrete . . . or the ground gets a little hard . . . so I get knots in my muscles." Chad stated, "You never really find like constant shelter. You never know where you're going to stay most of the time."

Lack of specific resources (e.g., telephones, transportation, money) prevented some participants from getting recommended follow-up care for injuries they had sustained while traveling (e.g., Bev broke both ankles jumping from a train).

The major obstacle to caring for oneself and staying healthy was expressed by Cody who said, "It's just hard to be out here on the streets and be sober. It's just that trying to handle my problems in a soberly manner is not easy. You get high together—that's basically how you establish friendships." Chad agreed, "That's pretty much what [using alcohol and drugs] everybody passes their time doing. It's a big problem." Hal and Roy thought the major obstacle to taking care of oneself on the street was that kids just "do stupid things that are unhealthy." Roy elaborated, "A lot of kids do a lot of very, very stupid things, I mean getting drunk . . . they don't know how to control like to slow down . . . and that can be very unhealthy for them."

■ Discussion

Homeless youths described how they cared for themselves in an environment that was stressful and full of serious threats to their health and safety. For many, the decision to leave home came from experiences of abuse and neglect. These findings were similar to those of Leenerts and Magilvy (2000) who found that homeless women developed self-care attitudes and practices after first valuing and caring about themselves.

Becoming aware of oneself through the processes of gaining self-respect and increasing self-reliance support Orem's (2001) conceptualization of functioning with integrity and self-awareness as a criterion behavior for positive mental health. Statements from participants indicated that through these processes they were less fearful and felt both happier and healthier living on the streets than in their homes of origin. These findings are similar to those of Rew, Taylor-Seehafer, Thomas, and Yockey (2001) who found that homeless youths who perceived themselves as resilient exhibited less life-threatening behaviors than those who were not resilient. McCormack and MacIntosh (2001) also found that homeless individuals living in shelters had self-confidence and self-images that allowed them to speak for themselves and perform tasks to promote their health.

Staying alive with limited resources through the processes of engaging in self-preservation and planning for self-protection may be unique to the high-risk environments in which these participants lived. Previous studies of the influence of sociocultural factors on self-care practices in adolescents have focused on those living at home with biological parents and attending public schools (McCaleb & Cull, 2000; McCaleb & Edgil, 1994). However, many of the behaviors these participants described as self-preservation reflect the universal self-care requisites identified by Orem (1985) such as maintaining sufficient intake of air, food, and water and preventing hazards. These self-care requisites have been measured in numerous studies of self-care practices in household children and adolescents (Denyes, 1988; McCaleb & Cull, 2000; McCaleb & Edgil, 1994). Other behaviors such as carrying weapons would not be viewed as self-care strategies for the general population. However, given that these youths believe they have no protection other than themselves, it represents another type of caring for oneself.

Handling one's own health through the processes of interacting with other people and confronting obstacles supports Orem's (1985) conceptualization of self-care agency as the person taking action on their own behalf to "maintain life, health, and well-being" (p. 84). These findings also reflect some of the suggestions made by Ervin (1998) on teaching self-care to delinquent adolescents. Noting that learning to care for oneself is a critical step in developing independence in adolescence, Ervin adds that it is even more important for adolescents who lack family support. Homeless youth lack positive role models for self-care behaviors. Participants in this study recognized the simultaneous benefit and risk of interacting with others where alcohol and other drugs were the focus of social interactions, and led youths to do "dumb things" that compromised their health.

The majority of homeless adolescents had few positive role models and knowledge of self-care came from experience with their peers in the street environment.

Homeless adolescents who participated in this study are strong agents of self-care attitudes and behaviors. They have faced numerous adversities in their lives and have shown remarkable courage to redirect their lives toward healthy growth and development. Findings suggest that programs that support healthy growth and development in homeless youths are needed. Such programs can build on the self-care attitudes and behaviors the adolescents learned from taking care of themselves in a high-risk environment.

Lynn Rew, EdD, RNC, FAAN is Denton and Louise Cooley and Family Centennial Professor in Nursing, The University of Texas at Austin.

Accepted for publication February 10, 2003.

This study was supported by a research award from the American Holistic Nurses' Association.

The author thanks the staff and clients at Project PHASE, Austin, Texas, for their assistance and David Kahn, PhD, Associate Professor, and Sharon Horner, PhD, Associate Professor, School of Nursing at The University of Texas at Austin, for their invaluable consultations.

Corresponding author: Lynn Rew, EdD, RNC, FAAN, The University of Texas at Austin, 1700 Red River, Austin, TX 78701 (e-mail: ellerew@mail.utexas.edu).

REFERENCES

Bailey, S. L., Camlin, C.S., Ennett, S. T. (1998). Substance use and risky sexual behavior among homeless and runaway youth. *Journal of Adolescent Health, 23*, 379–388.

Benson, P. L., & Pittman, K. J. (2001). *Trends in youth development: Visions, realities and challenges.* Boston: Kluwer Academic Publishers.

Canty-Mitchell, J. (2001). Life change events, hope, and self-care agency in inner-city adolescents. *Journal of Child and Adolescent Psychiatric Nursing, 14*(1), 18–31.

Christian, B.J., D'Auria, J.P., & Fox, L.C. (1999). Gaining freedom: Self-responsibility in adolescents with diabetes. *Pediatric Nursing, 25*, 255–260.

Craft-Rosenberg, M., Powell, S. R., Culp, K., & Iowa Homeless Research Team (2000). Health status and resources of rural homeless women and children. *Western Journal of Nursing Research, 22*, 863–878.

Ervin, M. H. (1998). Teaching self-care to delinquent adolescents. *Journal of Pediatric Health Care, 12*(1), 20–26.

Greene, J. M., Ennett, S. T., & Ringwalt, C. L. (1997). Substance use among runaway and homeless youth in three samples. *American Journal of Public Health, 87*, 229–235.

Koopman, C., Rosario, M., & Rotheram-Borus, M. J. (1994). Alcohol and drug use and sexual behaviors placing runaways at risk for HIV infection. *Addictive Behaviors, 19*, 95–103.

Leenerts, M. H., & Magilvy, J. K. (2000). Investing in self-care: A midrange theory of self-care grounded in the lived experience of low-income HIV-positive white women. *Advances in Nursing Science, 22*(3), 58–75.

McCaleb, A., & Cull, V. V. (2000). Sociocultural influences and self-care practices of middle adolescents. *Journal of Pediatric Nursing, 15*(1), 30–35.

McCormack, D., & MacIntosh, J. (2001). Research with homeless people uncovers a model of health. *Western Journal of Nursing Research, 23*, 679–697.

McNabb, W. L., Quinn, M. T., Murphy, D. M., Thorp, F. K., & Cook, S. (1994). Increasing children's responsibility for diabetes self-care: The In Control study. *Diabetes Educator, 20*, 121–124.

Montogomery, C. (1994). Swimming upstream: The strengths of women who survive homelessness. *Advances in Nursing Science, 16*(3), 34–45.

Moore, J. B. (1995). Measuring the self-care practice of children and adolescents: Instrument development. *Maternal-Child Nursing Journal, 23*(3), 101–108.

Morse, J. M. (1998) Designing funded qualitative research. In N. K. Denzin, & Y. S. Lincoln (Eds.). *Strategies of qualitative inquiry* (pp. 56–85). Thousand Oaks, CA: Sage Publications.

Nightingale, F. (1859/1946). *Notes on nursing: What it is, and what it is not.* London: Harrison and Sons.

Orem, D. E. (1971). *Nursing: Concepts of practice.* New York: McGraw-Hill Book Company.

Orem, D. E. (2001). *Nursing: Concepts of practice* (6th ed.). St. Louis: Mosby.

Rew, L. (1987). The relationship between self-care behaviors and selected psychosocial variables in children with asthma. *Journal of Pediatric Nursing, 2*, 333–341.

Rew, L. (1996). Health risks of homeless adolescents: Implications for holistic nursing. *Journal of Holistic Nursing, 14*, 348–359.

Rew, L. (2000). Friends and pets as companions: Strategies for coping with loneliness among homeless youth, *Journal of Child and Adolescent Psychiatric Nursing, 13*, 125–140.

Rew, L., Chambers, K. B., & Kulkarni, S. (2002). Planning a sexual health promotion intervention with homeless adolescents. *Nursing Research, 51*, 168–174.

Rew, L., Taylor-Seehafer, M., & Fitzgerald, M. L. (2001). Sexual abuse, alcohol and other drug use, and suicidal behaviors in homeless adolescents. *Issues in Comprehensive Pediatric Nursing, 24*, 225–240.

Rew, L., Taylor-Seehafer, M., Thomas, N. Y., & Yockey, R. D. (2001). Correlates of resilience in homeless adolescents. *Journal of Nursing Scholarship, 33*(1), 33–40.

Richards, T. J., & Richards, I. (1998). Using computers in qualitative research. In N. K. Denzin, & Y. S. Lincoln (Eds.). *Collecting and interpreting qualitative materials.* Thousand Oaks, CA: Sage Publishers.

Rotheram-Borus, M. J., Mahler, K. A., Koopman. C., & Langabeer, K. (1996). Sexual abuse history and associated multiple risk behavior in adolescent runaways. *American Journal of Orthopsychiatry, 66*, 390–400.

Shilling, L. S., Grey, M., & Knafl, K. (2002). The concept of self-management of type 1 diabetes in children and adolescents: An evolutionary concept analysis. *Journal of Advanced Nursing, 37*(1), 87–99.

Steiger, N. J., & Lipson, J. G. (1985). *Self-care nursing theory and practice.* Bowie, MD: Brady Communications Company, Inc.

Strauss, A., & Corbin, J. (1994). *Basics of qualitative research; Grounded theory procedures and techniques.* Newbury Park: Sage Publications.

Strauss, A., & Corbin, J. (1998). Grounded theory methodology. In N. K. Denzin, & Y. S. Lincoln (Eds.). *Strategies of qualitative inquiry* (pp. 158–183). Thousand Oaks, CA: Sage Publications.

Sullivan, T. R. (1996). The challenge of HIV prevention among high-risk adolescents. *Health & Social Work, 21*(1), 58–65.

Yoder, K. A., Hoyt., D. R., & Whitbeck, L. B. (1998). Suicidal behavior among homeless and runaway adolescents. *Journal of Youth & Adolescence, 27*, 753–771.

APPENDIX C

Culturally Tailored Diabetes Education Program for Chinese Americans

A Pilot Study

Chen-Yen Wang • Siu Ming Alain Chan

- ***Background:*** The prevalence of type 2 diabetes among Chinese Americans is rising, and cultural and socioeconomic factors prevent this population from achieving optimal diabetes management.
- ***Objectives:*** To assess the feasibility and acceptability of a culturally appropriate diabetes management program tailored to Chinese Americans with type 2 diabetes and the preliminary outcomes of the intervention.
- ***Method:*** Forty eligible subjects were recruited from the community to participate in this 10-session program developed by integrating Chinese cultural values into an established Western diabetes management program. Feasibility and acceptability of the program were evaluated by the percentage of participants meeting the course objectives and satisfaction with the program. Outcomes measures included the Diabetes Quality-of-Life (DQOL) survey, body weight, blood pressure, and HbA1c levels measured before, after, and 3 months after the intervention.
- ***Results:*** Thirty-three participants completed all 10 sessions and the outcome measurements. Attrition rate was 17.5%. The majority of the participants understood the course content (75%) and identified and demonstrated various diabetes management skills (70% and 82.5%, respectively). All participants who completed the program were "very satisfied" with the program. With regard to the outcome variables, 43.6% of the participants lost more than 5 pounds and most had a reduction in blood pressure at 3 months after completion of the program. Mean HbA1c decreased from 7.11 to 6.12 postintervention. Significant improvements on the DQOL also were reported.
- ***Discussion:*** Culturally tailored diabetes management may be effective in Chinese Americans with type 2 diabetes. Further study, with a larger sample size and a control group, is recommended.

- ***Key Words:*** American · Chinese · cultural · diabetes · management · tailored

Type 2 diabetes among Chinese Americans is rising. Statistics have shown that diabetes prevalence rates in the Asia-Pacific region already exceed 8% in 12 countries and areas within the region (Cockram, 2000). A study of progression to diabetes in 657 Chinese showed that the crude annual rate of progression to diabetes in participants with impaired fasting glucose was 8.38% per year (Ko, Chan, & Cockram, 2001), whereas the conversion rate in most Western countries was 1.5–13.8% per year. The prevalence of diabetes in Chinese people in Hawaii in 1993 was four times higher than in 1989 (Centers for Disease Control, 1993; Shim, 1995).

The literature regarding obstacles to achieving optimal diabetes management in Chinese Americans indicates that traditional American diabetes management strategies remain difficult for Chinese Americans to access, largely due to language barriers, difficulty in lifestyle transitions (Fujimoto, 1996), financial constraints (Cockram, 2000), and incomplete acculturation (Jang, Lee, & Woo, 1998).

Culturally tailored interventions have been successful for diabetes management in African American and Latino adults. In a study of 23 adult African Americans, culturally competent dietary education significantly improved fat intake, HbA1c and fasting blood glucose levels, and frequency of acute care visits (Anderson-Loftin, Barnett, Sullivan, Bunn, & Tavakoli, 2002). In a prospective study (Brown, Garcia, Kouzekanani, & Hanis, 2002) of 256 Mexican Americans, culturally tailored diet, social emphasis, family participation, and cultural health beliefs were incorporated into the intervention. The intervention consisted of 52 contact hours over 12 months provided by bilingual Mexican American nurses, dietitians, and community workers. At 6 months, participants in the experimental group had significantly lower levels of HbA1c and fasting blood glucose levels (1.4% below the control group mean).

The preferred learning style of Chinese American adults is similar to other American adults, who prefer to learn by attaching meaning to their experience (Cranton, 1994) and practice (Wlodkowski, 1985). Group classes (Jiang et al., 1999) are culturally appropriate for educating Chinese adults. Various studies (Arseneau, Mason, Bennett-Wood, Schwab, & Green, 1994; Gagliardino & Etchegoyen, 2001) using adult Latin Americans with type 2 diabetes have shown that participants in group classes had a significantly greater reduction in HbA1c levels than the control group who received individual consultations.

However, the literature regarding diabetes mellitus management in Chinese Americans in the United States is limited. A study of diabetes knowledge and compliance among 52 Chinese with type 2 diabetes (Chan & Molassiotis, 1999) showed no association between diabetes knowledge and compliance with treatment regimen. There was a gap between what the patients were taught and what they were doing. Strategies are needed to close this "knowledge–action gap" in this population. Therefore, the purpose of this pilot study was to assess the feasibility and acceptability of a culturally appropriate diabetes management program tailored to Chinese American with type 2 diabetes and to evaluate the preliminary efficacy of the interventions.

■ Methods

THEORETICAL FRAMEWORK

The *empowerment model* guided the development of this study. The empowerment model was used to help a patient explore and develop his or her inherent ability to manage his or her life and disease (Funnell, Nwankwo, Gillard, Anderson, & Tang, 2005). The empowerment model was used in this study to provide culturally tailored diabetes management information to equip patients with the knowledge to make informed decisions regarding lifestyle choices, diabetes control, and consequences. Therefore, patients became responsible to manage diabetes in a way that best fit their lives (Funnell et al., 2005).

DESIGN

A single group pretest and posttest quasiexperimental design was used to meet the objectives of this study. Course content was adapted from the American Diabetes Association's Standards of Medical Care of Diabetes guideline (American Diabetes Association, 2004).

SETTING AND SAMPLE

Forty participants were recruited from Chinese American social clubs, religious organizations, clinics, referrals from private physician offices, and newspaper advertisements. The participants had not received any organized diabetes education prior to this program. All of the participants were (a) previously diagnosed with type 2 diabetes and managing the diabetes with diet, oral hypoglycemic agents or insulin, or both, (b) 44–87 years of age, (c) residents of Hawaii, and (d) speakers of Mandarin, Cantonese, or Taiwanese. Exclusion criteria included persons who had self-reported cardiac conditions or cancer.

During the 10 weeks of the program, four sessions were offered on different days of the week to accommodate participants' schedules. The investigator and a registered nurse delivered the group sessions. A maximum of 10 persons was allowed for each session to enhance the interaction between the program leader and the participants. Information presented in each session strictly adhered to a predetermined agenda and was delivered in a standardized manner to minimize variations between different sessions.

FEASIBILITY AND ACCEPTABILITY MEASURES

Feasibility of this program was determined by the ability to recruit and retain participants, the ability to deliver the materials in 10 weeks, and the ability of participants to meet the in-class objectives. Ability to meet in-class objectives was assessed at the end of each lesson by skills demonstration and questions and answers; each participant used the same set of evaluation criteria. An investigator-developed tool utilizing Chinese languages was used to measure acceptability. At the 3-month follow-up interview, participants were asked to respond to three questions that served as single-item measures of their satisfaction with the culturally tailored intervention. Responding on a 5-point scale (1 = Very satisfied to 5 = Very dissatisfied), participants were asked the following questions: "In general, how satisfied were you with the culturally tailored intervention?" and "How satisfied were you with the integration of Chinese medicine, exercise, and diet into your diabetes management?" Participants were asked to offer a *yes* or *no* answer for the following question: "If you had the opportunity, would you recommend this intervention to a friend or relative?" These questions were used previously to assess patients' satisfaction with automated telephone disease management (Piette, 2000). The satisfaction scales had a Cronbach's alpha of .82 on content validity.

OUTCOME MEASURES

The Diabetes Quality of Life (DQOL) survey was administered before and immediately after the intervention program. The DQOL was originally created for the Diabetes Control and Complications Trial, but it was culturally adapted (Cheng, Tsui, Hanley, & Zinman, 1999) for an elderly Chinese population. The Chinese version of DQOL is a 42-item, multiple-choice tool with three primary scales including satisfaction, impact, and diabetes-related worry. Test–retest reliabilities of three subscales ranged from .94 to .99 (Cheng et al., 1999). Content validity (Cronbach's α = .76−.92) was performed with an expert panel (Cheng et al., 1999). Questions on the DQOL survey are related to diabetes management and how it affects an individual's life. A low score on the DQOL survey is indicative of high quality of life.

Glycosylated hemoglobin levels (HbA1c) were analyzed before and 3 months after the group sessions using the Metrika A1cNow test kits. Due to budget limitations, participants' HbA1c levels were not evaluated at the 10-week course completion time. The Metrika A1cNow test kit the certified by the National Glycohemoglobin Standardization Program as a viable method in testing a client's HbA1c value (Metrika, 2003; National (Glyohemoglobin Standardization Program, 2003).

Body weight was measured before, immediately after, and 3 months after the program using an upright scale in light indoor clothing to the nearest 10th of a pound. In accordance to the American Heart Association recommendations (Pickering et al., 2004), blood pressure was taken twice after sitting in a quiet room for 5 min. If the difference between two readings was larger than 2 mmHg, a third blood pressure reading was taken. Palpable obliterated pressure plus 30 mmHg was used to measure systolic blood pressure and the pressure at first heard muffling sound was used as the diastolic pressure.

PROCEDURES

Human subject approval was received from the Internal Review Board of the university. Written permission of participation was obtained from each participant at the first session. Baseline data (e.g., questionnaires, HbA1c, weight, and blood pressure) were collected at the first session. Participants then participated in 10 educational sessions (once a week). Questionnaires (except demographics) and outcome measures were collected again at the end of program and at 3 months after the program. A certified diabetes educator taught the group sessions in Mandarin, Cantonese, or Taiwanese as required by the participants. Each group session lasted for 60 min and was held at the primary investigator's clinic in Chinatown, Hawaii. The group session agenda is shown in Table 1. A monetary incentive was given to the participants at the third month follow-up visit. Handouts of lecture notes in Chinese were given to all participants. Cultural values in dietary practice, exercise, medication, and diabetes-related self-care behavior were integrated into handouts.

To facilitate effective communications for clients with low literacy skills, the investigators included hands-on activities and presented information using videos and Microsoft PowerPoint slides. Participants with low literacy were encouraged to ask questions as needed during class; however, no additional time was offered to this group, to maintain treatment integrity across all of the participants. In addition, participants were encouraged to involve their family in the learning process outside of the classroom setting. Peer-to-peer assistance was an unexpected phenomenon during the course, as participants enthusiastically helped each other to understand the course content. This type of mutual support was another way to overcome the literacy barriers.

DIETARY EDUCATION

During the first session, the investigators introduced participants to the food guide pyramid and then explained the nature of carbohydrates and their impact on blood glucose levels. A comprehensive list of carbohydrate and nutrition content of common Chinese foods was provided for the participants; this list was intended to assist them in making appropriate food selection. In addition, a placemat printed with common Chinese food nutritional values written in Chinese, a handy nutrition guide during meal times, was offered to clients. Other Chinese-oriented tools such as rice bowls, soup bowls, and Chinese-style dining utensils were used to illustrate serving sizes. Measuring cups and spoons were given to participants to assist them with food serving measurements. A knowledge empowerment and self-determination approach was used to facilitate participants' dietary changes. Throughout the program, participants engaged in hands-on activities such as packing their own lunch boxes and measuring food serving sizes.

EXERCISE

The second component of the program was to encourage participants to develop a regular exercise routine. The energy expenditure of various types of exercise, including Taichi and Chi-gong, was discussed with the participants, which empowered them with the knowledge to select types of exercise suitable for individual conditions and interests. Tudor-Locke, Bell, Myers, Harris, Lauzon, and Rodger (2002) demonstrated that the pedometer is a valid tool in quantifying the levels of physical activities for adults with type 2 diabetes. An activity log and pedometer were provided for each participant to record their exercise quantity.

Table 1. Objectives and Content for the Culturally Tailored Diabetes Intervention Program

Objectives	Content
1. Verbalize understanding of this program	a) Introduce the Chinese recipe books, exercise books, and some Chinese pamphlets regarding diabetes b) Give handout in Chinese about this program
2. Verbalize understanding of research findings	a) Translate the research findings into Chinese b) Application of research findings within Chinese culture c) Ask participants to bring their favorite recipes to the next session
3. Demonstrate healthy food choice	a) Explain Chinese dietary patterns with detailed analysis on the starch food group in terms of rice, noodle, yam, and dumpling b) Analyze 5 recipes brought by the participants
4. Demonstrate self-monitoring blood glucose (SMBG) with accurate skills	a) Recognize the uneasiness doing self monitoring in the Chinese b) Describe the relationship between SMBG and changes in serum glucose levels c) Ask participants to bring in information about their preferred exercise in the next session
5. Verbalize benefits of exercise	a) Analyze pros and cons of five common Chinese exercises b) Explain the calorie utilization of each listed exercise and their relationships with blood glucose control c) Ask participants to bring in medicine taken in the next session.
6. Verbalize understanding of oral agents	a) Analyze pros and cons of the Chinese medicine and the Western medicine used by participants b) Ask participants to bring in list of symptoms and complications they experienced in the next session
7. Develop plans for preventing/ treating diabetic complications	a) Compile symptoms and complications brought by the participants on the clipboard b) Explain the possible methods of prevention c) Help participants to develop individualized plans
8. Develop plans for sick days/ traveling	a) Compile the treatment plans used by the participants b) Explain the principle of handling sick days and traveling
9. Verbalize plans of foot and skin care	a) Show a video on the foot/skin care and its importance b) Ask participants to bring in preferred stress management methods in the next session
10. Demonstrate skills of stress management	a) Group sharing about the benefits of each stress management b) Summarize the benefits of stress management

MEDICATION

Medication compliance was the third focus of this program, as many participants expressed concern about medication cost, efficacy, side effects, and compatibility with other Chinese medicines. Medication cost prohibited medication compliance for some participants, as many of them were retired and lived on a limited income. To lessen participants' financial burden, they were assisted in applying to medication assistance programs from various drug manufacturers or provided drug samples if it was deemed appropriate by the program's advanced practice registered nurse. However, no changes were made to participants' medication regimens until 3 months after the classes, in order to minimize variations in data. A detailed discussion on various types of insulin and oral agents was held to assist participants in understanding the purpose, actions, and potential side effects of these medications, and ways to deal with hypoglycemia induced by medications.

SELF-CARE

Chinese values were incorporated into the diabetes self-care education program. The program offered information on how to manage diabetes during sickness; the yin and yang concept was used to illustrate types of food to consume in the event of illness. Because many participants traveled to their native countries frequently, information was offered on synchronizing medications or an insulin regimen for a different time zone, managing blood glucose during flight, and converting different measurement units for blood glucose. Participants were also helped to explore methods of stress management; various types of Chinese-specific activities were suggested to the participants, such as meditation, Taichi, and Chi-gong. Foot and skin care activities were demonstrated to the participants.

DATA ANALYSIS

Descriptive statistics were used to describe and summarize central tendency and variability of demographic variables. Feasibility of this culturally tailored diabetes management program was evaluated by percentages of (a) educational sessions having more than 85% of participants attending, (b) participants who attended all 10 educational sessions, and (c) participants who met at least 9 of the 10 class objectives. The acceptability of the culturally tailored diabetes program was determined by program satisfaction. Percentiles were used to measure the variability of satisfaction and participation rate, and mode and median were used to describe central tendency.

The DQOL was measured on an ordinal scale. Difference in total score between pretest and posttest was computed with a Student's *t* test. Differences in means between pretest and posttest for each item were computed with a *t* test of paired sample statistics with SPSS software. Study outcome measures were determined by the percentage of persons showing a decrease of Hb1Ac levels, degree of weight loss in 3 months (if appropriate), and blood pressure reduction.

■ Results

The native language of most participants was Cantonese (57.6%) (Table 2). Most participants were married with a living partner (66.7%), retired (75.8%), had less than $1,001 combined monthly household income (81.8%), and had an education level of high school graduate and beyond (57.6%).

Thirty-three out of the 40 recruits completed the 10-session program. The attrition rate was 17.5%. The seven participants who departed cited that traveling plans were the primary reason for their inability to complete the program. However, it was interesting to note that the seven participants who did not complete the program had all returned for the 3-month postprogram evaluation appointments.

Upon the completion of this program, the 33 remaining participants were able to meet 4 to 10 ($M = 8.22$, $SD = 2.18$) course objectives. Most of the group members were able

Table 2. Frequency Distribution of Demographic Data (*n* = 33)

Demographic Data	Frequency
Gender	
Male	48.5%
Female	51.5%
Length of time (years) in the United States (*n* = 33), *M* (*SD*)	16.5 (9.3)
1–5 years	5.0%
6–10 years	25.0%
11–20 years	40.0%
21–30 years	22.5%
31–35 years	7.5%
Native language	
Cantonese	57.6%
Mandarin	36.4%
Taiwanese	6.1%
Preferred medical treatment	
Western medicine only	66.7%
Chinese medicine only	9.1%
Western medicine plus Chinese medicine	7.5%
Home remedies and self-treatment	3.0%
Travel to home country for care	3.5%
Duration of DM (years), *M* (*SD*) (range)	9.03 (8.74) [1–40]
Age (years), *M* (*SD*) (range)	68.8 (10.1) [44–87]

Note. DM = diabetes management.

to demonstrate healthy food choices (82.5%), tell the benefits of frequent exercise (90%), identify ways to prevent or treat diabetes complications (82.5%), demonstrate stress management skills (70%), verbalize plans for foot and skin care (90%), and verbalize plans for diabetes self-management on sick days or during travel (70%). On the other hand, only 57.5% of the participants were able to demonstrate accurate self-monitoring blood glucose skills, and only 55% of the group were able to verbalize understanding of oral hypoglycemic agents. According to the course evaluation, 100% of the participants were "very satisfied" with this culturally tailored diabetes program and would recommend this program to friends and family who have type 2 diabetes. Ninety-two percent of the group were "very satisfied" or "somewhat satisfied" with the Chinese-oriented course content and 8% remained neutral on this item.

Table 3 shows the participants' averages of HbAlc level, systolic blood pressure, diastolic blood pressure, and body weight at the start of the program, immediately after the intervention, and at 3 months after the program. Comparison of participants' weight revealed that 20.5% of the participants were able to lose 5 pounds or more during the course of the program, and this increased to 43.6% 3 months after the completion of the program. About two-thirds of the participants weighed over 128 pounds at baseline, and 53.6% of them were able to lose 5 pounds or more 3 months after the program. The weight loss was greater among those in the upper-third weight class (weight >148 pounds); 71% of the participants who weighed more than

Table 3. Physiological Variables of Participants (n = 33) at Baseline, at the End of Classes, and at 3 Months Following the Intervention

	M (*SD*)	Range
Weight at baseline (lbs)	139.3 (26.7)	77–210
Weight after classes (lbs)	122.8 (48.9)	80–207
Weight at the third month (lbs)	121.8 (48.6)	80–202
HbA1c at baseline (%)	7.11(1.1)	5.4–11.0
HbA1c at the third month (%)	6.12 (2.4)	5.4–8.4
Systolic BP at baseline (mmHg)	131.5 (13.6)	100–162
Systolic BP after classes (mmHg)	118.9 (42.1)	100–160
Systolic BP at 3rd month (mmHg)	113.7 (46.2)	100–190
Diastolic BP at baseline (mmHg)	69.4 (10.9)	48–90
Diastolic BP after classes (mmHg)	63.4 (23.4)	50–88
Diastolic BP at 3rd month (mmHg)	63.2 (25.9)	50–92

Note. HbA1c was not assessed at the end of class due to study design.

148 pounds at baseline were able to lose 5 pounds or more in 3 months. In contrast, only 12.6% of the participants reported weight gain during the program, of which only one participant was in the upper-third weight class at baseline. Body mass index (BMI) of the participants ranged 18.4–37.9 with a mean of 26.4 prior to the start of the program. At baseline, 18% of participants had a BMI less than 23 and 37% of participants had BMI more than 27. Forty-two percent of the participants had a reduction in BMI with the program; 24% of the participants achieved a BMI equal to or lesser than 23 at 3 months postintervention. The mean BMI reduced to 25.8 (n = 33; SD = 4.16) 3 months after the class. The mean HbA1c level decreased from 7.11 (SD = 1.1) to 6.12 (SD = 2.4) at 3 months after the completion of the program.

■ Discussion

This culturally tailored diabetes program was developed to address obstacles that prevent Chinese Americans from receiving optimal diabetes management. The results from this program confirmed that by approaching diabetes management from a culturally specific perspective, diabetes self-care can be effectively enhanced. It was hypothesized that by integrating Chinese cultural values into the diabetes regimen, there would be an improvement in compliance of Chinese Americans' self-care practices related to diabetes management. Findings of this culturally tailored diabetes management program were congruent with the outcomes of a structured group education mode, called Programa de Education de Diabéticos No Insulinodependientes en América Latina (PEDNID-LA), used in several Latin American countries (Gagliardino & Etchegoyen, 2001). Similarities between our diabetes management program and PEDNID-LA include: (a) the interactive group method was used; (b) general concepts about type 2 diabetes and physiological changes were introduced; (c) educational materials were provided in the native language; and (d) photographs of cultural foods were used.

An important feature of this program was the language of instruction. The classes were conducted in Cantonese, Mandarin, or

Taiwanese. The use of participants' native languages helped facilitate communication and the learning process. Due to the mixture of participants, some of the classes were conducted with a combination of the above languages. By coincidence, all of the Taiwanese-speaking participants were able to speak and understand Mandarin fluently, so the use of Taiwanese during class instruction was minimal. However, it was interesting to note that many participants were more open to discussions and interactions when the class consisted of only Cantonese speakers or Mandarin speakers. It appeared that a language divide existed among the participants. Some participants attended different group sessions because of a change in working hours. They still communicated openly with participants in the new group when all participants spoke the same dialect. Therefore, if resources permit, it would be optimal to set up classes based on participants' dialectical preference rather than grouping participants on their cultural background alone. Also such criteria may apply to other cultures; for example, it may be feasible to group Filipino clients based on their dialectical preference (e.g., Ilocano, Tagalog, or Visayan).

Appropriate diet selection is one of the keys to successful diabetes management. However, it is also one of the major obstacles for Chinese Americans. As mentioned previously, most of the diabetes education materials were developed for the Western cultures and the Chinese dietary habits varied greatly from their Western counterparts. Because the Chinese translation for diabetes is "sugar urine disease," many participants took the term literally and thought that they had to avoid only sweet-tasting foods. Many participants reported that their physicians instructed them to consume less rice; subsequently, some participants avoided rice but consumed other carbohydrates (e.g., noodles or buns). Hence, the dietary education component of the program emphasized the concept of carbohydrates.

In this program, participants were empowered by providing information about the nutrition content of common Chinese foods and appropriate serving sizes. The pedometer was a useful tool in encouraging participants to exercise, as evidenced by participants' enthusiasm in comparing the number of steps shown on the pedometer with their peers. This type of mutual comparison created a motivation to exercise. Findings supported previous studies in which understanding the determinants of exercise led to behavioral change (Plotnikoff, Brez, & Hotz, 2000).

Concurrent use of Western medicine and Chinese medicine to treat elevated serum blood glucose levels may affect patients' adherence in Western medicine treatments. The percentage of participants (7.5%) using Chinese medicine was slightly lower than the 9% in the study by Wai, Lan, and Donnan (1995). In 1999, percentages of Chinese Americans living in Houston and Los Angeles who used traditional Chinese clinics, used Western clinics in the United States, and traveled to origin country for care were 25.3%, 21.3%, and 32%, respectively (Ma, 1999).

Literacy was a limitation of the study. Although informative, the handouts provided for the participants were word-intensive, which may have created a problem for those with limited literacy skills. Some of the participants hesitated in revealing their limitations in reading comprehension skills. Various studies have shown that individuals with low health literacy incur as much as four times the healthcare cost over the individuals with adequate literacy skills (AMA-MSS Community Service Committee, 2004). Hence, it was imperative for this group of participants to be able to comprehend the course content.

Another obstacle that can affact health literacy is the use of different writing systems. In general, Mainland Chinese use simplified Chinese characters, whereas clients from Taiwan and Hong Kong use traditional Chinese characters. Because most of the participants originated from Taiwan or Hong Kong, the course handouts comprised traditional Chinese characters. Fortunately, most of the participants from Mainland China were able to comprehend the course materials, as they were an older generation educated prior to the era of simplified Chinese characters. However, as Mainland China becomes the major source of Chinese immigration to the United States, it will be necessary to have simplified Chinese educational materials available.

The timing of the education sessions was another potential limitation to the study. The classes were held during a holiday season, and the seven participants who did not complete the classes left because of their travel plans. Therefore, it would be optimal to hold classes during a period with minimal holidays. In the case of the Chinese population, program coordinators should avoid holding classes during the Chinese New Year, because it is a period of frequent travel and festivities for many Chinese, which may affect the overall attendance rate and blood glucose control.

Language barriers, difficulty in lifestyle transitions (Fujimoto, 1996), financial constraints (Cockram, 2000), and incomplete acculturation (Jang, Lee, & Woo, 1998) were some of the obstacles preventing Chinese Americans from accessing optimal diabetes care. This culturally tailored diabetes education program was developed to address these concerns by integrating Eastern values into Western diabetes management strategies. Results indicated that most of the participants were able to decrease their body weight, blood pressure, and HbA1c values. Course materials were delivered in participants' native languages. Most of the participants were able to gain knowledge about diabetes, medications, prevention strategies, and self-care skills. Participants also formed a support network with some of their peers through this program. Results indicated that this culturally tailored diabetes management pilot study could be an effective tool in reducing the health disparities in the Chinese American population.

***Chen-Yen Wang, PhD, APRN, CDE,** is Associate Professor; and **Siu Ming Alain Chan, RN, MSN,** is Graduate Student, School of Nursing and Dental Hygiene, University of Hawaii at Manoa, Honolulu.*

Accepted for publication May 18, 2005.

This project was funded by the University of Washington, Center for Women's Health Research (NR04001).

Authors would like to give appreciation to Margaret Heitkemper, PhD, RN, FAAN, Chairperson and Professor of University of Washington, Department of Biobehavioral Nursing and Health Systems, for mentoring and finalizing this manuscript.

Corresponding author: Chen-Yen Wang, PhD, APRN, CDE, 1702 Kewalo Street, Apt. 1103, Honolulu, HI 96822 (e-mail: chenwang@hawaii.edu).

REFERENCES

American Diabetes Association. (2004). Standards of medical care of diabetes. *Diabetes Care, 27,* 15S–35S.

AMA-MSS Community Service Committee. (2004). *The abc of health literacy. A proposal for the ama-mss2004-2006 national service project.* Retrieved August 14, 2005, from http://www.ama-assn.org/ama1/pub/upload/mm/15/health_literacy.doc.

Anderson-Loftin, W., Barnert, S., Sullihvan, P., Bunn, P. S., & Tavakoli, A. (2002). Culturally competent dietary education for southern rural African Americans with diabetes. *Diabetes Educator, 28,* 245–257.

Arseneau, D. I., Mason, A. C., Bennett-Wood, O., Schwab, E., & Green, D. (1994). A comparison of learning activity packages and classroom instruction for diet management of patients with NIDDM. *Diabetes Educator, 20,* 509–514.

Brown, S. A., Garcia, A. A., Kouzekanani, K., & Hanis, C. L. (2002). Culturally competent diabetes self-management education for Mexican Americans: The Starr County border health initiative. *Diabetes Care, 25,* 259–268.

Center for Disease Control and Prevention. (1993). *Diabetes surveillance, 1991.* Washington, DC: US Government Printing Office.

Chan, Y. M., & Molassiotis, A. (1999). The relationship between diabetes knowledge and compliance among Chinese with non-insulin dependent diabetes mellitus in Hong Kong. *Journal of Advanced Nursing, 30,* 431–438.

Cheng, A. Y., Tsui, E. Y., Hanley, A. J., & Zinman, B. (1999). Cultral adaptation of the diabetes quality-of-life measure for Chinese patients. *Diabetes Care, 22,* 1216–1217.

Cockram, C. S. (2000). Diabetes mellitus: Perspective from the Asia-Pacific region. *Diabetes Research and Clinical Practice, 50*(Suppl. 2), S3–S7.

Cronton, P. (1994). *Transformative learning: A guide for educators of adults.* San Francisco, CA: Jossey-Bass.

Fujimoto, W. Y. (1996). Overview of non-insulin-dependent diabetes mellitus (NIDDM) in different population groups. *Diabetes Medicine, 13*(9 Suppl. 6), S7–S10.

Funnell, M. M., Nwankwo, R., Gillard, M. L., Anderson, R. M., & Tang, T. S. (2005). Implementing an empowerment-based diabetes self-management education program. *Diabetes Educator, 31*(1), 53, 55–56,61.

Gagliardino, J. J., & Etchegoyen, G. (2001). A model educational program for people with type 2 diabetes: A cooperative Latin American implementation study (PEDNID-LA). *Diabetes Care, 24*, 1001–1007.

Jang, M., Lee, E., & Woo, K. (1998). Income, language, and citizenship status: Factors affecting the health care access and utilization of Chinese Americans. *Health & Social Work, 23*, 136–145.

Jiang, Y. D., Chuang, L. M., Wu, H. P, Shiau, S. J., Wang, C. H., Lee, Y. J., Juang, J. H., Lin, B. J., & Tai, T. Y. (1999). Assessment of the function and effect of diabetes education programs in Taiwan. *Diabetes Research and Clinical Practice, 46*(2), 177–182.

Ko, G. T., Chan, J. C., & Cockram, C. S. (2001). Change of glycaemic status in Chinese subjects with impaired fasting glycaemia. *Diabetic Medicine, 18*, 745–748.

Ma, G. X. (1999). Between two worlds: The use of traditional and Western health services by Chinese immigrants. *Journal of Community Health, 24*, 421–437.

Metrika, Inc. (2003). *Clinical accuracy.* Retrieved July 20, 2003, from http://www.metrika.com/3medical/accuracy.html.

National Glycohemoglobin Standardization Program. (2003). *List of NGSP certified methods.* Retrieved July 22, 2003, from http://web.missouri.edu/~diabetes/ngsp/index.html.

Pickering, T. G., Hall, J. E., Appel, L. J., Falkner, B. E., Graves, J., Hill, M. N., Jones, D. W., Kurtz, T., Sheps, S. G., & Roccela, E. J. (2004). *Recommendations for blood pressure measurement in humans and experimental animals. Part 1: Blood pressure measurement in humans: A statement for professionals from the Subcommittee of Professional and Public Education of the American Heart Association Council on High Blood Pressure Research.* Retrieved February 28, 2005, from http://hyper.ahajournals.org/cgi/content/full/45/1/142.

Piette, J. D. (2000). Satisfaction with automated telephone disease management calls and its relationship to their use. *Diabetes Educator, 26*, 1003–1010.

Plotnikoff, R. C., Brez, S., & Hotz, S. B. (2000). Exercise behavior in a community sample with diabetes: Understanding the determinants of exercise behavior change. *Diabetes Educator, 26*, 450–459.

Shim, M. J. (1995). *Self-reported diabetes in Hawaii* (pp. 1988–1993). Manoa, HI: University of Hawaii at Manoa.

Tudor-Locke, C. E., Bell, R. C., Myers, A. M., Harris, S. B., Lauzon, N., & Rodger, N. W. (2002). Pedometer-determined ambulatory activity in individuals with type 2 diabetes. *Diabetes Research and Clinical Practice, 55*(3), 191–199.

Wai, W. T., Lan, W. S., & Donnan, S. P. (1995). Prevalence and determinants of the use of traditional Chinese medicine in Hong Kong. *Asian Pacific Journal of Public Health, 8*, 167–170.

Wlodlkowski, R. J. (1985). *Enhancing adult motivation to learn: A guide to improving instruction and increasing learner achievement.* San Francisco, CA: Jossey-Bass.

APPENDIX D

POST-TRAUMATIC STRESS DISORDER DUE TO CHILDBIRTH

The Aftermath

Cheryl Tatano Beck

► **Background:** Childbirth qualifies as an extreme traumatic stressor that can result in post-traumatic stress disorder. The reported prevalence of post-traumatic stress disorder after childbirth ranges from 1.5% to 6%.

► **Objective:** The aim of this phenomenologic study was to describe the essence of mothers' experiences of post-traumatic stress disorder after childbirth.

► **Methods:** The qualitative research design used for this study was descriptive phenomenology. The main recruitment approach was via the Internet through the help of Trauma and Birth Stress, a charitable trust in New Zealand. Purposive sampling was used and resulted in 38 mothers participating from the countries of New Zealand, the United States, Australia, and the United Kingdom. The participants were asked to describe their experiences with post-traumatic stress disorder after childbirth. Their stories were analyzed using Colaizzi's method of data analysis.

► **Results:** Mothers with post-traumatic stress disorder attributable to childbirth struggle to survive each day while battling terrifying nightmares and flashbacks of the birth, anger, anxiety, depression, and painful isolation from the world of motherhood.

► **Conclusions:** This glimpse into the lives of mothers with post-traumatic stress disorder attributable to childbirth provides an impetus to increase research efforts in this neglected area.

► **Key Words:** birth trauma · phenomenology · post-traumatic stress disorder

In 1980, post-traumatic stress disorder (PTSD) was first listed in the *Diagnostic and Statistical Manual of Mental Disorders* (DSM-III) (American Psychiatric Association [APA], 1980). Vietnam War veterans were the first individuals to be identified as experiencing PTSD. For the diagnosis of PTSD, the DSM-III criteria require an event considered beyond the range of usual human experience. The DSM-IV provides an expanded view of what constitutes an extreme traumatic stressor. It has broadened the definition to include "direct personal experience of an event that involves actual or threatened death or serious injury, or a threat to the physical integrity of self or others" (APA, 1994, p. 424). The individual's response is one of extreme fear, helplessness, or horror. Although the DSM-IV does not specifically identify childbirth as an example of an extreme traumatic stressor, childbirth certainly can qualify as a traumatic event (Beck, 2004). The reported prevalence of diagnosed PTSD after childbirth ranges from 1.5% (Ayers & Pickering, 2001) to 6% (Menage, 1993).

In the most recent review of the literature on PTSD after childbirth, Bailham and Joseph

(2003) identified possible features of PTSD presentation in mothers after delivery, including sexual avoidance, fear of childbirth, and mother-infant attachment and parenting problems. They strongly cautioned that these features are speculative at this stage, calling for further research to investigate the clinical presentation of PTSD in mothers as a result of traumatic births.

The purpose of this phenomenologic study was to investigate the essence of mothers' experiences of PTSD after traumatic births. This study focused on sequelae of birth trauma as PTSD rather than the immediate experiences of birth trauma.

■ Literature Review

A few published studies have described the prevalence of diagnosed PTSD attributable to childbirth and the PTSD symptoms of women after delivery. Two qualitative studies have been conducted: a phenomenologic study on birth trauma (Beck, 2004) and a grounded theory study on the process and impact of traumatic childbirth (Allen, 1998).

Wijma, Soderquist, and Wijma (1997) assessed the prevalence of PTSD after childbirth in Sweden using the Traumatic Event Scale. Among 1,640 women, 28 (1.7%) met the criteria for PTSD. Compared with a group of women who had no diagnosis of PTSD after childbirth, the PTSD group had significantly more primiparous women ($p = .003$), reported a higher frequency of psychiatric counseling ($p = .003$), and rated their contact with the delivery staff as significantly ($p = .01$) more negative than did the non-PTSD group.

In Australia, Creedy, Shochet, and Horsfall (2000) reported a 5.6% prevalence of PTSD attributable to childbirth (28 of 499 women). They based their diagnosis on the Post Traumatic Stress Symptoms Interview (Foa, Riggs, Dancu, & Rothbaum, 1993), which was conducted 4 to 6 weeks postpartum. A high level of obstetric intervention during childbirth and the perception of inadequate labor and delivery care were associated significantly with the development of acute trauma symptoms.

Ayers and Pickering (2001) also used the Post Traumatic Stress Symptoms Interview (Foa et al., 1993) to measure the prevalence of PTSD at 6 weeks and 6 months post-partum. Among a sample of 218 mothers in the United Kingdom, 2.8% fulfilled criteria for PTSD at 6 weeks post-partum, and this number decreased to 1.5% at 6 months postpartum.

Menage (1993) reported a prevalence rate of 6% for PTSD after childbirth in the United Kingdom. The PTSD Interview (PTSD-I) of the Veterans Administration Medical Center in Minnesota (Watson, Juba, Manifold, Kucala, & Anderson, 1991) was used to diagnose PTSD. The DSM-III-R criteria for PTSD were satisfied by 30 of the 500 mothers. The only such study conducted in the United States to date identified a prevalence rate of 1.9% (Soet, Brack, & Dilorio, 2003). In a sample of 103 women, 2 received a diagnosis of PTSD attributable to childbirth trauma at approximately 4 weeks postpartum.

In other studies, post-traumatic stress symptoms were examined, but a formal diagnosis of PTSD was not included in the design. In Sweden, Ryding, Wijma, and Wijma (1998) compared the psychological impact of emergency cesarean delivery ($n = 71$) with that of elective cesarean delivery ($n = 70$), instrumental delivery ($n = 89$), and normal vaginal delivery ($n = 96$). Post-traumatic stress symptoms were measured using the Impact of Events Scale (Horowitz, Wilner, & Alvarez, 1979) 1 month after delivery. Mothers who had undergone an emergency cesarean delivery reported significantly more post-traumatic stress symptoms than those who had elective cesarean and normal spontaneous delivery, but not in comparison with the women who had instrumental vaginal deliveries.

Lyons (1998) also assessed post-traumatic stress symptoms 1 month after delivery using the Impact of Events Scale (Horowitz et al., 1979) with 42 primiparas in the United Kingdom. Higher post-traumatic stress symptoms were related significantly to the feeling of not being in control during delivery, of being induced, and of having an epidural.

Post-traumatic stress symptoms have been reported at a higher level for mothers of high-risk infants (Callahan & Hynan, 2002; DeMier, Hynan, Harris, & Manniello, 1996) than for mothers of healthy, full-term infants. Holditch-Davis, Bartlett, Blickman, and Miles (2003) examined post-traumatic stress symptoms in mothers of premature infants using a semistructured interview with 30 mothers at 6 months postpartum. The interviews were analyzed for three PTSD symptoms: re-experiencing, avoidance, and increased arousal. Of the 30 women studied, 24 reported that they avoided thinking about aspects of the birth and the neonatal intensive care unit and re-experienced the preterm birth of their infant through intrusive thoughts. Most of the mothers (n = 26) described increased arousal that focused on overprotection of their infant as a type of hypervigilance. The mothers reported difficulty sleeping, generalized anxiety, and persistent fears that their children might die or become ill again.

In her grounded theory study, Allen (1998) examined the processes that occurred during traumatic childbirth, the mediating variables in the development of PTSD symptoms, and the impact on postpartum adaptation. In her study, 20 mothers were interviewed 10 months after delivery. The Revised Impact of Event Scale (Horowitz et al., 1979) was used to measure PTSD symptoms. Six of the mothers reported scores above the cutoff point, indicating clinically significant levels of PTSD symptoms after childbirth. Their distress included panic and tearfulness caused by thoughts of the trauma, the anger directed at clinicians and their partners, the decreased closeness in their relationships with their partners, the emotional detachment from the baby, less patience with their other children, and fear of future pregnancy.

Beck (2004) conducted a phenomenologic study investigating women's experiences of birth trauma. The 40 women in this study participated via the Internet: 23 in New Zealand, 8 in the United States, 6 in Australia, and 3 in the United Kingdom. Women were recruited primarily through Trauma and Birth Stress (TABS), a charitable trust located in New Zealand. The essential components of a traumatic birth that emerged were the mothers' perceived lack of communication and caring by labor and delivery personnel, the provision of unsafe care, and an overshadowing of the trauma by the delivery outcome. Beck (2004) concluded that birth trauma lies in the eye of the beholder. Mothers perceived that their traumatic births often were viewed as routine by clinicians.

A review of the literature located one conceptual framework that focused on the role of PTSD in childbearing. Seng (2002) developed a conceptual framework for research on lifetime violence, post-traumatic stress, and childbearing. Women's lifetime abuse trauma and post-traumatic stress both are considered important factors for guiding future research. Post-traumatic stress disorder is emphasized as a potential factor contributing to adverse maternal and fetal outcomes via both behavioral and neuroendocrine pathways. Seng (2002) proposed three groups of factors that moderate the relation between violence trauma and adverse childbearing outcomes: nonmodifiable factors that affect pregnancy outcome, life event stress factors, and modifiable healthcare-related factors. This third group of modifying factors, including the quality and amount of obstetrical care, can and should be influenced by clinicians.

The limited quantitative research conducted shows that risk factors for the development of PTSD after childbirth can include emergency cesarean delivery, first pregnancy, high level of obstetric intervention, perception of inadequate care during labor and delivery, premature or high-risk infants, and psychiatric history. No phenomenologic studies were found that described the experience of PTSD attributable to birth trauma.

■ Methods

RESEARCH DESIGN

Phenomenology is an inductive method that describes a phenomenon as it is experienced by an individual instead of transforming it into operationally defined behavior (Colaizzi, 1978). In descriptive phenomenology, objectivity is faithfulness to the phenomenon under investigation. Objectivity is "a refusal to tell the phenomenon what it is, but a respectful listening to what the phenomenon speaks of itself" (Colaizzi, 1978, p.52).

To help ensure respectful listening, researchers using Colaizzi's (1978) phenomenologic method begin by carefully questioning presuppositions about the phenomenon under investigation. Sample questions could include these: Why am I interested in this topic? How might my presuppositions related to the research influence what I study? Once such questions are answered, the researcher then scrutinizes and examines these presuppositions. A researcher's personal inclinations and predispositions can never be completely eliminated, although Husserl (1970) calls for phenomenologists to eliminate all presuppositions through phenomenologic reduction. Colaizzi supports Merleau-Ponty's (1962) stance that "the most important lesson that the reduction teaches us is the impossibility of a complete reduction" (p. xiv). To "return to the things themselves," phenomenologists strive for descriptive identification of each phenomenon under study (Husserl, 1960). One assumption of descriptive phenomenology is that for any human experience there are essential structures that make it up regardless of individual differences.

Table 1. Demographic and Obstetric Characteristics of the Sample ($N = 38$)

Characteristic	n	%
Country		
New Zealand	22	58
United States	7	18
Australia	6	16
United Kingdom	3	8
Marital status		
Married	34	90
Single	2	5
Divorced	2	5
Education (N=17)		
Graduate	6	35
College	8	47
Partial college	2	12
High school	1	6
Parity		
Primipara	12	32
Multipara	26	68
Delivery		
Vaginal	21	55
Cesarean	17	45
Induction		
Yes	16	42
No	22	58

SAMPLE

The purposive sample included 38 mothers representing four countries (Table 1). The majority of these mothers lived in New Zealand. The mean age of the women at the time of their participation in the study was 33 years (range, 25–44 years). Of the 17 women who reported their education level, 15 had at least a college degree. Most of the mothers in this sample (n = 32) also had participated in another phenomenologic study evaluating the experience of birth trauma (Beck, 2004). The length of time from the mothers' birth trauma to their participation in this study ranged from 6 weeks to 14 years.

PROCEDURE

Approval was first obtained from the institutional review board. Data collection extended over a 24-month period and occurred via the Internet mainly through the assistance of the chairperson of TABS, a charitable trust in New Zealand. Five mothers who had experienced traumatic births founded TABS (Web site: www.tabs.org.nz; e-mail: ptsdtabs@ihug.co.nz) to support women who have experienced birth trauma and to educate healthcare professionals and the lay public about PTSD after childbirth.

The two criteria for inclusion in the sample required that woman had experienced PTSD attributable to birth trauma and that she was willing to articulate her experience. The diagnosis of PTSD was made by the mother's self-report that this disorder had been identified by a healthcare professional. Members of TABS were informed of the study through a letter written by the chairperson of the self-help organization. An announcement to recruit mothers also was printed in the TABS newsletter. Women interested in participating in the study contacted the researcher using her e-mail address. Directions for the study and an informed consent were sent by e-mail attachment to prospective participants. Women electronically signed the informed consent and returned it by attachment to the researcher.

Each mother was asked to describe her experience of PTSD after childbirth in as much detail as she wished and could remember. Two women handwrote their stories and sent them to the researcher by regular postal mail. Of the 38 mothers in the sample, 36 sent their PTSD stories over the Internet to the researcher as e-mail attachments.

After the researcher had read the mother's description of her PTSD attributable to birth trauma, she e-mailed the woman if she had questions about any part of the mother's story that needed clarification. At the same time, the researcher e-mailed the mother asking her to provide specific examples of a point she had made in her story. For example, the researcher once e-mailed the following back to a responding mother: "You mentioned that in terms of mothering, the playing of your traumatic birth nonstop for almost 6 weeks definitely had been a distraction. Could you please explain that to me in more detail?"

From the perspective of the mothers, the process of participating in this study via the Internet was beneficial to them. One mother wrote, "I feel by writing about it, my story is outside me and no longer inside filling me up with anxiety. It has taken a couple of months to get my story out, but it's been a very therapeutic exercise doing so." As another woman shared, "Writing about my experience has helped consolidate lots of things that happened during that time, and also has said to part of my memory 'forget about some of the details for awhile; have a rest—it's all written down if you want to come back to it.'"

Preliminary findings after 12 months of data collection were validated by nine mothers who had participated in the study. The researcher met with these mothers while speaking at a conference in New Zealand. The final results were reviewed over the Internet by four mothers and one father. All five persons agreed with the themes that had emerged from the mothers' stories.

DATA ANALYSIS

The mothers' (n = 38) stories of their PTSD after childbirth were analyzed using Colaizzi's (1978) method of phenomenologic analysis. Colaizzi's method begins with a reading and rereading of all the participants' descriptions of their PTSD after traumatic births and ends with a final description of the essence of that phenomenon. The middle steps of Colaizzi's thematic analysis focus on extracting significant statements that pertain directly to the experience of PTSD and formulating their meanings. Next, the formulated meanings are categorized into theme clusters and referred back to the mothers' original stories. At this point in the thematic analysis, the theme clusters are integrated into an exhaustive description of PTSD after childbirth. Colaizzi (1978) called participants in a phenomenologic study co-researchers. On the basis of this perception, the Colaizzi method involves asking some of the co-researchers to validate the exhaustive description.

■ Results

Analysis of the 38 stories describing PTSD after childbirth resulted in five themes that

Theme #	Theme
1	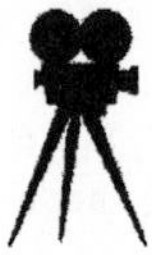 Going to the movies: Please don't make me go!
2	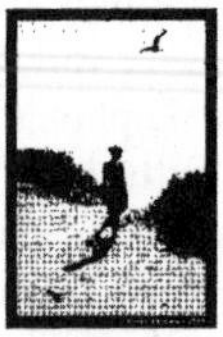 A shadow of myself: Too numb to try and change
3	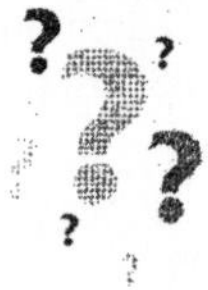 Seeking to have questions answered and wanting to talk, talk, talk
4	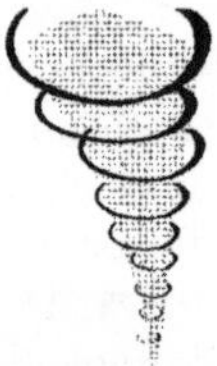 The dangerous trio of anger, anxiety, and depression: Spiraling downward
5	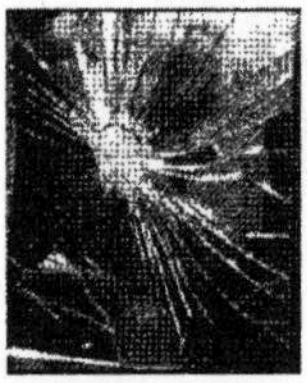 Isolation from the world of motherhood: Dreams shattered

Figure 1. Five essential themes of post-traumatic stress disorder due to childbirth.

described the essence of this experience for the mothers (Figure 1).

THEME 1. GOING TO THE MOVIES: PLEASE DON'T MAKE ME GO!

Mothers who experienced PTSD were bombarded not only during the day with flashbacks in which they relived their traumatic births, but also during the night with terrifying nightmares. These mothers repeatedly used the image of a video on automatic replay or loop tracks imprinted in their brains to describe how uncontrollable the distressing memories or "movies" of their traumatic childbirths were to them.

A primipara who had a failed vacuum extraction followed by a forceps delivery and a fourth-degree tear provided an illustration of these loop tracks that left her feeling as if she was "faking it" and stuck in the past, unable to enjoy the present with her infant:

> I lived in two worlds, the videotape of the birth and the "real" world. The videotape felt more real. I lived in my own bubble, not quite connecting with anyone. I could hear and communicate, but experienced interaction with others as a spectator. The "videotape" ran constantly for 4 months.

Another mother, who also had a failed vacuum extraction followed by a forceps delivery, desperately wanted to get out of the nightmare in which she was starring. She explained:

> I had nightmares of my delivery doctor as a rapist, coming knocking on my door. I also believed when my son was born that the doctor had ripped his head off. These two images were what affected my existence.

One woman who had been refused an epidural and subsequently experienced an "agonizing forceps delivery" experienced "extraordinarily realistic nightmares." She described her experience as follows:

> Like Lady MacBeth, I became terrified of sleeping! I would go without sleep for about 72 to 96 hours. I always knew I'd have to fight the nightmares again. I was scared that this time I wouldn't have the strength to fight it, that it would succeed in destroying me.

Flashbacks and nightmares of the traumatic births affected mothers' relationships not only with their children, but also with their husbands. One multipara who had experienced a high level of medical intervention during the delivery shared:

> After about 6 months, my husband and I still hadn't had sex since before the birth. When we began to try, I had flashbacks to the birth. At the moment of penetration, I would have a flashback to the instant when my body was pulled down the operating table during one of the failed forceps attempts.

THEME 2: A SHADOW OF MYSELF: TOO NUMB TO TRY AND CHANGE

Traumatized by their birth experience, mothers experiencing PTSD considered themselves only a shadow of their former selves. This numbing of self and actual dissociation experienced by some women can began immediately after delivery. One woman who had an emergency cesarean and postpartum hemorrhage vividly described that after delivery she was put in a room with two other mothers:

> I had a drip, a catheter, and was silent. I felt completely numb. I did what was required and I felt my head was floating way above my body. I struggled to bring it back onto my shoulders. I still feel dissociated like this sometimes.

Another mother who had hemorrhaged on the delivery table recalled that she was wheeled out to the recovery room:

> My parents were there, as was my sister. I did not cry or smile. I watched them looking happy. I was completely numb and could not remember any emotional context to do with my delivery day. The midwife pointed my baby out to me in the nursery as I was wheeled by. He was so big. I felt no recognition. I felt nothing.

Once home, the mothers reported that these feelings of numbness and detachment continued. One primipara who had undergone a terrifying experience with an epidural shared: "I'd wake up numb unable to feel a thing. I'd drag myself through the day. I am having the hardest time trying to overcome this feeling of being dead." Another woman poignantly described herself feeling as though her soul had left her and she was now only an empty shell:

> Mechanically I'd go through the motions of being a good mother. Inside I felt nothing. If the emotion did start to leak, I quickly suppressed it. I'd smack myself on the hand and put my "robot suit" back on.

THEME 3: SEEKING TO HAVE QUESTIONS ANSWERED AND WANTING TO TALK, TALK, TALK

Mothers who experienced PTSD had an intense need to know the details of their traumatic births and to get answers to their questions. These women obsessed over trying to understand what had happened and why it had happened. This obsession took on many different forms. For some women, it entailed making repeated appointments with the physicians or midwives who had delivered their infants to have their questions answered and to go over their hospital records. Others read obstetrical textbooks during their free time when they were not caring for their infants.

Revisiting the delivery room became necessary for some women even as long as a year after the birth. One multipara whose request for pain medications during labor had been denied, shared:

> At the first birthday of my little daughter, I had a horrible recurrence of the PTSD. I insisted that the hospital let me visit the delivery room and threatened them with a lawsuit if they didn't grant my request.

Women experiencing PTSD reported that they wanted to talk excessively about their traumatic births, but they quickly discovered that healthcare providers and family members became tired of listening. After a traumatic delivery a mother of multiples said:

> I was so devastated at people's lack of empathy. I told myself what a bad person I was for needing to talk. I felt like the Ancient Mariner doomed to forever be plucking at people's sleeves and trying to tell them my story which they didn't want to hear.

Eventually, some women stopped discussing their traumatic births, but this became detrimental to their mental health. As one woman explained, "I didn't communicate with anyone anymore. The room I was in became my cave. I was consumed by my birth demon." Their unasked, unanswered questions "gnawed away" at them.

One mother of multiples who had undergone an emergency cesarean poignantly tried to express in words what happened:

> Not only does PTSD isolate me from the outside world; it isolates me even from those I love. How do I explain the sort of blind terror that overtakes me without warning and without obvious logical cause? And what of my family and friends? They don't know how I feel. They don't know what to say, and they cannot make it better, so they end up feeling useless. That's the real problem with PTSD. It separates people at the time when love and understanding are most needed. It's like an invisible wall around the sufferer.

After repeated unsuccessful attempts to get satisfactory answers about their traumatic births or at least an apology from their healthcare providers and the hospital, some women took their quest to a higher level. Examples of this next step included taking their cause to the Health and Disability Commissioner, filing an accident compensation claim, and submitting a formal complaint to the State Medical Board. When, for instance, the State Medical Board sided with the physicians, women stated they were "retraumatized." One woman who had experienced an emergency cesarean delivery painfully shared that "the emotional pain of this secondary wounding was worse than the actual physical pain of labor."

THEME 4: THE DANGEROUS TRIO OF ANGER, ANXIETY, AND DEPRESSION: SPIRALING DOWNWARD

This trio of distressing emotions permeated the daily lives of mothers experiencing PTSD. The women experienced these emotions on a heightened level. Anger was rage; anxiety turned into panic attacks; and depression left many mothers suicidal. Anger was directed in multiple directions, lashing out at healthcare providers, family members, and self. Marital relationships were at times strained to the limit. As one mother whose firstborn infant had died explained:

> To live daily with the fact that you were like a time bomb ready to go off was dreadful. As time went on, I knew I was personally "too hot to handle" and not nice to be with, as invariably you could not help but have some of your inner state ooze or jump out at those who did come close.

Another woman stated:

> Powerful seething anger would overwhelm me without warning. To manage it I would go still and quiet, then eventually "come to," realizing that one or all of the children were crying and I had no idea for how long.

Mothers experiencing PTSD also turned their anger inward at times toward themselves. A mother who had given birth to twins shared that she was so full of anger at herself.

"How could I have let this happen? Why did I trust the doctors? How could I have been so stupid?"

Women were angry at the labor and delivery staff, who they perceived had betrayed their trust and let them down. This anger was not a fleeting emotion. A mother whose infant had sustained a skull fracture from a vacuum extraction 3 years earlier shared that she sometimes "relives" the traumatic birth and still is angry and mistrustful of doctors.

Anxiety also plagued women with PTSD attributable to birth trauma. For some mothers, the anxiety began on the delivery table. As a woman who had experienced "excruciating" pain once her membranes had been artificially ruptured shared: "I had intense pains in my chest from the first moment after the birth that have been extremely difficult to get rid of. They turned into anxiety." After a traumatic birth, one primipara became extremely anxious regarding intercourse, causing her to have a non-intimate relationship for most of the next 9 years. One mother was so anxious that she "made sores in my scalp and face." Women who had never experienced panic attacks before their birth trauma began to be plagued by them. One mother whose infant had received cuts and bruises attributable to a forceps delivery experienced panic attacks whenever she went to a hospital or doctor's office.

Depression at times became severe enough to lead some mothers to contemplate ending their own lives. A mother of multiples shared as follows:

> I wanted to kill myself. My life was a mess. Death seemed like a wonderful idea. I'd fight with myself while driving, "Put your foot on the brake, the light's red. No, don't put your foot on the brake," and so it went on.

THEME 5: ISOLATION FROM THE WORLD OF MOTHERHOOD: DREAMS SHATTERED

The tightening grip of PTSD after childbirth choked off three lifelines to the world of motherhood: the woman's infant, the supporting circle of other mothers, and hopes for any additional children. Concentrating first on the present, some women shared that much to their dismay, PTSD distanced them from their infants. As one mother who had an unplanned cesarean delivery painfully remembered:

> At night I tried to connect/acknowledge in my heart that this was my son and I cried. I knew that there were great layers of trauma around my heart. I wanted to feel motherhood. I wanted to experience and embrace it. Why was I chained up in the viselike grip of this pain? This was my Gethsemane—my agony in the garden.

The walls that the birth trauma erected between mother and infant did not appear to be temporary for some mothers. A multipara who had survived a severe postpartum hemorrhage 3 years earlier painfully shared that PTSD still holds a destructive grip on her relationship with her son:

> My child turned 3 years old a few weeks ago. I suppose the pain was not so acute this time. I actually made him a birthday cake and was grateful that I could go to work and not think about the significance of the day. The pain was less, but it was replaced by a numbness that still worries me. I hope that as time passes I can forge some kind of real closeness with this child. I am still unable to tell him I love him, but I can now hold him and have times when I am proud of him. I have come a long, long way.

Post-traumatic stress disorder also caused women to isolate themselves from other mothers and babies. Mothers with PTSD could not tolerate or cope with being around other women who had not experienced traumatic births. One mother would ask the nurse to schedule her baby's well child checkups 15 minutes before the clinic opened so she would not see or meet other mothers.

To have more children or not? What a heart wrenching decision this was for mothers experiencing PTSD. The only choice for three of the women was to have a tubal ligation, and one woman asked her husband to have a vasectomy. The following passage illustrates this:

> I couldn't envision *ever* having another baby. There was no way I could expose myself again to that degree of vulnerability and abandonment. My little girl was the most precious thing in my

life, but events that occurred at her birth mean that I will not be having any more children. I had a tubal ligation, and I grieved for the babies I thought I wouldn't have.

Other women, although terrified at the prospect of going through another childbirth, opted to have another child. Proactive planning and an "ironclad" birth plan helped prepare the PTSD mothers for a second childbirth. Throughout her second pregnancy, one mother kept a diary as she struggled with her PTSD. One entry from her diary vividly illustrates how vulnerable and fragile these women are as they bravely face another childbirth:

While I am trying to put my PTSD behind me, I am having to prepare for the birth of my second child. My reality is that I am scared, heart and womb. I need special care. My heart is fragile, and I am trying to protect it.

Another mother who had an emergency cesarean with her first delivery kept a list of questions to ask different midwives as a help in choosing a midwife she felt she could trust. A sampling of these questions from her diary includes the following:

Why are you a midwife? How would you describe your approach to women in labor? What is the difference between being delivered and giving birth? What do you do when a woman in labor starts saying "I'm scared" as you commence a procedure?

Of the 38 women in the study, 16 (42%) went on to have other children after experiencing traumatic births. Not all of these subsequent pregnancies, however, were planned. During these subsequent pregnancies, the mothers were terrified of having to go through another labor and delivery. One woman experienced panic attacks while pregnant. Another woman said, "I was in the most terrible state once I found out I was pregnant. I couldn't eat or sleep, crying all the time and having suicidal thoughts."

Two mothers described their subsequent births as positive experiences. As one of these women explained, "I felt cocooned and cared for this time in the hospital. My second pregnancy and birth helped me recover from my first traumatic experience." The second mother said, "Last year I had a home birth, the most amazing, healing, uplifting, empowering thing that has ever happened to me. That birth experience has given me the strength and confidence to do many things, including writing my birth trauma story."

In summary, the essence of mothers' experiences of PTSD attributable to childbirth can be portrayed as a life haunted by terrifying nightmares and flashbacks of the birth and at times consumed with seeking answers to questions about the traumatic birth. On a daily basis, anger, anxiety, and depression pervaded mothers' lives to the point that the women were only a shadow of their former selves. Mothers' dreams were shattered as they became isolated from the coveted world of motherhood.

■ Discussion

The themes that emerged from analysis of the mothers' gripping stories illustrate the characteristic symptoms of PTSD within the context of new motherhood (e.g., flashbacks and persistent avoidance of stimuli associated with the trauma). This study supports previous quantitative research regarding precipitating events of PTSD such as increased obstetric intervention and perceptions of inadequate care (Creedy et al., 2000), painful labors, and feelings of powerlessness (Soet et al., 2003). Themes 1, 4, and 5 confirm Allen's (1998) qualitative findings that women with severe PTSD symptoms after childbirth experience anxiety attributable to thoughts of the trauma, anger, and emotional detachment from their partners and babies, and to fear of future pregnancies.

For these women, the extreme traumatic stressor that triggered their PTSD was childbirth. Obviously, the best intervention is to prevent birth trauma in the first place so that PTSD will not develop. In addition to providing safe care, the basic skills that all healthcare professionals are taught need to come to the forefront with each and every mother: to be caring and to communicate effectively.

Clinicians should play a proactive role in helping to prevent PTSD attributable to birth trauma. Knowledge concerning predictors of PTSD after childbirth, such as high levels of obstetric intervention, is crucial for healthcare providers so they can be alert to these high-risk women. Clinicians also need to be vigilant in symptomatic recognition during the prenatal, intrapartum, and postpartum periods (Church & Scanlan, 2002). Symptoms of PTSD or previous trauma that clinicians should recognize during labor include: extreme fear and lack of trust of healthcare providers, flashbacks that may cause some women to cry or scream when a clinician can see no apparent reason for this extreme emotional behavior, dissociation as women psychologically escape from their current labor, and an intense need to control their labor (Crompton, 1996; Kennedy & MacDonald, 2002). The labor and delivery process can retraumatize women who have experienced previous trauma. Crompton (1996) urged clinicians to be aware of the suffering a woman may have endured already in her life. She believed that the best approach to ensure that fewer mothers are traumatized during childbirth is for clinicians to treat all women as if they all had been survivors of previous trauma (Crompton, 2003).

Debriefing sessions may be helpful in reducing trauma symptoms for women who perceive their delivery experiences as traumatic (Allen, 1998; Gamble, Creedy, Webster, & Moyle, 2002). Support and trauma counseling are essential for diminishing the impact of traumatic childbirth. Crompton (2003) suggested that access to a support group, such as TABS, composed of other women who have had birth trauma and PTSD attributable to childbirth is of primary importance.

The theme of isolation from the world of motherhood powerfully alerts clinicians to the specific effects of PTSD when the traumatic event is childbirth. Not only can PTSD have devastating effects on the mother; it also can affect the developing relationship with her child. Mother-infant attachment problems have been addressed in a few studies on PTSD after childbirth (Allen, 1998; Ballard, Stanley, & Brockington, 1995; Reynolds, 1997; Weaver, 1997). For some mothers, their infants were reminders of their traumatic births, and in keeping with one characteristic of PTSD, the women avoided any stimuli associated with the trauma. Further complicating these fragile mother-infant dyads was the numbness the women experienced. Functioning as only a shadow of their former selves took a heavy toll on the attachment some mothers felt with their infants. Routine assessment of mother-infant interaction during the postpartum period can provide one way to identify women struggling with PTSD.

Studies focusing on women who have gone on to have other children even after experiencing PTSD attributable to birth trauma are needed. A purposive study of women who had a healing experience with this subsequent labor and delivery could examine how this healing childbirth was different from the previous traumatic birth. Studies can be designed to evaluate the effectiveness of PTSD intervention using childbirth support groups or specific prevention strategies.

Cheryl Tatano Beck, DNSc, CNM, FAAN, is Professor of Nursing, University of Connecticut School of Nursing, Storrs, Connecticut.

Accepted for publication December 15, 2003.

The author thanks the Chairperson of Trauma and Birth Stress, Sue Watson, for her invaluable help and never-ending support. The author also thanks the four mothers and one father who thoughtfully revieved the final version of the manuscript. Most importantly, the author thanks the unselfish mothers who courageously shared their painful stories in the hopes of helping other women to avoid PTSD attributable to childbirth.

Corresponding author: Cheryl Tatano Beck, DNSc, CNM, FAAN, University of Connecticut School of Nursing, 231 Glenbrook Road, Storrs, CT 06269-2026 (e-mail: cheryl.beck@uconn.edu).

REFERENCES

Allen, S. (1998). A qualitative analysis of the process, mediating variables, and impact of traumatic childbirth. *Journal of Reproductive and Infant Psychology, 16*, 107–131.

American Psychiatric Association. (1980). *Diagnostic and statistical manual of mental disorders.* Washington DC: Author.

American Psychiatric Association (1994). *Diagnostic and statistical manual of mental disorders.* (4th ed.) Washington DC: Author.

Ayers, S., & Pickering, A. (2001). Do women get post-traumatic stress disorder as a result of childbirth? A prospective study of incidence. *Birth, 28*, 111–118.

Bailham, D., & Joseph, S. (2003). Post-traumatic stress following childbirth: A review of the emerging literature and directions for research and practice. *Psychology, Health, and Medicine, 8*, 159–168.

Ballard, C. G., Stanley, A. K., & Brockington, I. F., (1995). Post-traumatic stress disorder (**PTSD**) after childbirth. *British Journal of Psychiatry, 166*, 525–528.

Beck, C. T. (2004). Birth trauma: In the eye of the beholder. *Nursing Research, 53*, 28–35.

Callahan, J. L., & Hynan, M. T. (2002). Identifying mothers at risk for postnatal emotional distress: Further evidence for the validity of the Perinatal Post-traumatic Stress Disorder Questionnaire. *Journal of Perinatology, 22*, 448–454.

Church, S., & Scanlan, M. (2002). Post-traumatic stress disorder after childbirth. *The Practicing Midwife, 5*, 10–13.

Colaizzi, P. (1978). Psychological research as the phenomenologist views it. In R. Valle & M. King (Eds.). *Existential phenomenological alternatives for psychology* (pp. 48–71). New York: Oxford University Press.

Creedy, D. K., Shocher, I. M., & Horsfall, J. (2000). Childbirth and the development of acute trauma symptoms: Incidence and contributing factors. *Birth, 27*, 104–111.

Crompton, J. (1996). Post-traumatic stress disorder and childbirth: 2. *British Journal of Midwifery, 4*, 354–356.

Crompton, J. (2003). Post-traumatic stress disorder and childbirth. *Childbirth Educators New Zealand Education Effects*, summer, 25–31.

DeMier R. L., Hynan M. T., Harris H. B., & Manniello R. L. (1996). Perinatal stressors as predictors of symptoms of post-taumatic stress in mothers of infants at high risk. *Journal of Perinatology, 16*, 276–280.

Foa, E. B., Riggs, D. S, Dancu, C., & Rothbaum, B. O. (1993). Reliability and validity of a brief instrument for assessing post-taumatic stress disorder. *Journal of Trauma Stress, 6*, 459–473.

Gamble, J. A., Creedy, D. K., Webster, J., & Moyle, W. (2002). A review of the literature on debriefing or nondirective counseling to prevent postpartum emotional distress. *Midwifery, 18*, 72–79.

Holditch-Davis, D., Bartlett, T. R., Blickman, A. L., & Miles, M. S. (2003). Post-traumatic stress symptoms in mothers of premature infants. *Journal of Obstetric, Gynecologic, and Neonatal Nursing, 32*, 161–171.

Horowitz, M. J., Wilner, N., & Alvarez, W. (1979). Revised Impact of Event Scale: a measure of subjective stress. *Psychosomatic Medicine, 41*, 209–218.

Husserl, E. (1960). *Cartesian meditations* (D. Cairns, trans.). The Hague: Netherlands: Martineus Nijhoff.

Husserl, E. (1954/1970). *The crisis of European sciences and transcendental phenomenology: An introduction to phenomenological philosophy* (D. Carr, trans.). Evanston, IL: Northwestern University Press.

Kennedy, H. P., & MacDonald, E. L. (2002). "Altered consciousness" during childbirth: Potential clues to post-traumatic stress disorder? *Journal of Midwifery and Women's Health, 47*, 380–381.

Lyons, S. (1998). A prospective study of post-traumatic stress symptoms 1 month following childbirth in a group of 42 first-time mothers. *Journal of Reproductive and Infant Psychology, 16*, 91–105.

Menage, J. (1993). Post-traumatic stress disorder in women who have undergone obstetric or gynecological procedures. *Journal of Reproductive and Infant Psychology, 11*, 221–228.

Merleau-Ponty, M. (1962). *Phenomenology of perception.* New York: Humanities Press.

Reynolds, J. L. (1997). Post-traumatic stress disorder after childbirth: The phenomenon of traumatic birth. *Canadian Medical Association Journal, 156*, 831–835.

Ryding, E. L., Wijma, K., & Wijma, B. (1998). Psychological impact of emergency cesarean section in comparison with elective cesarean section, instrumental, and normal vaginal delivery. *Journal of Psychosomatic Obstetrics and Gynecology, 19*, 135–144.

Seng, J. S. (2002). A conceptual framework for research on lifetime violence, post-traumatic stress, and childbearing. *Journal of Midwifery and Women's Health, 47*, 337–346.

Soet, J. E., Brack, G. A., & Dilorio, C. (2003). Prevalence and predictors of women's experience of psychological trauma during childbirth. *Birth, 30*, 36–46.

Watson, C. C., Juba, M. P., Manifold, V., Kucala, T., & Anderson, E. D. (1991). The PTSD interview: Rationale, description, reliability, and concurrent validity of a DSM-III- based technique. *Journal of Clinical Psychology, 47*, 179–189.

Weaver, J. (1997). Childbirth: Preventing post-traumatic stress disorder. *Professional Care of Mother and Child, 7*, 2–3.

Wijma, K., Soderquist, M. A., & Wijma, B. (1997). Post-traumatic stress disorder after childbirth: A cross-sectional study. *Journal of Anxiety Disorders, 11*, 587–597.

APPENDIX E

Older Men's Health

Motivation, Self-Ratings, and Behaviors

Susan J. Loeb

- ***Background:*** There is a documented need to examine the complex motivational systems that lead individuals to adopt health-promoting behaviors and to evaluate the psychosocial aspects of male health. A study focused on health motivation as a determinant of self-rated health and health behaviors among older men was therefore undertaken.
- ***Objectives:*** This study aimed to explore the relations among health motivation, self-rated health, and health behaviors in community-dwelling older men.
- ***Methods:*** A descriptive, correlational survey design was used for this study of 135 community-dwelling men ages 55 years and older. The questionnaire packet included a demographic tool, the Older Men's Health Program and Screening Inventory, the Health-Promotion Activities of Older Adults Measure, and the Health Self-Determinism Index.
- ***Results:*** Older men with more intrinsic motivation rated their health as better ($p \leq .001$) and assessed their lifestyles as more healthy ($p \leq .001$) than did their counterparts with more extrinsic motivation. Whereas anticipated benefits (a potential motivator) were significantly related to health-promoting behaviors ($p \leq .001$), health program attendance ($p \leq .001$), and health screening participation ($p \leq .01$), the Health Self-Determinism Index score did not demonstrate significant relations with any of these three variables.
- ***Conclusions:*** The findings suggest that promoting self-motivation may be key to increasing older men's perceptions of health and well-being. Further exploration of anticipated benefits as a motivator of health-promotion activities is warranted, as well as intervention studies to promote older men's health screening and program attendance.

- ***Key Words:*** health-promoting behaviors · motivation · older men · self-rated health

The achievement and maintenance of higher well-being levels hold promise as ways for older adults, many of whom have limited incomes, to combat the ever-increasing cost of medical care and work toward the attainment of optimal health. Watson and Pulliam (2000) suggested that increasing older adults' well-being will serve not only to improve their quality of life and protect their financial resources, but also to decrease our nation's yearly healthcare costs significantly. Increased attention must be directed toward promoting the health of elders if an increase in healthy years is to be achieved rather than merely prolonged life expectancy (Minkler, Schauffler, & Clements-Nolle, 2000). Specifically, there is a need for more applied research addressing motivational strategies designed to increase participation in health-promotion activities, particularly by older men (Loeb, O'Neill, & Gueldner, 2001).

Elderly men are a population of extraordinary concern because males reportedly value health less (Felton, Parsons, & Bartoces, 1997), participate in fewer health screenings (Zabalegui, 1994), experience poorer health, have shorter life expectancies, and allow an illness to progress longer before consulting with a doctor than their female counterparts (Baker, 2001). Despite the clear necessity for addressing challenges to older men's health, elderly men have been described as both a forgotten minority (Kosberg & Kaye, 1997) and invisible in gerontology (Kosberg & Mangum, 2002). This concerning phenomenon may be attributed to older men's smaller numbers, their lack of advocacy by gerontologic organizations, and the mistaken perception that older men experience a better quality of life than older women (Kosberg & Mangum, 2002). It is important to include older men of diverse ethnic and cultural backgrounds in studies because prevalence of health conditions, risk factors for diseases, and factors impacting health may vary across individuals of different races, ethnicities, and cultures (Wrobel & Shapiro, 1999). A factor contributing to diversity in a population is geographic location of residence. Thus, efforts to include participants from both rural and urban areas are essential. Krout, McCulloch, and Kivett (1997) assert that few researchers actually have focused on comparing rural and urban older males.

In response to the need for research addressing older men's health, the current study focuses exclusively on elderly men. Additionally, this research represents an extension of prior investigations because a variety of health behaviors are explored simultaneously (i.e., health-promotion activities, health screening participation, and formal health-promotion program participation) and a variety of self-ratings of health are included.

■ Motivation and Attitudes in Relation to Healthy Behaviors

Earlier, Rosenstock (1960) reviewed the findings of studies within the disciplines of the social sciences to address determinants of individuals' participation in public health programs. However, the motivating factors for health-promoting behaviors among elderly individuals remain uncertain and may differ from those of middle-aged and young adults (Miller & Iris, 2002). In their focus group study of 45 older men and women, Miller and Iris (2002) found that motivators for health behaviors included a desire to feel better, gain social support and combat loneliness, substitute a positive health behavior for a prior negative behavior (i.e., drinking alcohol), take on a challenge (especially related to participation in physical activities), and continue with lifelong positive health habits. A supportive spouse was reported to be an especially important motivator for the older men in the study. Similarly, a focus group study of 37 community-dwelling elders living with multiple chronic health conditions found social support to be key in long-term adherence to an exercise program (Loeb, Penrod, Falkenstern, Gueldner, & Poon, 2003).

Frenn's (1996) grounded theory study investigating elders' perceptions of health behaviors identified two constructs of intrinsic motivation as important for health promotion: self-determination and perceived competence. Furthermore, the participants identified external forces, the way they were raised, and new awareness as important aspects of motivation for healthy behaviors. Haq and Griffin's (1996) survey of 156 elders found that more intrinsic health motivation was related to better health and greater participation in health-promoting behaviors. Also, interpersonal relationships and greater physical activity have been found to be significantly and positively related to more intrinsic health motivation (Lucas, Orshan, & Cook, 2000). Finally, a qualitative study (Gabhainn et al., 1999) explored sociodemographic variations in perspectives on cardiovascular disease. Older men were the least motivated for health behavior modifications and expressed an attitude that they were too old to change. In light of prior study findings, increased insights about how health motivation relates to various health behaviors in elderly males would guide nurses in planning health programs that better meet older men's needs.

■ Self-Rated Health

The early work of Maddox (1962) warned that self-rated health and physician-rated health may not be identical. However, more recently it has been established that elders' self-reports of health status are reliable indicators, as demonstrated through associations with objective measures of health (Riffle, Yoho, & Sams, 1989), and that these self-reports have significant relations with functional ability and numbers of prescription drugs (Idler & Kasl, 1995). Self-rated health also is useful for ascertaining patterns before and after sentinel health events (Diehr, Williamson, Patrick, Bild, & Burke, 2001). Borawski, Kinney, and Kahana (1996) reviewed a number of well-designed epidemiologic studies, all of which found a robust relation between self-rated health and mortality, even after control was used for a wide variety of potentially confounding variables.

■ Health Behaviors

Padula (1997a) indicated that health behaviors to be explored in older adults include attendance at formal health-promotion programs, participation in health screenings, and the following variety of health-promotion activities: exercising, avoiding health hazards, promoting one's safety, visiting healthcare providers on a regular basis, eating healthy foods, limiting alcohol intake, managing stress, seeking out health information, and ensuring adequate sleep and rest. Participation in such health behaviors is a means by which older men strive to meet the *Healthy People 2010* goal of increasing years of functional health (U. S. Department of Health and Human Services [USDHHS], 2001).

■ Theoretical Framework

The Health-Promoting Self-Care System Model was the conceptual framework chosen to guide this study because it links nursing with both the attitudinal and behavioral patterns of clients' health (Simmons, 1990) (Figure 1). This model synthesizes and expands upon facets of the Health Promotion Model (Pender, 1987), the Interaction Model of Client Health Behavior (Cox, 1982), and the Self-Care Deficit Nursing Theory (Orem, 1985). Simmons' (1990) model is based on the principles that health responsibility and self-care are central to health promotion and that people are able to gain the attitudes, knowledge, and skills necessary for participation in health-promoting behaviors. Finally, the model is useful for explicating the patterns among factors influencing health-promoting lifestyles (Simmons, 1990). Considering this model, the purpose of this study was to explore the relations among health motivation, self-ratings of health, and various health behaviors in a sample of community-dwelling older men.

■ Methods

SETTINGS AND SAMPLE

A convenience sample of older men were accessed at a "55-Alive" drivers' safety class held at a hospital, senior exercise classes that met in a church community room, seven senior citizen centers (5 rural and 2 urban), two McDonald's restaurants (only one yielded participants), and social groups of older men known by the investigator (i.e., neighbors and friends). Recruitment took place in both urban and rural regions of a Mid-Atlantic state to achieve a more ethnically diverse sample, because in that state, 97.9% of the rural dwellers are White (U. S. Census Bureau, 2000). In particular, urban recruitment sites facilitated access to more African American older men (n = 25, 18.5%). However, more elderly men were accessed from the rural locations (61%) because of greater success in gaining permission from the agencies/businesses. A rural McDonald's provided the researcher with almost as many participants (n = 34, 25.2%) as the second and third most participatory sites combined (an urban exercise class and an urban senior center yielding 19 and

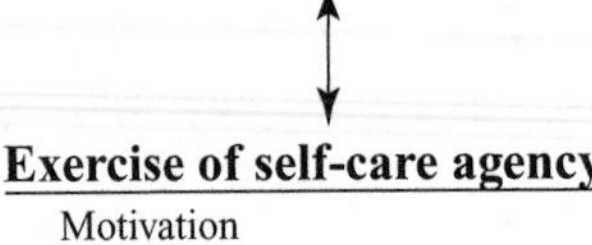

Figure 1. From The Health-Promoting Self-Care System Model: Directions for nursing research and practice by S. J. Simmons, 1990, *Journal of Advanced Nursing, 15,* 1164. Copyright 1990 by Blackwell Science. Adapted with permission.

16 participants, respectively), which was not surprising because McDonald's has targeted older men via television marketing (Bone, 1991). Convenience sampling was chosen because it is well suited for community settings, where limited space, time for recruitment, and data collection procedures are challenges.

The inclusion criteria for this study were the male gender; age of 55 years or older; ability to read, understand, and write English; and absence of obvious cognitive impairments. Originally, 139 men agreed to participate. However, two questionnaires were excluded because of unacceptable amounts of missing data, and two other men excused themselves and never returned, resulting in a total of 135 participants.

Power was computed for regression analysis, the most sophisticated level of statistics. Therefore, the conventional standards of .05 for committing a Type 1 error (alpha) and .20 for committing a Type 2 error (beta), as well as an effect size of .10, which Cohen (1988) identified as a small to moderate effect size for regression analysis, were chosen, resulting in a minimum sample size of 130 participants needed to achieve a power level of .80.

DESIGN AND PROCEDURES

A descriptive, correlational survey design was used. Approval for research involving human subjects was obtained through the office for regulatory compliance at a major research university. A written Explanation of Study Form and an oral explanation were provided to all participants. Participants were informed that completion of the pencil and paper questionnaire packet implied consent to participate in the study. Anonymity of participant responses was ensured. All questionnaires were stored in a locked file cabinet in the investigator's office.

When the data collection site was either a facility or organization, contact people at each location were asked to alert potential participants that the researcher would be coming on a particular day and time. For example, at the McDonald's restaurant, the researcher observed a large group of elder male patrons between the hours of 6:30 AM and 10:30 AM. To begin data collection, the researcher struck up a conversation with one group, explaining the purpose and procedures of the study, and then circulated throughout the restaurant over the ensuing 4-hour period soliciting participation. In contrast, when social groups (i.e., friends and neighbors) known to the investigator were accessed, the men were contacted by telephone, with the investigator ascertaining whether they were interested in participating, and then arrangements were made to meet. On the days of data collection at the senior centers, exercise class, and driving class, the investigator met with each group of potential participants and distributed the explanation of the study form. The form, including the purpose and procedures of the study, was explained. Surveys were self-administered by the participants, with the investigator present to answer questions. Each participant received a token gift of appreciation (a $5.00 restaurant gift certificate).

INSTRUMENTS

The four measures used were compiled into a questionnaire packet in the following order: a 6-item demographics instrument, the 8-item Older Men's Health Program and Screening Inventory (Loeb, 2003), the 44-item Health-Promotion Activities of Older Adults Measure (Padula, 1997a), and the 17-item Health Self-Determinism Index (Cox, 1985). The required reading levels for the instruments ranged from a grade 5.7 to grade 7.9. All were typed in 14-point font with sufficient white space.

DEMOGRAPHICS INSTRUMENT

The demographics instrument, the first instrument in the questionnaire packet, inquired about participants' age, ethnicity/race, marital status, education, income, and the presence of others in the same residence. These demographic variables were chosen for inclusion because prior research (Cox, 1986; Haq & Griffin, 1996) had determined that different combinations of these variables are related significantly to health motivation.

OLDER MEN'S HEALTH PROGRAM AND SCREENING INVENTORY

The Older Men's Health Program and Screening Inventory (Loeb, 2003) inquires about older men's attendance at formal health-promotion programs, participation in age- and gender-appropriate health screenings, current health conditions, barriers to and anticipated benefits of health-promotion behaviors, and self-ratings of health, healthiness of lifestyle, and satisfaction with current health-promoting behaviors. The first five items are structured as checklists, and participants are to check all responses that apply. The final three questions use 4-point Likert-type scales. One question asks participants to evaluate their health status (poor to excellent). The second question has them rate how healthy their current lifestyle is (never healthy to always healthy), and the third asks them to rate how satisfied they are with their health-promoting behaviors (never satisfied to always satisfied). Reliability testing for these three scaled items yielded a Cronbach alpha of .78 (Loeb, 2003).

HEALTH-PROMOTION ACTIVITIES OF OLDER ADULTS MEASURE

The Health-Promotion Activities of Older Adults Measure (HPAOAM) was chosen for this study because it is designed specifically to measure health-promoting behaviors (lifestyle practices) in older adults. Total scores for the tool are obtained by tallying responses to the 4-point Likert-type items that range from 1 (never) to 4 (always). Possible scores range from 44 to 176, with higher scores indicating greater participation in health-promoting behaviors. Padula (1997a) reported Cronbach's alpha reliability estimates of .87 to .93 for the HPAOAM. In the current investigation, the coefficient alpha was .91.

HEALTH SELF-DETERMINISM INDEX

The Health Self-Determinism Index (HSDI) (Cox, 1985) is a Likert-type survey in which the total score on the instrument is used to measure health motivation. Each item is scored on a scale ranging from 1 (strongly disagree) to 5 (strongly agree). Possible total scores on the HSDI range from 17 to 85, with lower scores indicating more extrinsic motivation and higher scores indicating more intrinsic motivation for health (Cox, 1985). The Cronbach alpha reliability estimates for the HSDI have varied from .82 (Cox, 1985) to .78 (Cox, Miller, & Mull, 1987) to .64 (Loeb et al., 2001) to .61 in the current study.

STATISTICAL ANALYSIS

The Statistical Package for the Social Sciences (SPSS) was used to compute frequency distributions, descriptive statistics, Pearson's product-moment correlations, and stepwise multiple regression analysis. Data were inspected for normalcy. No evidence of multicollinearity was present. Significant differences across data collection sites were found to exist, so a dummy control variable for recruitment site was used in the regression analysis. Because age was significantly different at the rural senior centers, it also was included in the regression equation. The challenge of missing data was addressed by replacing missing values with means for the cases in which variables were scaled in nature. Only one item, anticipated benefits of health-promoting behaviors, had a concerning amount of missing data (10, 7.5%). Other items in the packet were rarely missed.

■ Results

DESCRIPTION OF PARTICIPANTS

The men ranged in age from 55 to 91 years (mean, 70 years). The majority were White (78.5%), rural (60.7%), and married (66.7%). Levels of education ranged from completion of the fourth grade through completion of doctoral degrees (both MD and PhD), with the most frequently reported level being a high school diploma (21.6%). The participants lived with at least one other person (70.7%) and reported incomes that were "about the same as others my age" (49.3%). Although interval level data on income arguably could have provided more valuable information about the effects of socioeconomic status on health behaviors, categorical data were collected to ensure that participants did not skip the income question.

BIVARIATE ANALYSES

The Pearson product-moment correlation analyses were computed to assess the relations between health motivation and various perceptions regarding health. Total scores on the HSDI were significantly and positively related to self-rated health status ($p \leq .001$), self-rated healthiness of lifestyle ($p \leq .001$), satisfaction with health-promoting behaviors ($p \leq .01$), and total anticipated benefits of health-promoting behaviors ($p \leq .05$). After the Bonferroni adjustment for multiple testing (Munro, 1997) was computed, only self-rated health and self-rated healthiness of lifestyle remained significantly correlated with total HSDI scores (Table 1). More intrinsically motivated elderly men assessed their health to be better and their lifestyles to be more healthy.

Table 1. Bivariate Correlation Results

Variable		1	2	3	4	5	6	
1 Health motivation (HSDI)	r	1.00						
	Significant							
2 Health-protmoting behaviors (HPAOAM)	r	.130	1.00					
	Significant	.132						
3 Personal evaluation of health (self-rated)	r	.320***[a]	.321***[a]	1.00				
	Significant	.000	.000					
4 Healthiness of lifestyle	r	.325***[a]	.368***[a]	.470***[a]	1.00			
	Significant	.000	.000	.000				
5 Satisfaction with health behaviors	r	.232**	.564***[a]	.470***[a]	.665***[a]	1.00		
	Significant	.007	.000	.000	.000			
6 Total benefits	r	.181*	.485***[a]	.155	.149	.291**[a]	1.00	
	Significant	.043	.000	.085	.098	.001		
7 Total screenings	r	−.064	.265**[a]	−.046	−.069	.008	.272**[a]	1.00
	Significant	.463	.002	.596	.428	.924	.002	
8 Total programs	r	.057	.374***[a]	.005	.049	.170*	.344***[a]	.156
	Significant	.515	.000	.957	.571	.049	.000	.071

Note. HSDI = Health Self-Determinism Index; HPAOAM = Health Promotion Activities of Older Adults Measure.
[a]Those still significant after Bonferroni correction for multiple testing; $p \le .004$. $n = 135$, except in the correlations with total benefits; there, $n = 124$.
$^{*}p \le .05$ level (two-tailed). $^{**}p \le .01$ level (two-tailed). $^{***}p \le .001$ level (two-tailed).

Table 2. Stepwise Multiple Regression Analysis for Variance in HPAOAM Scores

Step Variable Entered	R^2	F Change	Beta	df_1	df_2
1 Satisfaction	.298	53.153***	.442	1	123
2 Benefits	.414	24.296***	.357	1	122

Note. HPAOAM = Health Promotion Activities of Older Adults Measure; satisfaction = satisfaction with health-promoting behaviors; benefits = total anticipated benefits of health-promoting behaviors.
***$p \leq .001$ level (two-tailed).

Through correlation analyses, health motivation was found to have had no significant relation to health-promotion activities, health screening attendance, or health-promotion program attendance. However, health-promotion activities were significantly and positively related to health-promotion program attendance ($p \leq .001$) and health screening attendance ($p \leq .01$), both withstood the Bonferroni adjustment. Therefore, older men who practiced more health-promotion activities attended significantly more formal health-promotion programs.

Total scores on the HPAOAM were significantly (even with the Bonferroni correction) and positively related to self-rated health status ($p \leq .001$), self-rated healthiness of lifestyle ($p \leq .001$), satisfaction with health-promoting behaviors ($p \leq .001$), and total anticipated benefits from health-promoting behaviors ($p \leq .001$). Older men who practiced more health-promotion activities reported better health, more healthy lifestyles, greater satisfaction with their health-promoting behaviors, and more anticipated benefits from health-promoting behaviors. Also, older men who anticipated more benefits from health-promotion behaviors participated in significantly more health screenings ($p \leq .01$), a relation that withstood the Bonferroni adjustment.

MULTIPLE REGRESSION

A stepwise multiple regression analysis was conducted to determine the most predictive equation for health-promotion activities. In addition to the six initially proposed variables, the data collection site variable was compressed into two categories (rural and urban) and entered into the equation, along with age. Only two variables entered the final equation (Table 2). Satisfaction with health-promoting behaviors entered the equation first, explaining 29.8% of the variance. Anticipated benefits of health-promoting behaviors entered second, contributing another 11.6%. Thus, these two variables together explained 41% of the total variance in HPAOAM scores.

Multicollinearity was examined before the stepwise multiple regression analysis. Specifically, the highest correlation coefficient between any two predictor variables was only 0.47. After computation of the step-wise regression, the collinearity tolerances for the two-predictor variables were calculated, with a result of 0.916, which indicated a high level of tolerance and thus low collinearity (Munro, 1997).

DIFFERENCES BETWEEN GROUPS

Independent sample *t*-tests were computed to compare Whites with non-Whites (Blacks not of Hispanic origin, Hispanics, Asians/Pacific Islanders, and Native Americans/Alaskan Natives) for differences in mean scores on the major study variables. Three significant differences were noted, and all withstood the Bonferroni adjustment (Table 3). The non-White older men had greater numbers of current health conditions, anticipated more benefits from health-promoting behaviors, and participated in more screening programs. Similarly, rural and urban older men also

Table 3. Comparison of White and Nonwhite Older Men

	White, $n = 106$	Nonwhite, $n = 29$			
Variable	Mean (SD)	Mean (SD)	t	df	p^a
HPAOAM	140.94 (16.91)	145.55 (20.27)	−1.246[b]	133	.215
HSDI	53.18 (6.54)	52.34 (7.11)	0.603[b]	133	.547
Total benefits	4.49 (2.62)	6.00 (2.24)	−2.813[b]	123	.006**[d]
Income	3.11 (0.98)	2.90 (.77)	−1.104[b]	133	.272
Total barriers	0.54 (0.85)	0.97 (1.11)	−1.915[c]	133	.063
Total health conditions	3.40 (2.11)	4.97 (2.41)	−3.440[b]	133	.001**[d]
Total screenings	3.83 (1.62)	4.86 (1.51)	−3.078[b]	133	.003**[d]
Total programs	2.44 (2.13)	2.34 (1.82)	0.227[b]	133	.820

Note. HSDI = Health Self-Determinism Index; HPAOAM = Health Promotion Activities of Older Adults Measure.
[a]Two-tailed significance.
[b]Equal variance formula.
[c]Unequal variance formula.
[d]Those still significant after Bonferroni correction for multiple testing ($p \leq .006$).
*$p \leq .05$. **$p \leq .01$. ***$p \leq .001$.

were assessed for differences in these same variables of interest. Significant differences were found for three of the variables. However, when the Bonferroni value was computed, only two remained statistically significant (Table 4). Urban men were found to anticipate more benefits from health-promoting behaviors and to have participated in a greater number of screenings than their rural counterparts.

Table 4. Comparison of White and Nonwhite Older Men

	Rural, $n = 82$	Urban, $n = 53$			
Variable	Mean (SD)	Mean (SD)	t	df	p^a
HPAOAM	139.39 (16.52)	145.83 (18.89)	−2.100[b]	133	.038*
HSDI	53.39 (7.01)	52.41 (6.07)	0.830[b]	133	.408
Total benefits	4.19 (2.64)	5.82 (2.23)	−3.597[c]	123	.000***[d]
Income	3.11 (1.01)	3.00 (0.83)	0.666[b]	133	.507
Total barriers	0.66 (0.92)	0.58 (0.95)	0.449[b]	133	.654
Total health conditions	3.44 (2.10)	4.19 (2.44)	−1.897[b]	133	.060
Total screenings	3.62 (1.63)	4.72 (1.46)	−3.968[b]	133	.000***[d]
Total programs	2.22 (2.13)	2.74 (1.93)	−1.427[b]	133	.156

Note. HSDI = Health Self-Determinism Index; HPAOAM = Health Promotion Activities of Older Adults Measure.
[a]Two-tailed significance.
[b]Equal variance formula.
[c]Unequal variance formula.
[d]Those still significant after Bonferroni correction for multiple testing ($p \leq .006$).
*$p \leq .05$. **$p \leq .01$. ***$p \leq .001$.

Morin, Professor of Nursing, Bronson School of Nursing, Western Michigan University; and Dr. Diana Morris, Associate Professor of Nursing and Associate Director of the University Center on Aging and Health, Frances Payne Bolton School of Nursing, Case Western Reserve University.

Corresponding author: Susan J. Loeb, PhD, RN, Department of Nursing, 367 McDowell Hall, University of Delaware, Newark, DE 19716 (e-mail: sloeb@udel.edu).

REFERENCES

Armer, J. M., & Conn, V. S. (2001). Exploration of spirituality and health among diverse rural elderly individuals. *Journal of Gerontological Nursing, 27*(6), 28–37.

Baker, P. (2001). *Sex and gender matter: From boys to men: The future of men's health*. Conference report. Accessed June 13, 2003 at http://www.medscape.com/viewarticle/415037_2/

Barber, K. R., Shaw, R., Folts, M., & Taylor, K. (1998). Differences between African American and Caucasian men participating in a community-based prostate cancer screening program. *Journal of Community Health, 23*, 441–451.

Bone, P. F. (1991). Identifying mature segments. *The Journal of Services Marketing, 5*(1), 47–60.

Borawski, E. A., Kinney, J. M., & Kahana, E. (1996). The meaning of older adults' health appraisals: Congruence with health status and determinant of mortality. *Journal of Gerontology: Social Sciences, 51B*, S157–S170.

Cohen, J. (1988). *Statistical power analysis for the behavior sciences* (2nd ed.). Hillsdale, NJ: Lawrence Erlbaum Associates.

Cox, C. L. (1982). An interaction model of client health behavior: Theoretical prescription for nursing. *Advances in Nursing Science, 5*(1), 41–56.

Cox, C. L. (1985). The health self-determinism index. *Nursing Research, 34*(3), 177–183.

Cox, C. L. (1986). The interaction model of client health behavior: Application to the study of community-based elders. *Advances in Nursing Science, 9*(1), 40–57.

Cox, C. L., Miller, E. H., & Mull, C. S. (1987). Motivation in health behavior: Measurements, antecedents, and correlates. *Advances in Nursing Science, 9*(4), 1–15.

Diehr, P., Williamson, J., Patrick, D. L., Bild, D. E., & Burke, G. L. (2001). Patterns of self-rated health in older adults before and after sentinel health events. *Journal of the American Geriatrics Society, 49*, 36–44.

Felton, G. M., Parsons, M. A., & Bartoces, M. G. (1997). Demographic factors: Interaction effects on health-promoting behavior and health-related factors. *Public Health Nursing, 14*, 361–367.

Fischera, S. D., & Frank, D. I. (1994). The health belief model as a predictor of mammography screening. *Health Values: Achieving High Level Wellness, 18*(4), 3–9.

Frenn, M. (1996). Older adults' experience of health promotion: A theory for nursing practice. *Public Health Nursing 13*(1), 65–71.

Gabhainn, S. N., Kelleher, C. C., Naughton, A. M., Carter, F., Flanagan, M., & McGrath, M. J. (1999). Sociodemographic variations in perspectives on cardiovascular disease and associated risk factors. *Health Education Research, 14*, 619–628.

Haq, M. B., & Griffin, M. (1996). Health motivation: Key to health-promoting behavior? *The Nurse Practitioner, 21*(11), 155–156.

Idler, E. L., & Kasl, S. V. (1995). Self-ratings of health: Do they also predict change in functional ability? *Journal of Gerontology: Series B: Psychological Sciences & Social Sciences, 50B*, S344–S353.

Kaufmann, J. E. (1996). Personal definitions of health among elderly people: A link to effective health promotion. *Family Community Health, 19*(2), 58–68.

Kosberg, J. I., & Kaye, L. W. (1997). The status of older men: Current perspectives and future projections. In J. I. Kosberg, & L. W. Kaye (Eds.), *Elderly men: Special problems and professional challenges* (pp. 295–307). New York: Springer.

Kosberg, J. I., & Mangum, W. P. (2002). The invisibility of older men in gerontology. *Gerontology and Geriatrics Education, 22*(4), 27–42.

Krout, J. A., McCulloch, B. J., & Kivett, V. R. (1997). Rural older men: A neglected elderly population. In J. I. Kosberg, & L. W. Kaye (Eds.), *Elderly men: Special problems and professional challenges* (pp. 113–130). New York: Springer.

Loeb, S. J. (2003). The older men's health program and screening inventory: A tool for assessing health practices and beliefs. *Geriatric Nursing, 24*, 278–285.

Loeb, S. J., O'Neill, J., & Gueldner, S. H. (2001). Health motivation: A determinant of older adults' attendance at health promotion programs. *Journal of Community Health Nursing, 18*, 151–165.

Loeb, S. J., Penrod, J., Falkenstern, S., Gueldner, S. H., & Poon, L. W. (2003). Supporting older adults living with multiple chronic conditions. *Western Journal of Nursing Research, 25*(1), 8–29.

Lucas, J. A., Orshan, S. A., & Cook, F. (2000). Determinants of health-promoting behavior among women ages 65 and above living in the community. *Scholarly Inquiry for Nursing Practice, 14*(1), 77–109.

Maddox, G. L. (1962). Some correlates of differences in self-assessments of health status among the elderly. *Journal of Gerontology, 17*, 180–185.

Miller, A. M., & Iris, M. (2002). Health promotion attitudes and strategies in older adults. *Health Education and Behavior, 29*, 249–267.

Minkler, M., Schauffler, H., & Clements-Nolle, K. (2000). Health promotion for older Americans in the 21st century. *American Journal of Health Promotion, 14*, 371–379.

Morgan, K., Armstrong, G. K., Huppert, F. A., Brayne, C., & Solomou, W. (2000). Research papers. Healthy ageing in urban and rural Britain: A comparison of exercise and diet. *Age and Ageing, 29*, 341–349.

Munro, B. H. (1997). *Statistical methods for health care research* (3rd ed.). Philadelphia: Lippincott.

Orem, D. E. (1985). *Nursing: Concepts of practice* (3rd ed.). New York: McGraw-Hill.

Padula, C. A. (1997a). Development of the health promotion activities of older adults measure. *Public Health Nursing, 14*(2), 123–128.

Padula, C. A. (1997b). Predictors of participation in health promotion activities by elderly couples. *Journal of Family Nursing, 3*(1), 88–106.

Pender, N. J. (1987). *Health promotion in nursing practice* (2nd ed.). Norwalk, CT: Appleton & Lange.

Ratner, P. A., Bottorff, J. L., Johnson, J. L., & Hayduk, L. A. (1994). The interaction effects of gender within the Health Promotion Model. *Research in Nursing and Health, 17*, 341–350.

Riffle, K. L., Yoho, J., & Sams, J. (1989). Health-promoting behaviors, perceived social support, and self-reported health of Appalachian elderly. *Public Health Nursing, 6*(4), 204–211.

Rosenstock, I. M. (1960). What research in motivation suggests for public health. *American Journal of Public Health, 50*, 295–302.

Simmons, S. J. (1990). The Health-Promoting Self-Care System Model: Directions for nursing research and practice. *Journal of Advanced Nursing 15*, 1162–1166.

U. S. Census Bureau. (2000). Race and Hispanic or Latino. Geographic area: Pennsylvania: Urban/rural and inside/outside metropolitan area. Accessed September 7, 2003 at http://factfinder.census.gov/servlet/GCTTable?_ts 5 81015591484.

U. S. Department of Health and Human Services. (2001). *Healthy People 2010*. Boston: Jones and Bartlett.

Walker, S. N., Sechrist, K. R., & Pender, N. J. (1987). The health-promoting lifestyle profile: Development and psychometric characteristics. *Nursing Research, 36*(2), 76–81.

Watson, N., & Pulliam, L. (2000). Transgenerational health promotion. *Holistic Nursing Practice, 14*(4), 1–11.

Wieck, K. L. (2000). Health promotion for inner-city minority elders. *Journal of Community Health Nursing, 17*(3), 131–139.

Wrobel, A. J., & Shapiro, N. E. K. (1999). Conducting research with urban elders: Issues of recruitment, data collection, and home visits. *Alzheimer Disease and Associated Disorders, 13*(Suppl 1), S34–S38.

Zabalegui, A. (1994). Aging matters: Barriers to health. *Nursing Times, 90*(1), 58–61.

APPENDIX F

Health Disparities, Social Injustice, and the Culture of Nursing

Lynne S. Giddings

- ▶ ***Background:*** Nurses are well positioned to challenge institutionalized social injustices that lead to health disparities.
- ▶ ***Objective:*** The aim of this cross-cultural study was to collect stories of difference and fairness within nursing.
- ▶ ***Methods:*** The study used a life history methodology informed by feminist theory and critical social theory. Life story interviews were conducted with 26 women nurses of varying racial, cultural, sexual identity, and specialty backgrounds in the United States ($n = 13$) and Aotearoa New Zealand ($n = 13$). Participants reported having some understanding of social justice issues. They were asked to reflect on their experience of difference and fairness in their lives and specifically within nursing. Their stories were analyzed using a life history immersion method.
- ▶ ***Results:*** Nursing remains attached to the ideological construction of the "White good nurse." Taken-for-granted ideals privilege those who fit in and marginalize those who do not. The nurses experienced discrimination and unfairness, survived by living in two worlds, learned to live in contradiction, and worked surreptitiously for social justice.
- ▶ ***Discussion:*** For nurses to contribute to changing the systems and structures that maintain health disparities, the privilege of not seeing difference and the processes of mainstream violence that support the construction of the "White good nurse" must be challenged. Nurses need skills to deconstruct the marginalizing social processes that sustain inequalities in nursing and healthcare. These hidden realities—racism, sexism, heterosexism, and other forms of discrimination—will then be made visible and open to challenge.

- ▶ ***Key Words:*** discrimination · health disparities · health status · horizontal violence · marginalization · social justice

In 1978, the World Health Organization's (WHO) Constitution stated that "health is one of the fundamental rights of every human being" (WHO, 2004), but since that time the gap has widened in the health status between those who are marginalized by their social identities and those who are privileged (Ajwani, Blakely, Robson, Tobias, & Bonne, 2003; Ministry of Health, 2002; U.S. Department of Health and Human Services, 2003). Although nurses are well positioned to challenge the institutionalized social injustices within the healthcare system, discriminatory and marginalizing practices continue. Few inroads have been made into decreasing the disparities. The purpose of this cross-cultural life history study was to investigate the culture of nursing by collecting nurses' stories of difference and fairness.

Nursing has led the way in promoting awareness of cross-cultural issues (Peplau, 1952). The two movements that have most influenced nursing education, practice, and policies concerning cultural care of clients worldwide are transcultural nursing, which originated in the United States (Leininger, 1991), and cultural safety, which originated in

Aotearoa New Zealand (Ramsden, 1990; Wepa, 2005).

The theoretical positions of transcultural nursing were derived from social anthropology and the work of Madeleine Leininger. The central purpose is to use research-based knowledge to help nurses give safe, responsible, and meaningful care to people from culturally different backgrounds (Leininger, 1991). Nurses are assumed to form a politically neutral and homogeneous group; their client populations are diverse with culturally specific needs.

The cultural safety movement, in contrast, began as a political movement in the late 1980s. Nurses who were Maori (indigenous people) wished to draw attention to the place of racism in perpetuating the many social and health disparities between their cultural group and the dominant Pakeha (White) culture (Ramsden, 1993). Rather than assuming the homogeneity of nurses, cultural safety promotes their cultural self-awareness and places racism at the center of its processes. Nurses are expected to give clients culturally safe care as determined by that person or family. Although initially focused on racial cultural identity, in 2002 the definition was extended to include "but is not restricted to age or generation; gender; sexual orientation; occupation and socio-economic status; ethnic origin or migrant experience; religious or spiritual belief; and disability" (Nursing Council of New Zealand, 2002, p. 7). Similarly in the United States, other forms of discrimination have been acknowledged (Abrums & Leppa, 2001; Eliason, 1993, 1998; McDonald & Anderson, 2003); the focus, however, remains primarily on racial and ethnic differences and how cross-cultural issues affect clients and their care. The role of nursing in perpetuating discrimination in healthcare has been noted (Eliason, 1999; Taylor, 1998), and studies have been undertaken concerning the attitudes and education processes of students (Boutain & Olivares, 1999; Eliason, 1998). Studies on the many differences and related social injustices among nurses themselves were not found. This lack of critique, and the primary focus on race, creates a space in nursing for discriminatory and marginalizing practices.

Feminist scholars have critiqued internal patterns of oppression in nursing (Freshwater, 2000; Roberts, 1994; Street, 1995) linking them to its oppressed position within the hierarchy of the patriarchal healthcare system (Doering, 1992; Muff, 1982). Discriminatory practices such as stereotyping and horizontal violence have been analyzed also (Glass, 1997; McKenna, Smith, Poole, & Coverdale, 2003). Black feminist scholars in particular (Banks-Wallace, 2000; Boutain, 1999; Taylor, 1998) have drawn attention to the Anglocentric nature of nursing theory and research. What has not been explored in detail is the culture of nursing itself. The questions explored in this study were: What happens to nurses who are part of a marginalised cultural or social group? What are their experiences of difference and fairness? What happens to nurses who take a stand on social justice issues? Is there a culture of discrimination?

A LIFE HISTORY STUDY OF SOCIAL INJUSTICE WITHIN NURSING

This cross-cultural, participatory, life history study was focused on the experience of nurses who reported that they acted from an awareness of social injustice. Three assumptions underpinned this study: (a) social group differences do exist, some groups are more privileged and others are oppressed; (b) all people experience a complex interweaving of privilege and oppression; and (c) nurses' experience is a microcosm of the larger structures and systems in society. The final assumption links social injustice with its base in societal structures and the development of social consciousness, which is related to continuing political and social disparities.

■ Method

The life history methodology, an adaptation of oral history (Gluck & Patai, 1991), incorporated storytelling in the form of life story, and it was informed by feminism and critical social theory. Paulo Freire's (1972) pedagogy of empowerment influenced the participatory approach used, particularly the notion of the formation of critical consciousness (conscientization) by the process of questioning the nature of historical and social conditions. Such processes can lead to social transformation for groups as well as individuals. The interviews, therefore, were structured so the women could reflect on their lives in relation to issues of oppression, power, and social action that may have led to personal and social change (Lather, 1991).

A feminist life story approach (Gluck & Patai, 1991) was useful in capturing the women's voices and the meaning they gave to their experience of being a nurse, and it made possible the construction and analysis of narratives. The narrative accounts revealed the women as active subjects in their own stories. Also revealed were the social nature of their life experiences, the work they did to position themselves in their social world, and the value judgments that helped them make sense of it all (Chanfrault-Duchet, 1991). The personal narratives and the meaning the women gave them differed, depending on how their lives intersected with social and cultural representations of their identities. This methodological approach, therefore, was not only useful in exploring the women's experience of difference in their lives, but in showing difference.

PARTICIPANT PROFILES AND LIFE HISTORY INTERVIEWS

Life history interviews (two to three each) ranging 45–90 minutes were conducted with 26 articulate women nurses of varying racial, cultural, sexual identity, and specialty backgrounds in the United States (n = 13) and Aotearoa New Zealand (n = 13). Ages ranged 24–57 years, and years as a registered nurse ranged 1–40 years. Study procedures were approved by ethical review committees in the United States and Aotearoa New Zealand. Written consent was obtained from each participant. Standards of rigor for qualitative research were applied: specifically dependability, reflexivity, credibility, consensus, and complexity (Hall & Stevens, 1991), as reflected in the following description of the study's design.

The semistructured interviews were tape recorded in duplicate and structured to elicit stories about women's experience of difference and fairness in their lives. Initially broad open-ended questions were asked (e.g., "What has it been like for you being a nurse?") to encourage the women to follow their own thoughts and tell the stories that mattered. Conversations developed and became more focused as ideas evolved reflecting the narrative process of making joint meaning (Riessman, 2002).

Cultural and social differences between the researcher and the researched create unequal relations of power (Smith, 1999). Prior to receiving consent, the researcher acknowledged her identity as nurse and midwife, Pakeha New Zealander, lesbian-identified, and middle-aged woman. At the first interview, cultural and identity differences were acknowledged. These were "the elephants sleeping in the room," influencing what was said and how it was perceived. Our *cultural filters* led us to avoid trigger statements known to produce cross-cultural misunderstandings or prejudiced responses. Despite this, some 'elephants' woke up. The energy change was instantaneous, recognized by both people, the talk moving to firmer ground. A few times there was re-engagement, negotiating to return to controversial terrain, a gift from generous participants, patient in their effort to assist the researcher's conscientization (Freire, 1972). The women's stories were further filtered through the situated relationship, the conversation structured by a generalized culture, reflecting the power relationships within it (Spender, 1980). Therefore it is acknowledged that the use of an interview rather than another form of communication (e.g., dance or art) structured this study to reflect the dominant discourse of the cultures in which the women were immersed.

Prior to the second interview, tapes were transcribed and an initial analysis undertaken to determine the predominant stories. The women listened to their first interview on a duplicate tape. This enabled their independent reflection and knowledge of their own story. Reflections were shared at the second interview. Listening to their voices tell their stories "was an unbelievably deep emotional experience" (Anna-NZ, Maori); "I had to stop driving because I couldn't stop crying" (Beverly-US, European).

DATA ANALYSIS AND INTERPRETATION

The mutual review of the women's stories began the first level analysis. Focused life stories or snippets were constructed to ensure the women's voices were not lost during thematic analysis. These included demographic details, stories from the women's early years (early life story), and of their experiences in nursing (nurse-story). The focus here is on the women's nurse-stories, but it is acknowledged that the early life stories contributed to their framing. Biographical notes were kept sparse for reasons of confidentiality. Each woman reviewed her story to provide affirmation and approval of the content. They told how this process altered their understandings, challenged assumptions, and contributed to personal change. As a consequence of this analysis, categorizing themes became apparent. A second level of analysis substantiated a meta-story, *not fitting-in to nursing*. Here "meta-story" does not refer to an all-encompassing archetype, but to an umbrella story incorporating the meta-themes of the life story experiences that had meaning for the women (Chase, 2003).

An immersion analysis style was used. This involved a cyclical process of listening and relistening to the tapes while reading transcripts on-screen. Life story snippets were constructed, then data were coded for life story themes and beginning categorizes were made. Memos were made throughout the process. The coding and categorization continued until there was confidence that the meta-themes had captured recurring similarities and differences within the women's stories. Focus groups in both countries provided a third level of analysis. The majority of the women attended and with laughter and tears, discussed, argued, verified, and "troubled" the interpretation. Changes were made. Since completion of the study, a fourth level of analysis has been carried out using a dialectical reasoning process (Gadow, 1995) to construct a three-position theoretical inclusive model of social consciousness (Giddings, 2005).

■ Findings

Analysis of the 26 nurses' stories resulted in the meta-story, *not fitting-in to nursing*. The life story meta-themes and subthemes focus on their experience of unfairness and their responses. Narrative exemplars of each theme are given in Tables 1 and 2. Excerpts are indexed with pseudonym, country (United States or New Zealand), and cultural identity as agreed by the participants (African American = AA; European = E; Hispanic = H; Asian = A; Pakeha = P; Maori = M). To discuss the findings, two life story meta-themes are used, *experiencing unfairness* and *trying to survive*.

LIFE STORY META-THEME I: EXPERIENCING UNFAIRNESS

How the women experienced unfairness was linked in part to how they were perceived as different, the period in which they began their nursing education, and their cultural and nursing practice contexts. Though these layered contexts created complexity and differences of experience, there were shared meanings and understandings.

Theme 1: Difficulties Getting into Nursing. Women of color, from working class backgrounds, or with a disability felt the unfairness of the nursing system even prior to "being admitted." Molly (USA-AA) tells of being rejected by a nursing school in a southern state in 1956. Her story captures the blatant discrimination faced by African Americans wanting to become registered nurses at that time (Table 1). Accepted into "a more liberal college," Molly has had a successful career in nursing and is now a professor, "not that it has been easy." Nearly 40 years later Lisa (USA-AA) felt more subtle discrimination: "I had high grades in a previous degree . . . and the concern about the health and healthcare of minorities got me in, but that first day, I was sure shocked to find I was the only black face in my class . . . I felt like I was *their* success story!"

Theme 2: Most Suitable (But Not Quite) for Nursing. Even though Ariel (USA-AA) graduated with honors, she was enrolled into a diploma rather than a baccalaureate program because it was "more suitable." The dominant culture career advisor knew Ariel's proper place. Although Ariel experienced blocks and barriers at "every step on the way" she went on to get a baccalaureate degree and PhD. "I have survived," she says, "and I am still surviving in a system that says I can't." The stories of Jo (USA-H) and Anna (NZ-M) capture how academic achievement does not necessarily determine career choice (Table 1).

Theme 3: Assumptions of Sameness. All the African American women noted it was assumed they were the same, knew each other, and got along well together. The heterogeneity within was ignored. Maori women agreed (Maj, Table 1). Homogenizing of identity was reported by all the minority women. "Know one, know them all," chuckled Fiona (USA-E) who identified as lesbian. By creating a generalized *other*, stereotypes developed that not only served to reinforce negative images but also rendered difference invisible.

Related to "sameness" was an assumption that all women deemed of minority status had the cultural perspective on health issues. Recently graduated students talked of "fearing the liberal teacher who tries to be inclusive" and how they were expected to be experts on the health issues of their cultural group. Lisa's story illustrates these hegemonic and racist-based assumptions (Table 1).

Theme 4: Differences Take on Symbolic Meaning. Women whose differences were overt told stories of how people responded to their appearance before anything else (Table 1). Molly's stories demonstrate how skin color is the first thing people respond to. Visitors coming to see "the professor" would "initially walk right past me with barely a glance"; ask her if "the professor was in"; ask her for a cup of coffee; or shake the hand of her White professional assistant saying, "hello professor."

Although openly identifying as lesbian created some risks for Shadow, it was living in a wheelchair that elicited "blatant stereotyping and discrimination." Her acceptance *into* nursing did not mean acceptance *in* nursing. "Some nurses would hover, talk about me in front of me as though I was deaf, and make it clear they expected me to not succeed in doing nursing work."

Theme 5: It's a Level Playing Field—They are Advantaged by Their Minority Status. Women of color in both countries told stories of mainstream nursing culture's lack of awareness of privilege and internalized racism. This was made visible in their mainstream colleagues' notions about minority status. The African American teachers with official responsibility to support minority students told how students' retention and success became their problem. For Maori women it was the success of cultural safety: "we Maori nurses have become its visible face." Negative attitudes toward cultural safety were most often expressed indirectly. Anna (NZ-M), who was successfully working with Maori families in her community, was challenged by her supervisor when she was talking about her work and asked, "Is this about community health or that Maori thing?" The Maori women also noted that joking was often used to "put down" and dismiss serious issues pertaining to being Maori. Not joining in the laughter was interpreted as "not having a sense of humor" or "being oversensitive." Jo, who believed a "glass ceiling" exists for minority groups, told a story that captured the dominant culture belief of a level playing field (Table 1).

Women of color experienced the effects of a related assumption: any success was because of their minority status, not their ability. Jo's story illustrates how racist assumptions can be embedded in a person's thinking (Table 1).

Theme 6: What Happens If You Do Not Obey the Rules? Some White, heterosexual, and middle-class women were surprised when they found themselves marginalized. This occurred when they "stepped out of line" by standing up for an issue or a socially marginalized person, did not take part in negatively criticizing or labeling colleagues or clients, challenged "bullying," or questioned a policy or a person who was in authority. They were accused of being "disrespectful," "inappropriate," "uncaring," and "not nice." The punishments included being "watched" or "checked up on." They "had to work with the senior nurse on afternoon shift," were "kept working late," were "reported to the teacher," and were "not spoken to by the other nurses." The privilege accorded their color, sexual identity, and class had become secondary to the interpretation of their behavior. These women told many stories of *horizontal violence:* "It is everywhere in nursing."

The women's stories also highlighted the contradictions experienced within the various nursing contexts and the consequences of nonconformity and independent thinking. Jeanine (US-E), a student, made a suggestion during a staff meeting. Following it, a nurse told her, "You just don't fit in to nursing. That's not the way nurses think ... you just have to learn to obey the rules."

When Louisa (NZ-P) tried to advocate for her patients, her teachers told her to "tone it down and fit in" or she would not pass her clinical. Miriam's (NZ-P) story of being labeled a "trouble maker" highlights the pressure on students to conform. It also demonstrates how horizontal violence is not confined within nursing but extends to patients (Table 1).

All the women in the study told stories of blatant and subtle marginalization (see Table 1). They gave many examples of violence from mainstream nursing in their everyday work, including the withholding of information by other nurses in positions of authority, not being heard at meetings when offering information or ideas that were later credited to a dominant culture person, and not receiving relevant information or material to assist in their work. Anna (NZ-M) tried to set up a clinic for Maori families. She was given "hand-me-downs from other clinics" and her initiatives to improve the services to Maori were blocked by nurses in authority.

A response to nurses who were perceived to be breaking the rules was the "scurrying" between dominant and outsider groups. The women of color told stories of what happened when two or more of them got together in the presence of White nurses. "Someone would always come and ask 'What's going on here?'" Molly noticed. "I would make a joke about it. When it's a thousand of them it's a group thing; when it's two or three of us, it's a conspiracy!" Ginny (NZ-E) reflected, "We scurry to deal with our differences. I used to think it was my job to uphold the status quo. The outcome of a shift in power would be upsetting." The pressure to "conform and be nice" came from all quarters—peers, senior nurses, classroom and clinical teachers, managers, and the medical staff. This theme threaded through all the women's stories.

LIFE STORY META-THEME II: TRYING TO SURVIVE

The women's stories showed how social consciousness shifted as they experienced being marginalized. They developed different ways of coping and working.

Theme 1: Trying to Survive by Leading Two Lives. The women of color told stories of surviving by denying their cultural identity and keeping their two lives separate. As a student, Sue did not identify as Maori. "I never took my classmates home," she said, "It was like I had two lives." Maj was so

Table 1. Life Story Meta-Theme 1: Experiencing Unfairness

Experiencing Unfairness	Life Story Subthemes With Narrative Exemplars
Theme 1	Difficulties getting into nursing • *I wrote the school, "I realize the reason you didn't accept me was because of my color. I did meet the criteria. I was valedictorian of my class. I surpassed some of the White students whom you're accepting, but I wanted to let you know, it's OK." It was not really OK, but I wanted to let them know I was aware of the racism.* Molly (US-AA) • *I had to push for a second much more in-depth interview after being rejected on my first application. The person the first time around saw my disability—saw my wheelchair, that's all she saw.* Shadow (US-E)
Theme 2	Most suitable (but not quite) for nursing • *I was encouraged by an Hispanic teacher to apply for a scholarship. My grades were high enough for other professional careers such as medicine, but being Hispanic and my own lack of expectations made nursing the most suitable choice.* Jo (US-H) • *I was a Maori with brains—that was the problem. There was a tendency to believe that Maori were stupid. I was told I was going nursing. I never quite fitted. I find myself becoming very angry about the fact that I wasn't encouraged to look at other alternatives.* Anna (NZ-M)
Theme 3	Assumptions of sameness • *I was employed to teach my clinical specialty but I became associated with Maori issues and cultural safety. . . . I was not prepared for all the expectations. . . . Many of the Pakeha teachers assumed that we* [Maj and Maori teachers] *were joined at the hip.* Maj (NZ-M) • *I could sense it coming, "Now Lisa, what is the Black perspective on such and such?" In my third year I plucked up courage and challenged the content of a course because African American perspectives were invisible. The instructor barked at me and said, "Well I gave you the opportunity to do that."* Lisa (US-(A))
Theme 4	Differences take on symbolic meaning • *This doctor asked if I "could find the nurse on the floor?" I stood in front of him in my RN uniform. I watched as he became more and more agitated with what he saw as my noncompliance with his request. "Look at my name tag," I said quietly. He responded with confusion and embarrassment but he never made that mistake again.* Rebecca (US-AA) • *I was in my full RN uniform and working with another African American nurse in the recovery room and this doctor told the supervisor that he didn't think it was right that two nurse aides should be working back there.* Rebecca (US-AA)
Theme 5	It's a level playing field—"they" are advantaged by their minority status • *I set up promotion support groups for all staff. They were going well with some success and then came complaints from dominant culture*

(*continued*)

Table 1. (continued)

Experiencing Unfairness	Life Story Subthemes With Narrative Exemplars
	people in the administrative hierarchy and I was attacked for "spoon feeding" minority workers. Jo (US-H) • *People often only see my minority identity and ignore my academic success. I was truly shocked when a colleague in my postgraduate class said: "Oh, you are so lucky you are one of the few minority people in the program. . . . Anything that you would do, the school would see to it that you're still going to graduate."* Jo (US-H)
Theme 6	What happens if you don't obey the rules: • *I stopped to talk with a patient during a "pan round": We didn't talk for long and I got back to my duties. But the Charge Nurse yelled, "We don't have time to sit and talk with patients" and refused to give all the patients their dessert that night!* Miriam (NZ-P) • *I read this research paper that oil and "meths" is not helpful for back rubs and I went to the Charge Nurse in the orthopedic ward and I said, "Guess what, I have got this fantastic information we can change how we do things, we don't have to do these 4 hourly rubs. . . . " And she was furious at me, and sent me down to the Matron for insubordination!* Irene (NZ-P, Lesbian)

"Pakehafied" that she was not aware she had two lives. Her parents ensured she spoke English at home and she was educated in the White school system. She noticed that at times she was treated differently from other nurses but did not think it was because she was Maori. Anna worked hard to keep her "Maoriness" invisible at work and only relaxed when she returned home. In contrast, Ariel was very aware of her cultural identity and worked hard to hide it. From an early age she learned to mimic a White person's accent and associated mostly with "White blue-eyed girl friends." Though Ariel reclaimed her identity in her twenties, she was continually "shocked" when other nurses discriminated against her. All the women talked about how slow they were to realize that it was their difference and its related stereotype that people responded to, not them personally.

The women of color in both countries told of how at first they tried to survive by fitting in. They carefully watched and copied the dominant culture nurses and made sure they adhered rigidly to the rules. Molly noted that "White dominant culture folk can break the rules . . . and it isn't seen. A Black person is assumed to have broken the rules. Just by being there, we're guilty" (Table 2).

All the lesbian-identified women in the study were White. They could maintain their privilege and lead separate lives by passing as heterosexual. Closeting to survive was a common theme in nearly all their stories but the cost involved was exemplified by Kate (USA-E) who told how she "flip flopped" between bouts of drinking, going to bars, attending church, and denying her lesbian identity (see Table 2). In contrast, Maureen (NZ-E) survived for many years by being a "chameleon." "I only presented that which fitted in with the cardboard cut-out nurse. I would be reasonable and nice when I really wanted to scratch their eyes out." The cost of Maureen's niceness

Table 2. Life Story Meta-Theme 2: Trying to Survive

Trying to Survive	Life Story Theme With Narrative Exemplars
Theme 1: Trying to survive by leading two lives	• *I felt I was always coming from the back foot. There were huge assumptions made about my knowledge of the dominant culture and how I should operate in it. Consequently I found myself continuously worried that I was going to do something wrong. I was always a bit frightened to say anything or do anything in case I put my foot in it. I only felt safe when I walked through my door. And that still happens even now.* Anna (NZ-M) • *When I first came "out" I felt incredibly liberated. All the pieces were falling together. It made total sense. Then the guilt started in. I had heard all this stuff about gay people. I thought that all I needed was to just choose not to do it and pray myself out of it. So if I wasn't a good Mormon person, then I must have been in this other category—a horrible person. So it didn't matter what I did, drugs, drinking, sex. It didn't matter because I had already crossed over the line.* Kate (USA-E)
Theme 2: Trying to survive by living and transiting between two worlds	• *I'll shave down and survive in their world and as soon as 5:00 comes, I unshave and get into my world where I am my own self. So I show two faces. That's why we [AAs] are so hypertensive. It's because we have to deal in two worlds. White folks don't. It's their world. They operate the same way in their work world, their home, and in their environment. For us it's like wearing "two hats." I become another person when I walk out my door.* Molly (US-AA)
Theme 3: Living in contradiction and working surreptitiously	• *Straddling two worlds is positive to me. Not being part of the privileged group makes me a privileged person. People in the dominant culture can't slip over into my culture but I move freely within theirs . . . you can't give that to somebody—I live it. . . . My more White features allow me to pass so I do not get the same discriminatory treatment as some of my minority friends. Also I'm highly skilled at not disclosing a lot about myself unless I purposefully intend to do that. . . . I can talk to you probably for a whole year and you will know maybe five facts about me!* Jo (US-H) • *A Maori man was dying and his family wanted to take him home. The doctors wouldn't let him go. . . . So I kept opening his window because his spirit had to go and people kept shutting his window. We had a battle with this window. His family would look at me and go "Oh aye," because they knew what I was doing. . . . It is things like that that I try to do. But you never let on why you are doing them.* Sue (NZ-M)

was repeated episodes of depression and the label "mentally ill." Her involvement in the study led her to reflect on why she stayed in nursing "putting up with the bullying and all that."

Other women survived by trying to conform. Participant 3 (NZ-A), for example, worked to assimilate by "trying to fit in" and trying to "do better than they did." She found that when she let go of trying to please, she became more authentic with her colleagues and clients. No matter how hard some of these women tried to "fit in," their difference meant they never quite made it. The cost of *leading two lives* was struggling with guilt, being self-blaming, and feeling inauthentic.

Theme 2: Trying to Survive by Living and Transiting Between Two Worlds. The majority of women talked of the demands and costs of moving between multiple worlds. Molly illustrates the process well (see Table 2). The women of color reported their automatic "little rituals" as they transited between home and work. Lisa has "Black music blasting from my car radio and I'm usually singing. By the time I get there I'm ready." Rebecca dresses up, applies make-up, and makes sure that when she gets to work "everything's just perfect." Lesbian women talked about "re-positioning" and getting into "het-speak" as they walked on duty so they did not "out" themselves. "We have to be careful to say 'I' and not 'we' and not be specific about what 'we' did at the weekend," said Louisa.

The transiting process between worlds was recognized by nearly all of the women. One White, heterosexual woman, however, was mystified by this concept. She lived in a world not divided into parts, seeing herself as part of the mainstream.

Theme 3: Living in Contradiction and Working Surreptitiously. A number of women talked of the contradictory and tenuous nature of their relationship with nursing. Their attention shifted from focusing on the mainstream culture to looking after themselves and they tended to work with marginal groups of clients. The women described the process of *living in contradiction* in various ways. Jo took seriously the responsibility that came with having an education, seeing her ability to straddle two cultures as positive. She could maintain a private and a public self (Table 2). Beverly, in contrast, was open about who she was and what she thought and chose when *not* to be "out." Unlike the other lesbian women in the study, she was "out" to most of her clients and all her students. "It's often the first time that the conversation has been in the room," she declared. "If it's not acknowledged from the front of the room, it ain't in the room, you know!" Beverly had been a social activist for many years, openly challenging everything that she saw as unfair, but learned to conserve her energy and choose her fights.

Working surreptitiously was the way women of color worked with their own people. They "made space" for clients and colleagues who were "not treated right." Maori women talked of how they would give culturally appropriate care "out of sight" of Pakeha managers and colleagues. Sue's story illustrates this (Table 2).

White heterosexual women marginalized by their stand on social injustice directed their energies toward making each action "count for something." They could practice with integrity by *working surreptitiously.* White women also talked of the responsibility to take a stand on social justice issues because of the privilege of their color. Fiona argued that diversity directly challenges White, middle class, and academic nursing. "It's threatening to you and me. We would not be having this conversation if we truly valued diversity in nursing. Not only because of the subject matter, but because you and I wouldn't be in our privileged positions."

■ Discussion

The feminist participatory approach and three levels of analysis made visible the diversity of the women's experiences and gave a richness and depth to the data that supported the meta-story: *not fitting-in to nursing.* Transferability of the findings to other settings was strengthened by the inclusion of a variety of socially recognized marginalized groups from two countries, and within the purposive sample, a range of ages and nursing specialties. Limitations were the inclusion of women who reported that they acted from an awareness of social injustice, the noninclusion of men, and the predominance of women with advanced nursing education. Life story interviews with mainstream nurses and men would usefully uncover further complexities of issues of difference within nursing.

According to the study's findings, there were assumptions made within nursing as to who could and who could not be a "good nurse." It became evident that in Aotearoa New Zealand and the United States, the stereotypical ideal nurse was female, White, middle class, heterosexual, able bodied, and nice, with the added qualities of the mythical Nightingale nurse, obedient and nurturing (Reverby, 1987; Roberts & Group, 1995). The problem with this taken-for-granted ideal was that it served to privilege those who fitted in and marginalized those who did not.

The hegemonic construction most evident in the stories was the ideal of the "White good nurse." Nurses of color in both countries talked of how they were confronted everyday with denial of their right to be a "real" nurse. They could not pass the ideological barrier no matter how hard they tried to fit in. Though different historical and political contexts created some differences in expression, all women of color in Aotearoa New Zealand and the United States experienced structural, ideological, and personal manifestations of racism within nursing. They instantly recognized each other's stories of discrimination and survival, such as the assumptions of homogeneity: they are "all the same" and are "all" advantaged by their marginalized status. Shared too were the stories of off-hand or joking dismissal of their efforts to improve the health status of their people. The tears shed during the interviews were often not for themselves but for the generic, global experience of racism. The hegemonic nature of the archetypal ideal of the "White good nurse," however, was not limited to women of color. It extended to women who, although White, were marginalized for other ideological transgressions. Openly identifying as lesbian or challenging hierarchical authority was viewed as the ideal's antithesis. The ideological assumptions and associated discriminatory practices captured in the construction of the "White good nurse" are so integrated within the routines of everyday mainstream nursing that they are normalized. It is the normalization of social injustice within the constructed meanings and everyday routines of nursing practice that makes discrimination invisible.

It could be assumed that nurses who are marginalized advocate for marginalized clients and promote self-determining policies. This is not necessarily so. Many in the study were silenced by their efforts to conform and fit in. Some worked surreptitiously within mainstream systems; others worked openly for social justice and social change, but often on the margins of mainstream nursing. The nurses who were different and who survived in nursing knowingly stood on the margins of their profession. Aware they would never fit in with the cultural ideals captured in the construction of the "White good nurse," they developed unique ways of dealing with their everyday experiences of social injustice. They recognized the contradictions of their position and worked alongside mainstream nursing, not in it.

The unjust expectation that marginalized groups provide the solution for problems caused by nursing's discriminatory systems and processes was apparent in this study. Maori nurses were expected to be the cultural safety experts, students who belonged to "ethnic groups" were responsible for the visibility of their specific health issues, and lesbians in their work context were expected to deal with all issues relating to lesbianism. The popular solution to the "minority nurse problem" in both countries to increase the intake of racial minority people into nursing, teaching, and research (Andrews, 2003; Leeman,

Goeppinger, Funk, & Roland, 2003), without first establishing strategies to counter institutionalized racism, reflects this "let them fix it" approach. The emphasis on "the minority nurse" also keeps the focus on racial differences, inadvertently reinforcing a hierarchy of "-isms." Differences and related social injustices, such as sexism and heterosexism, can become relegated to the margins. Social consciousness can remain culturally specific rather than broad based and inclusive.

Mainstream violence made visible within this study affects all nurses, but not all are its direct recipients and not all see it. By not seeing or naming the violence embedded in the everyday social injustices within nursing, mainstream nurses collude with exploitation and abuse, including their own (Glass, 1997). It is also apparent from the women's stories that they do not see the benefits they derive from maintaining the status quo of injustice. As Frye (1983) described, they are privileged not to see; when a person is part of the mainstream they can ignore differences, which are normalized as "that's the way it is."

The stories of everyday violence were not confined within nursing's professional boundaries as the more commonly used descriptor "horizontal violence" would indicate. It affects all within the healthcare system, especially those with least power, the clients. Socially marginalized clients are the most vulnerable to discriminatory practices of nurses (Cartwright, 1988; Gamble, 1997). The everyday realities of marginalization within nursing intersect with the everyday reality of health disparities within the client population; both are sustained by mainstream violence.

The findings of this study, though highlighting the importance of challenging racism, support the use of inclusive rather than specific definitions of social consciousness. A primary focus on one "-ism" not only dismisses people's reality; it ignores the multiplicity of oppression. Whether an act is seen as discriminatory depends on where one is standing. It is the hidden nature of discrimination within the nursing profession that maintains the privilege of those who fit the ideal of "White good nurse" and the marginalization of those who do not.

Lynne S. Giddings, PhD, RN, is Associate Professor, Auckland University of Technology, New Zealand.

Accepted for publication May 6, 2005.

Thank you to the 26 courageous women who dare to acknowledge and make visible their difference in nursing. They are the everyday leaders and heroes who challenge the institutionalized systems and processes of discrimination that underpin healthcare disparities. Thanks to my partner Kate Prebble and many friends who said "just do it."

Corresponding author: Lynne S. Giddings, PhD, RN, Auckland University of Technology, Private Bag 92006, Auckland 1020, New Zealand (e-mail: lynne.giddings@aut.ac.nz).

REFERENCES

Abrums, M. E., & Leppa, C. (2001). Beyond cultural competence: Teaching about race, gender, class, and sexual orientation. *Journal of Nursing Education, 40*(6), 270–275.

Ajwani, S., Blakely, T., Robson, B., Tobias, M., & Bonne, M. (2003). *Decades of disparity: Ethnic mortality trends in New Zealand 1980–1999.* Wellington, NZ.: Ministry of Health & University of Otago.

Andrews, D. R. (2003). Lessons from the past: Confronting past discriminatory practices to alleviate the nursing shortage through increased professional diversity. *Journal of Professional Nursing, 19*(5), 289–294.

Banks-Wallace, J. (2000). Womanist ways of knowing: Theoretical considerations for research with African American women. *ANS: Advances in Nursing Science, 22*(3), 33–45.

Boutain, D. M. (1999). Critical nursing scholarship: Exploring critical social theory with African American studies. *ANS: Advances in Nursing Science, 21*(4), 37–47.

Boutain, D. M., & Olivares, S. A. (1999). Nurturing educational multiculturalism in psychosocial nursing: Creating new possibilities through inclusive conversations. *Archives of Psychiatric Nursing, 13*(5), 234–239.

Cartwright, S. R. (1988). *The report of the Committee of Inquiry into Allegations Concerning the Treatment of Cervical Cancer at the National Women's Hospital and into Other Related Matters.* Auckland, NZ: Government Printing Office.

Chanfrault-Duchet, M. F. (1991). Narrative structures, social models, and symbolic representation in the life story. In S. B. Gluck & D. Patai (Eds.), *Women's words: The feminist practice of oral history* (pp. 77–92). New York: Routledge.

Chase, S. E. (2003). Learning to listen: Narrative principles in a qualitative research methods course. In R. Josselson, A. Lieblich, & D. P. McAdams (Eds.), *Up close and personal: The teaching and learning of narrative research* (pp. 79–99). Washington, DC: American Psychological Association.

Doering, L. (1992). Power and knowledge in nursing: A feminist poststructuralist view. *ANS: Advances in Nursing Science, 14*(4), 24–33.

Eliason, M. J. (1993). Cultural diversity in nursing care: The lesbian, gay, or bisexual client. *Journal of Transcultural Nursing, 5*(1), 14–20.

Eliason, M. J. (1998). Correlates of prejudice in nursing students. *Journal of Nursing Education, 37*(1), 27–29.

Eliason, M. J. (1999). Nursing's role in racism and African American women's health. *Health Care for Women International, 20*(2), 209–219.

Freire, P. (1972). *Pedagogy of the oppressed.* Hammondsworth: Penguin Books.

Freshwater, D. (2000). Crosscurrents: Against cultural narration in nursing. *Journal of Advanced Nursing, 32*, 481–484.

Frye, M. (1983). *The politics of reality: Essays in feminist theory.* Trumansburg, New York: The Crossing Press.

Gadow, S. (1995). Clinical epistemology: A dialectic of nursing assessment. *Canadian Journal of Nursing Research, 27*(2), 25–34.

Gamble, V. N. (1997). Under the shadow of Tuskegee: African Americans and health care. *American Journal of Public Health, 87*, 1773–1778.

Giddings, L. S. (2005). A theoretical model of social conciousness. *Advances in Nursing Science, 28*(3), 224–239.

Glass, N. (1997). Horizontal violence in nursing: Celebrating conscious healing strategies. *The Australian Journal of Holistic Nursing, 4*(2), 15–23.

Gluck, S. B., & Patai, D. (Eds.). (1991). *Women's words: The feminist practice of oral history.* New York: Routledge.

Hall, J. M., & Stevens, P. E. (1991). Rigor in feminist research. *ANS: Advances in Nursing Science, 13*(3), 16–29.

Lather, P. (1991). *Getting smart: Feminist research and pedagogy with/in the postmodern.* New York: Routledge.

Leeman, J., Goeppinger, J., Funk, S., & Roland, E. J. (2003). An enriched research experience for minority undergraduates: A step toward increasing the number of minority nurse researchers. *Nursing Outlook, 51*(1), 20–24.

Leininger, M. M. (Ed.). (1991). *Culture care diversity & universality: A theory of nursing.* New York: National League for Nursing Press.

McDonald, C., & Anderson, B. (2003). The view from somewhere: Locating lesbian experience in women's health. *Health Care for Women International, 24*(8), 697–711.

McKenna, B. G., Smith, N. A., Poole, S. J., & Coverdale, J. H. (2003). Horizontal violence: Experiences of registered nurses in their first year of practice. *Journal of Advanced Nursing, 42*(1), 90–96.

Ministry of Health. (2002). *Reducing inequalities in health.* Wellington, NZ: Author.

Muff, J. (1982). *Socialization, sexism, and stereotyping: Women's issues in nursing.* St. Louis: Mosby.

Nursing Council of New Zealand. (2002). *Guidelines for cultural safety, the Treaty of Waitangi, and Maori health in nursing and midwifery education and practice.* Wellington, NZ: Author.

Peplau, H. E. (1952). *Interpersonal relations in nursing: A conceptual frame of reference for psychodynamic nursing.* New York: Putnam.

Ramsden, I. (1990). *Kawa Whakaruruhau: Cultural safety in nursing education in Aotearoa.* Wellington, NZ: Ministry of Education.

Ramsden, I. (1993). Cultural safety in nursing education in Aotearoa. *Nursing Praxis in New Zealand, 8*(3), 4–10.

Reverby, S. M. (1987). *Ordered to care: The dilemma of American nursing 1850–1945.* New York: Cambridge University Press.

Riessman, C. K. (2002). Doing justice: positioning the interpreter in narrative work. In W. Patterson (Ed.), *Strategic narrative: New perspectives on the power of personal and cultural stories* (pp. 195–216). Lanham, MA: Lexington Books.

Roberts, J. I., & Group, T. M. (1995). *Feminism and nursing: An historical perspective on power, status, and political activism in the nursing profession.* Westport, CT: Praeger.

Roberts, S. J. (1994). Oppressed group behavior: Implications for nursing. *Revolution–Journal of Nurse Empowerment, 4*(3), 28–35.

Smith, L. T. (1999). *Decolonizing methodologies: Research and indigenous peoples.* Dunedin, NZ: University of Otago Press.

Spender, D. (1980). *Man made language.* Thetford, Norfolk: Routledge & Kegan Paul.

Street, A. F. (1995). *Nursing replay: Researching nursing culture together.* Melbourne, Australia: Churchill Livingstone.

Taylor, J. Y. (1998). Womanism: A methodologic framework for African American women. *ANS: Advances in Nursing Science, 21*(1), 53–64.

U.S. Department of Health and Human Services. (2003). *National healthcare disparities report.* Rockville, MD: Agency for Healthcare Research and Quality.

Wepa, D. (Ed.). (2005). *Cultural safety in Aotearoa New Zealand.* Auckland, NZ: Pearson Education New Zealand.

World Health Organization. (2004). Health and human rights. Retrieved November 27, 2004, from http://www.who.int/hhr/en/.

APPENDIX G

Postoperative Arm Massage: A Support for Women With Lymph Node Dissection

Cheryl Forchuk • Pat Baruth • Monique Prendergast
Ronald Holliday • Ruth Bareham • Susan Brimner
Valerie Schulz • Yee Ching Lilian Chan • Nadine Yammine

- ***Purpose/objective:*** To evaluate the usefulness of arm massage from a significant other following lymph node dissection surgery.
- ***Design:*** Randomized clinical trial with a pretest-posttest design. Data were collected prior to surgery, within 24 hours post surgery, within 10 to 14 days post surgery, and 4 months post surgery.
- ***Sample:*** 59 women, aged 21 to 78 undergoing lymph node dissection surgery and who had a significant other with them during the postoperative period.
- ***Methods:*** Subjects were randomly assigned to intervention and control groups. Subjects' significant others in the intervention group were first taught, then performed arm massage as a postoperative support measure.
- ***Research main variables:*** Variables included postoperative pain, family strengths and stressors, range of motion, and health related costs.
- ***Findings:*** Participants reported a reduction in pain in the immediate postoperative period and better shoulder function.
- ***Conclusion:*** Arm massage decreased pain and discomfort related to surgery, and promoted a sense of closeness and support amongst subjects and their significant other.
- ***Implication for nursing practice:*** Postoperative massage therapy for women with lymph node dissection provided therapeutic benefits for patients and their significant other. Nurses can offer effective alternative interventions along with standard procedures in promoting optimal health.

- ***Key Words:*** Arm massage · Lymph node dissection · Pain reduction

Women diagnosed with breast cancer frequently undergo lymph node surgery to assist in the staging of the disease. The pain and discomfort from this surgery can create an additional burden at this point in their journey. In addition to the immediate postsurgical pain, women may experience longer-term sequelae, such as reduced range of motion (ROM) and function in the affected arm, and/or lymphedema.[1–4] The purpose of this investigation was to examine the usefulness of arm massage by a significant other in the immediate postoperative period.

■ Current Knowledge

Breast cancer is a serious disease with an estimated lifetime risk of around 1 in 9 for every woman in Canada and the United States. Breast cancer is the most common cancer to affect women (excluding nonmelanoma skin cancer).[5,6] Although the mortality rate from breast cancer has been consistently decreasing, the rate of detection of breast cancer has steadily risen; this pattern is occurring due to the screening programs and improved treatment methods.[5] For those women diagnosed with the disease, current management includes some type of breast surgery and/or adjuvant therapy. Surgical options include a partial mastectomy/lumpectomy with axillary node dissection, or modified radical mastectomy with axillary node dissection. Emotionally, both surgeries can be devastating for women and their significant others. Following surgery, women work through the turmoil of the cancer diagnosis, as well as disturbances to body image, pain, and altered sensation, including numbness/tingling to the underside of the affected arm.[2–4]

LYMPH NODE DISSECTION

During lymph node dissection surgery, the woman's arm is draped and abducted as needed throughout the procedure. The positioning of the arm during surgery can cause pain from muscle cramping and stiffness in the immediate postoperative period. Discomfort may lead to a reluctance or difficulty in moving the arm. Further complications may include reduced range of motion and fluid accumulation.[1,2,4,7] In studies investigating weakness, stiffness, pain, and ROM restriction of the arm following breast surgery, pain and loss of sensation were reported by greater than 50% of patients.[1,2,8–10]

MASSAGE

Massage has been used for breast cancer patients who develop lymphedema. Lymphedema or swelling of the affected arm is a potential complication related specifically to lymph node removal. Lymphedema is a complication found in about 12% of all women who have undergone breast surgery and lymph dissection[2] and can constitute a handicap for patients and impede their daily functional abilities[1,2,10,11]; massage therapy or manual lymph drainage may be recommended.[9,12,13] Physiotherapists generally accept the notion of gentle massage, or effleurage strokes. Self-administered retrograde massage and backward massage strokes have been routinely prescribed to patients and have been included in a multidisciplinary treatment approach for lymphedema.[9]

Nurses, physical therapists, and massage therapists commonly practice a technique using hand strokes from the distal portion of the limb to the proximal in a circular pattern[14]; this helps to redirect fluid from one area of the body to another. Furthermore, effleurage, light manual rubbing,[12] a classical type of massage, retrograde self-massage, and gentle, rhythmic stroking may result in a mild pressure gradient, assisting in removing edema from the affected limb; these techniques may be administered by a properly trained therapist, nurse, or by the patient's significant other following adequate instructions and proper demonstrations.[15]

Massage therapy has been well documented in the literature as an effective treatment intervention for lymphedema secondary to breast surgery.[9,12,14,16,17] However, the concept of massage therapy as a preventative measure to the development of lymphedema has not been described in the literature.

PAIN

Massage therapy has also been used frequently as a nonpharmacological alternative to reduce pain.[12,18,19] Bredin[20] determined that massage therapy reduced numbness and pain of the affected arm. Weinrich and Weinrich[21] found that massage decreased the intensity of pain in male cancer patients. Gibson[22] and Joachim[23] concluded that massage assisted in providing better control over pain.

RANGE OF MOTION

Le Vu et al[1] concluded that massage therapy improved the range of motion in the shoulder of the affected arm. Patients that were subjected to circular massage and mobilization of their arm experienced a 15% improvement in shoulder extension and an 18% improvement in abducting their affected shoulder. Consequently, Le Vu et al[1] recommend initiation of massage therapy and mobilization of the affected limb on the first day postoperatively.

▪ Hypotheses

It was hypothesized that individuals receiving arm massage from a significant other following lymph node dissection surgery would have greater immediate comfort and fewer functional constraints compared to women receiving the standard postoperative treatment. Functional constraints were defined as constraints that affect women's ability to use their arm and shoulder in activities of daily living.

SUBHYPOTHESES

Specific subhypotheses considered in addressing immediate comfort examined differences between individuals receiving arm massage from a significant other following lymph node dissection surgery and control groups, receiving standard postoperative treatment, in relation to

1. reduction of pain; and
2. perceived control and comfort of significant other.

Subhypotheses associated with fewer functional constraints in individuals receiving arm massage from a significant other following lymph node dissection surgery at 2 weeks and 4 months considered

1. swelling;
2. range of motion;
3. shoulder function; and
4. costs.

▪ Design

The design was a randomized clinical trial with measures taken (1) prior to surgery, (2) within 24 hours post surgery, (3) within 10 to 14 days post surgery, and (4) four months post surgery.

SAMPLING

Sampling was initially completed with 14 individuals in order to pilot the procedure, test the instruments and determine the power required for a final sample. Based on a power of .80 and $P < .05$, a minimum of 25 participants per group would be required. There were 30 participants per group recruited to allow for dropouts. Only one person dropped out (due to death). There were no refusals to participate.

INCLUSION CRITERIA

Inclusion criteria were

1. 18 years of age or older;
2. diagnosed with breast cancer, and scheduled for lymph node dissection;
3. planning on having significant other (spouse, family, or friend) present in post surgical period (at least 1 hour immediately after leaving post anesthesia care unit);
4. both woman with breast cancer and significant other consent to participate and able to make informed consent by understanding the nature of participation; and
5. proficient in English to the degree necessary to participate in interviews.

EXCLUSION CRITERIA

The following would exclude potential subjects from participation in the study:

1. Diagnosed with an organic brain disease; and
2. Preexisting disorder affecting functional ability of affected arm or lymphatic system.

DEMOGRAPHICS

Demographic data were collected, including age, marital status, and educational level.

141 patients' reports on laboratory tests compared to clinical records. Observed agreement ranged from 0.72 to 0.99. When this was adjusted for chance agreement the Kappa statistic was 0.48 to 0.89.

■ Analysis

Descriptive statistics were completed for all variables. *T*-tests were carried out comparing responses of women in the control group to women in the intervention group for the following measures: pain control, family strengths and stressors, shoulder function, ROM, and girth measurement. The stated measures tested hypotheses related to comparing the intervention group to the control group. The Statistical Package for Social Sciences was used in the data analysis.

■ Results

SAMPLE CHARACTERISTICS

The study included 59 women diagnosed with breast cancer. Thirty were in the intervention group and 29 were in the control group. Slightly more than half ($n = 33$, 55%) of the women had a lumpectomy/partial mastectomy with axillary node dissection, 13 (21.7%) had a total mastectomy and axillary node dissection, 10 (16.7%) had a modified radical mastectomy and axillary node dissection, 3 (5%) had axillary node dissection alone, and 1 (1.7%) reported other. Their ages ranged from 21 to 78 with a mean of 56.19. The majority were married or had a common law partner (88.1%). Three women had an education level of primary school or less, 12 had some secondary, 15 had completed secondary, 13 had a community college diploma, and 14 had a university degree. The majority of women ($n = 48$, 80%) reported previous experience with massage therapy.

The majority of significant others were spouses ($n = 49$, 83.1%), 4 (6.8%) were parents, 2 (3.4%) were other relatives, 1 (1.7%) was a friend, and 3 (5.1%) were reported as "other." Significant others' educational level included 9 individuals with university degrees (15.3%) and 18 who had completed secondary school (30.5%). Eight (14.8%) of the significant others had previous experience with massage therapy.

POSTOPERATIVE PAIN CONTROL AND PAIN CONTROL

Pain was recorded on a daily record, provided to subjects at the time of enrollment. Subjects were asked to complete this record each day, as long as they had pain. Pain records were then collected at 2 weeks postsurgery or could be mailed in to the researchers.

Pain control in the immediate postoperative period for both the intervention and control group is described in Table 2. On the first day postoperation, women in the intervention group reported significantly greater [$t(40) = 2.31$, $P < .05$] pain control than reported by the control group. On the second day postoperation, women in the intervention group reported significantly lower [$t(36) = 2.38$, $P < .05$] pain *when pain was at its least* than reported by the control group. On the third day postoperation, women in the intervention group reported significantly lower [$t(36) = 2.68$, $P < .05$] pain *when pain was at its least* than reported by the control group. Past the third day postoperation, there were no significant differences in terms of pain control between the two groups.

FREQUENCY OF MASSAGE

The average number of massages varied over the first 3 days post-operatively (see Table 2). The number of massages peaked on Day 4, with an average of 2.69, and a range of 0 to 10. One of the participants in the intervention group never received massage. After Day 4 women reported progressively less use of massage.

FAMILY STRESS AND STRENGTHS

Overall, there were some differences between the groups' ratings of family strengths and

Table 2. Postoperative Pain Control in the Intervention and Control Group

	Day 1	Day 2	Day 3
Intervention group			
Average number of massages			
Mean	1.72	2.28	2.44
Range	0–5	0–6	0–8
SD	1.41	1.45	2.13
Pain control from massage			
Mean (%)	39.5	57.06	54.44
Range (%)	0–100	0–100	0–100
SD	39.19	39.5	37.31
Pain control from medication			
Mean (%)	83.18	88	87.81
Range (%)	0–100	50–100	60–100
SD	28.64	14.62	13.29
Control group			
Pain control from medication			
Mean SD (%)	84.74	84.38	80.31
Range (%)	50–100	50–100	50–100
SD	16.45	13.02	12.44

stressors. During the preoperative interview, women in the control group ($M = 4.28$, SD = 0.75) rated the overall physical health of their families significantly higher [$t(46.73) = 2.07$, $P < .05$] than women in the intervention group ($M = 4.23$, SD = 0.91). At the second follow-up visit, 10 to 14 days post surgery, women in the control group ($M = 4.68$, SD = 0.67) rated overall family functioning significantly higher [$t(43.65) = 2.06$, $P < 0.05$] than women in the intervention group ($M = 4.24$, SD = 0.88). At the third follow up, 4 months after surgery, women in the intervention group ($M = 4.57$, SD = 0.60) rated fostering family table time and conversation significantly higher [$t(37.48) = 2.78$, $P < 0.05$] than women in the control group ($M = 3.91$, SD = 0.95).

SHOULDER FUNCTION

At the initial measurement prior to surgery, there were no significant differences between the groups on the SPADI disability scale. At the second follow-up visit, women in the intervention group reported significantly less difficulty than the women in the control group with the following tasks:

1. washing their back;
2. putting on an undershirt or a pullover;
3. placing an object on a high shelf; and
4. removing something from their back pocket (see Table 3).

By the third follow-up there were no significant differences between the intervention and control groups on the disability scale.

RANGE OF MOTION

ROM measurement was not performed at the first follow-up, 24 hours post surgery. There were no statistical differences in ROM between the intervention and control groups at the second and third follow-up visits.

Table 3. Significant Shoulder Function Differences Between the Intervention and Control Group

	Intervention Group		Control Group		
Task	**Mean**	**SD**	**Mean**	**SD**	***T* value ($p < .05$)**
Washing their back	2.86	2.98	4.89	3.48	53
Putting on an undershirt or pullover	2.2	3	4.04	3.36	52
Placing an object on a high shelf	3.03	3.4	5	3.56	52
Removing something from their back pocket	1.23	2.32	2.94	3.04	49

SWELLING

At the second follow-up, women in the intervention group had significantly higher (20 cm) proximal girth measurements than women in the control group (see Table 4). Similarly, women in the intervention group had significantly higher base of ulnar styloid measurements than women in the control group. These differences remained significant during the third follow-up. The difference seemed to be based on a single outlier. When the outliers from follow-up 2 (30.5 cm for 20 cm proximal girth measurement and 20 cm for ulnar styloid measurement) were removed the differences between the intervention and the control group became nonsignificant [proximal girth measurements: $t(52) = 1.80$, $P = .078$; ulnar styloid measurements $t(51) = 1.81$, $P = .077$]. Similarly, when the outliers from follow-up 3 (22.20 cm for 20 cm proximal girth measurement and 38.50 cm for the ulnar styloid) were removed from the analysis, the difference between the control and the intervention became nonsignificant [proximal girth measurements: $t(48) = 1.91$, $P = .062$; ulnar styloid measurements: $t(48) = 1.98$; $P = .053$].

COSTS/UTILIZATION OF HEALTH CARE SERVICES

There were no significant differences between the groups in terms of costs related to health care utilization. In general, patients in both groups had 1 to 2 appointments with their surgeons after surgery. They were also seen by their family physicians once and some had more consultations with nurses ($t = 0.996$, $P = .324$). Since patients in both groups had similar diagnoses, the type and quantity of postoperative tests done in hospital and out

Table 4. Girth Measurements for Intervention and Control Groups at Follow-up 2

	Intervention Group	Control Group	*t*, P values
Proximal girth measurements			
Mean	16.95 cm	16.20 cm	$t(53) = 2.02$, $P < .05$
SD	1.49	1.15	
Ulnar styloid measurements			
Mean	2.38	26.20 cm	$t(52) = 2.07$, $P < .05$
SD	2.37	25.27 cm	

of hospital were similar (t = 1.655, P = 1.104).

In addition to the specific medication prescribed by their physicians, painkillers and vitamins were the common medication taken by patients of both groups (t = .716, P = .477). Thus, the costs related to health care utilization for both groups are similar. On the other hand, the insignificant difference (t = 1.423, P = .161) amongst groups in social costs (eg, loss of income of patients and significant others) may be partially attributed to the large amount of missing data (almost half) for this section of the questionnaire. Missing data was attributable to discomfort of participants in disclosing financial information.

FEEDBACK FROM INTERVENTION GROUP

Participants in the intervention group reported a sense of closeness and support they have felt with their partners while receiving the massage. Subjects described how the massage was something "lighthearted" to do in a stressful time. Another report stated that the massage was more effective in dealing with pain in the postoperative period than medication and that an added factor was that there are no "side effects" to deal with in massage. Several other descriptors included "relaxing," "enjoyable," and "fostering intimacy." Negative feedback received was related to the massage ending too soon. Participants felt that 10-minute massages, as it was suggested by the study, were not long enough.

■ Limitations

This study demonstrates some encouraging trends regarding massage as a therapeutic intervention for women following surgery for breast cancer. However, one of the prerequisites to participate in the study was the availability of a significant other; therefore, women with no significant other are not represented in this study. An additional limitation of this study was related to incomplete data sets. In particular, women tended to stop filling out the pain measurement instrument after the first week postoperatively and felt uncomfortable about disclosing financial information. Furthermore, more than one research assistant completed measurement of ROM and girth width, which could have contributed to the insignificant difference in ROM and girth width between the intervention and the control group. The sample size of 59 may not have been sufficient to determine differences.

■ Discussion

The average number of received massages varied amongst the women; massage was performed when women felt they needed it, with no prescribed time and duration. Nonetheless, the number of received massages consistently increased to reach a peak on the fourth postoperative day, with an average of 2.69 massages, and a range of 0 to 10. Benefits of massage in the immediate postoperative period was evident with a significant improvement of shoulder function in the intervention group. Although there were no significant differences between the groups in their ROM, women in the intervention group experience significant improvement of their shoulder function as identified on the SPADI scale (see Table 3). Essentially, the questions on the SPADI scale tested the women's range of motion in carrying out daily activities. LeVu[1] concluded similar findings in their study. After determining the positive effects of massage on ROM, LeVu[1] recommended the initiation of massage on the first postoperative day.

Moreover, the use of massage was accompanied by some pain relief. Both women in the intervention and the control group experienced similar ranges of pain relief from medication. However, women in the intervention group endured less pain (39.5% less pain on the first postoperative day, 56.07% on second postoperative day, and 54.44% on third postoperative day) after receiving arm massage from a significant other. It appears that the positive effects of massage are transient, but do help during the initial stages of recovery in terms of pain management and return to normal function. These results concur with the findings of Bredin[33] who concluded that massage following breast mastectomy reduced pain and discomfort associated with the affected side. Additionally, Ferrell-Torry and Glick[34] declared that following 15 minutes of massage for cancer patients, their perception of pain decreased significantly.

In addition to the physiological benefits of postoperative arm massage by a significant other, women experienced a range or emotional and mental benefits. Women reported being comfortable and relaxed during massage. Bredin[33] determined that massage assisted her subject in relaxing and generated a "great" feeling. Women and their significant other felt that massage promoted a sense of closeness and support during a stressful time. Arm massage promoted the involvement of a significant other in the treatment. Bredin[33] described the touch of a massage as a method of communication that expresses the other person's willingness to tolerate and accept the woman after her disfiguring surgery.

■ Implications for Nursing Practice

The majority of studies completed by both physiotherapy and nursing describe chronic management of lymphedema and ongoing range of motion difficulties. The notion of health prevention and recommendations for the need to study alternate prevention strategies has been suggested. An opportunity to explore the effects of massage therapy in the early postoperative period following breast related surgery exists. The National Cancer Institute (NCI) of Canada suggests a list of exercises appropriate for the immediate, early, and late postoperative period following mastectomies.[16] While much of the NCI teaching focuses on preventative strategies, the notion of gentle massage therapy is excluded; the effect of the addition of massage to the usual exercise program is another area of interest. Furthermore, teaching the significant other the simple massage technique may provide a tangible helping role that traditionally has not existed.

■ Conclusion

Breast cancer and mastectomy inflict an extensive range of problems that women and their families are forced to endure. Often after surgery, the women's daily living activities are affected by the complications. Simple activities such as mobilizing the arm and putting on clothes can become very difficult. Massage therapy, in this study, helped minimize some of these restrictions.

Teaching significant others to perform a simple massage on the affected arm after lymph node surgery has several benefits. Women in the intervention group expressed great satisfaction and beneficence from massage. Arm massage decreased pain and discomfort and improved their shoulder function in the immediate period after surgery. Additionally, massage was a way that significant others could demonstrate support. Many women found the massage relaxing and fostering a sense of closeness at a difficult juncture.

REFERENCES

1. Le Vu B, Dumortier A, Guillaume MV, Mouriesse H, Barreau-Pouhaer L. Efficacité du massage et de la mobilisation du member supérieur après treatement chirurgical du cancer du sein. *Bull Cancer.* 1997;84:957–961.
2. Voogd AC, Ververs JMMA, Vingerhoets AJJM, Roumen RMH, Coebergh JWW, Crommelin MA. Lymphoedema and reduced shoulder function as indicators of quality of life axillary lymph node dissection for invasive breast cancer. *Br J Surg Soc.* 2003;90:76–81.
3. Kuehn T, Klauss W, Darsow M, et al. Long-term morbidity following axillary dissection in breast cancer patients-clinical assessment, significance for life quality and the impact of demographic, oncologic and therapeutic factors. *Breast Cancer Res Treat.* 2000;64:275–286.
4. Erickson VS, Pearson ML, Ganz PA, Adams J, Kahn KL. Arm edema in breast cancer patients. *J Natl Cancer Inst.* 2001;93(2):96–111.

5. National Cancer Institute of Canada. *Canadian Cancer Statistics 2000*: Toronto, Canada: National Cancer Institute of Canada; 2000.
6. National Alliance of Breast Cancer Organization. NABCO: fact sheets about breast cancer in the USA 2002. New York. Available at: www.nabco.org/index.php/7/rl-sections/1/39. Accessed June 21, 2002.
7. Brennan M, DePompolo R, Garden F. Focused review: postmastectomy lymphedema. *Arch Phys Med Rehabil.* 1996;77:S74–S80.
8. Maunsell E, Brisson J, Deschenes L. Arm problems and psychological distress after surgery for breast cancer. *Can J Surg*, 1993:36:315–320.
9. Bass SS, Cox CE, Salud CJ, et al. The effects of postinjection massage on the sensitivity of lymphatic mapping in breast cancer. *Am Coll Surg.* 2001;192(1):9–16.
10. Brennan MJ, Miller LT. Overview of treatment options and review of the current role and use of compression garments, intermittent pumps, and exercise in the management of lymphedema. *Am Cancer Soc.* 1998;83(12):2821–2827.
11. Schijven MP, Vingerhoets AJJM, Rutten HJT, et al. Comparison of morbidity between axillary lymph node dissection and sentinel node biopsy. *Eur J Surg Oncol.* 2003;29:34l–350.
12. Billhult A, Dahlberg K. A meaningful relief from suffering. *Cancer Nurs.* 2001;24(3):180–184.
13. Williams AF, Vadgama A, Franks PJ, Mortimer PS. A randomized controlled crossover study of manual lymphatic drainage therapy in women with breast cancer-related lymphoedema. *Eur J Cancer Care.* 2002;11: 254–261.
14. Humble CA. Lymphedema: incidence, pathophysiology, management, and nursing care. *Oncol Nurs Forum.* 1955;22:1503–1509.
15. Brennan M, Miller L. Overview of treatment options and review of the current role and use of compression garments, intermittent pumps, and exercise in the management of lymphedema. *Cancer Suppl.* 1998;83:2821–2827.
16. Granda C. Nursing management of patients with lymphedema associated with breast cancer therapy. *Cancer Nurs.* 1994;17:229–235.
17. Kirshbaum M. Using massage in the relief of lymphedema. *Prof Nurse.* 1996;11(4):230–232.
18. Dicken SC, Lerncr R, Klose G, Cosimi AB. Effective treatment of lymphedema of the extremities. *Am Med Assoc.* 1998;133:452–458.
19. Gillham L. Lymphoedema and physiotherapists: control not cure. *Physiotherapy.* 1994;80:835–843.
20. Boone DC, Azen S, Lin CM. Reliability of goniometric measurements. *Phys Ther.* 1978;58:1355–1360.
21. Riddle DL, Rothstein JM, Lamb RL. Goniometric reliability in a clinical setting. *Phys Ther.* 1987;67: 668–673.
22. Stranden E, Oslo J. A comparison between surface measurements and water displacement volumetry for the quantification of lymphedema. *City Hosp.* 1981;31:153–155.
23. Farncombe M, Daniels G, Cross L. Lymphedema: the seemingly forgotten complication. *J Pain Symptom Manage.* 1994;9(4):269–276.
24. Kremer E, Atkinson JH, Ingelzi RJ. Measurement of pain: patient preference does not confound pain measurement. *Pain.* 1981;10:24l–248.
25. Paice JA, Cohen FL. Validity of a verbally administered numeric rating scale to measure cancer pain intensity. *Cancer Nurs.* 1997;20(2):88–97.
26. Jensen MP, Turner JA, Romano JM. What is the maximum number of levels needed in pain intensity measurement? *Pain.* 1994;58:387–392.
27. Mischke KB, Hanson SM. *Pocket Guide to family Assessment and Intervention.* St Louis: Mosby; 1991.
28. Hanson SMH. Family assessment and intervention. In: Hanson SMH, Boyd ST, ed. *Family Health Care Nursing: Theory, Practice, and Research.* Philadelphia: FA Davis Co; 1996:147–172.
29. Williams JW Jr, Holleman DR Jr, Simel DL. Measuring shoulder function with the shoulder pain and disability index. *J Rheumatol.* 1995;22:727–732.
30. Roach KE, Budiman-Mak E, Songsiridej N, Lertratanak Y. Development of a Shoulder Pain and Disability Index. *Arthritis Care Res.* 1991;4(4):143–149.
31. Norkin CC, White DJ. *Measurement of Joint Motion: A Guide to Goniometry.* Philadelphia: FA Davis Co; 1985.
32. Browne G, Arpin K, Corey P, Fitch M, Gafni A. Individual correlates of health services utilization and the cost of poor adjustment to chronic illness. *Med Care.* 1990;28(l):43–58.
33. Bredin M. Mastectomy, body image and therapeutic massage: a qualitative study of women's experience. *J Adv Nurs.* 1999;29:1113–1120.
34. Ferrell-Torry A, Glick OJ. The use of therapeutic massage as a nursing intervention to modify anxiety and the perception of cancer pain. *Cancer Nurs.* 1993;16(2):93–101.

■ Appendix: Instructions for Massage

POSITIONING

It is important that the patient is comfortable and her arm is fully supported. She can lay on her side with her arm supported on 1 or 2 pillows.

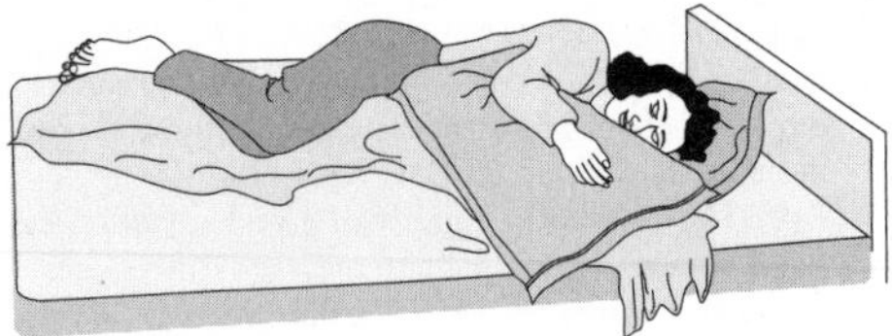

Or she can lay on her back with her arm on 1 or 2 pillows.

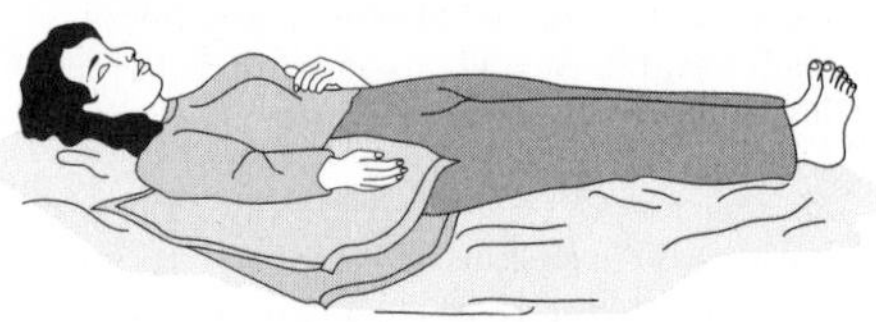

Her clothing should be loose so that her arm and shoulder are free. A sleeveless night gown or loose T-shirt would be okay. You should not use any creams, lotions, or powders.

TECHNIQUE

The first stroke uses light pressure under your palm. Start at her hand and gently glide your hand over her shoulder. Keeping your fingertips in contact with her skin, follow the same path down to her hand. Repeat the stroke again in a smooth rhythm. The pressure may be increased gradually as is comfortable.

Another stroke is done with only your fingertips. Starting at her hand, glide your fingertips over her shoulder. Return, following the same path. Repeat the stroke again in a smooth rhythm.

The third stroke is called *kneading* and is done in circles. You can use your whole hand or just your fingertips. Use gentle pressure in the upward circle and less on the way down. This stroke is good for the shoulder or neck muscles.

You can use these strokes on her arm, shoulder, or neck. Do not massage the underarm area. If she is uncomfortable, try changing your position or the amount of pressure you are using.

Cheryl Forchuk*, RN, PhD;* ***Pat Baruth****, RN, MScN; Monique Prendergast, BScPT;* ***Ronald Holliday****, MD, FRCS, FACS;* ***Ruth Bareham; Susan Brimner****, RMT, CLDT;* ***Valerie Schulz****, MD, FRCPC (Anaesth), MPH;* ***Yee Ching Lilian Chan****, PhD;* ***Nadine Yammine****, RN, BScN, BSc, MScN (candidate)*

From the University of Western Ontario (Dr Forchuk), Lawson Health Research Institute (London Health Sciences Centre) (Drs Forchuk and Holliday, Ms Baruth and Prendergast), London, Ontario, Canada; Department of Family Medicine, London Regional Cancer Centre/London Health Sciences Centre, University of Western Ontario, London, Ontario, Canada (Dr Schulz); Michael G. DeGroote School of Business, McMaster University, Hamilton, Ontario, Canada (Dr Chan); and the Faculty of Health Sciences, School of Nursing, University of Western Ontario, London, Ontario, Canada (Ms Yammine). Ms Bareham is a Breast Cancer Survivor and Ms Brimmer is in Private Practice.

We thank the Canadian Breast Cancer Research Initiative and the National Cancer Institute of Canada for the funding to conduct this study, and the London Health Sciences Centre Research Inc for the funds for the pilot work.

Corresponding author: Cheryl Forchuk, RN, PhD, Lawson Health Research Institute, 375 South St, Rm C201 NR, London, Ontario, Canada N6A 4G5 (e-mail: cforchuk@uwo.ca).

Accepted for publication October 16, 2003.

Critique of Forchuk et al.'s Study, "Postoperative Arm Massage: A Support for Women With Lymph Node Dissection"

■ Overall Summary

Overall, this was a good study that used a strong (experimental) research design to test a promising intervention that could easily be adopted by nurses to promote better patient outcomes among women with lymph node dissection. The small sample size, however, undermined study validity in a number of ways, including its internal validity (the experimental and control group were not equivalent at the outset, which is more likely to happen with a small sample), external validity, and, especially, statistical conclusion validity. The absence of statistical controls for pre-existing group differences in the analysis and the erratic pattern of findings make interpretation of the results difficult—especially in the absence of a guiding conceptual framework. The study can be construed as a good preliminary study of an intervention of great relevance to nursing that merits additional refinement and testing.

■ Title

The title of this report indicates the independent variable (postoperative arm massage) and the population of interest (women with lymph node dissection), but it does not communicate that the study was a test of an intervention, nor that the intervention involved a significant other. (In fact, the title does not make it clear that this was an empirical investigation.) Also, the title does not indicate what the outcome variables were—perhaps because there were so many of them. Nevertheless, a more informative (albeit wordy) title might be something like the following: "The effect of postoperative arm massage by a significant other on pain and functional constraints in women with lymph node dissection."

■ Abstract

The abstract was, in general, excellent, summarizing all major features of the study in a succinct but thorough fashion. There was, however, one problem with the abstract. The claim that the arm massage "*promoted* a sense of closeness and support amongst subjects and their significant other" is not supported by experimental data. Information about the subjects' emotional responses was gathered qualitatively from women in the experimental group only—that is, the emotional and mental benefits were not evaluated as part of the experimental design, and therefore the implied causal connection needs further verification. It would have been better to say that the intervention "was perceived to be helpful in promoting closeness and support by the women and their significant other."

■ Introduction

The introduction to this study was well organized. There were several sections, including an introductory paragraph that provided a statement of the problem and purpose statement, a section on "Current Knowledge," and a section labeled "Hypotheses."

PROBLEM STATEMENT

The first paragraph set the stage for the rest of the report by articulating the problem: Women who undergo lymph node surgery experience postsurgical pain and other consequences. The purpose of the study ("to examine the usefulness of arm massage by significant other in the immediate postoperative period") was then presented at the end of the first paragraph. This was a judicious, easily locatable placement for the statement of purpose—although a bit more could have been said here about what the researchers meant by "usefulness". Nevertheless, the researchers targeted a problem of considerable clinical significance to nursing and this was communicated early in the report.

LITERATURE REVIEW

The literature was reviewed in a section labeled "Current Knowledge." The review was organized into four subsections that provided background information on the following: lymph node dissection, massage, pain, and range of motion. The section on lymph node dissection summarized research on the consequences and complications of lymph node dissection, providing support for the researchers' statement of the problem. The next section summarized research on the effectiveness of massage as a treatment for lymphedema; the researchers noted the absence of studies on the use of massage as a preventive measure, thereby providing a rationale for conducting this study. The last two sections described research on massage in relation to two key outcomes, pain and range of motion.

Overall, the literature review was brief, but it was well-written, organized, and up-to-date, with many studies published after the year 2000 cited (its thoroughness could not be determined without undertaking our own review, of course). One concern is that the researchers overstated the confidence that can be placed in findings from non-experimental studies. The review indicated that "Bredin determined that massage therapy reduced numbness and pain of the affected arm," but Bredin's study was not experimental (primarily qualitative) and so it should not have been the basis for drawing conclusions about the effectiveness of massage as an intervention. Also, the literature review provided little information about the confidence we can place on the findings from earlier studies (i.e., the review did not comment on the *quality* of existing evidence).

Another concern is that the review did not describe any literature relating to the effect of massage on psychosocial variables such as family stress, which was one of the outcome variables. Indeed, the researchers did not offer a rationale for including this outcome in their study. Evidence tying massage interventions to the use of health care services and to costs—two other outcomes of interest in this study—also was not summarized, and we do not know if this is because there *is* no existing literature on these topics, or if the review failed to cover these topics because of an oversight or journal page constraints.

One final issue is that it would have been useful for the researchers to conclude their literature review section with a brief summary statement that laid out what is known or not known and why their study would contribute to knowledge.

HYPOTHESES

In addition to providing a purpose statement in the first paragraph, the researchers devoted one section of the introduction to a statement of their hypotheses. Their overall hypothesis was well-stated: "Individuals receiving arm massage from a significant other would have greater immediate comfort and fewer functional constraints compared to women receiving the standard postoperative treatment."

The researchers also present subhypotheses, which are elaborations of the main hypothesis. For example, they indicated that "greater immediate comfort" would be tested as the effect of the intervention on "reduction of pain" and "perceived control and comfort of the significant other." It is not clear, however, what was meant by "comfort of the significant other." Both pain and pain control were outcomes that were measured and described in the subsection called "Measures," but "comfort of the significant other" does not appear to have been measured and tested in this study—unless this "comfort" variable was operationalized as "family stress and strengths." This needs clarification.

One other point is that the subhypotheses elaborating on the effect of the intervention on functional constraints listed "cost" as one of the outcomes to be considered. It could be argued that this is not really a subset of the hypothesis on functional constraints, and could have been elevated to a higher status in their hypothesis hierarchy.

FRAMEWORK

Forchuk and her colleagues did not include any discussion of the conceptual or theoretical underpinnings of their study. It would have been useful for the researchers to discuss what it is about the intervention that might be expected to result in "greater immediate comfort" and "fewer functional constraints." Did the researchers envision the massage as having its expected effects primarily as a physiological response? (This is suggested but not elaborated on with the statement in the subsection labeled *Massage:* "this helps to redirect fluid from one area of the body to another"). Or did they conceptualize the massage as having beneficial effects primarily through an emotional/psychological mechanism? An emotional mechanism must have been partly envisioned, given that the researchers examined the effects of the intervention on a psychological variable, family stress and strengths.

This concern about the study's conceptual framework is not merely about the absence of an intellectual context—there are methodological implications. The intervention can be thought of as having multiple components, the effects of which are hard to disentangle. Is the key ingredient in the intervention the presence and concern of the significant other? Is *touch* the key ingredient? Or is it the actual massage? This is the very common "black box" problem that many tests of interventions face. If the researchers had paid more attention to potential underlying causal mechanism, they might have designed a somewhat different study (e.g., with multiple comparison groups, as discussed later in this critique).

The study's conceptual framework should also influence the researchers' choice of outcome variables, but in this study the underlying rationale for the choice of outcomes is not always clear. For example, the rationale for concluding that the intervention might affect family stress was not articulated. Indeed, it might be wondered if a measure of marital relationships or marital satisfaction would have been a better choice, inasmuch as the great majority of significant others were husbands.

■ Method

The method section was nicely organized, with numerous subheadings so that readers could easily locate specific elements of the design and methods.

RESEARCH DESIGN

Forchuk and colleagues chose a very strong design to test the effectiveness of the arm massage by a significant other—a pretest-posttest experimental design that involved random assignment of study participants to an experimental (E) group or a control (C) group. The

participants were told about the study, but perhaps the C group members (and E group members for that matter) altered their behavior based on their expectations about the study, regardless of the intervention itself. Significant others in the C group, for example, may have been more vigilant and solicitous of the patients than they otherwise would have been. The report did not mention whether the research assistants responsible for measuring girth width (swelling) and range of motion were blinded to the patients' group assignments, as would ideally be the case. In the absence of an explicit assurance, we must conservatively conclude that blinding did not occur. (Since the differences between the groups on these measures were not statistically significant, there is less of a concern of bias than would be true if an intervention effect had been found, because expectations would tend to bias observers in the direction of the hypotheses.)

MEASURES

The section on "Measures" included many laudable features, as well as some shortcomings. Of particular note, the section lacked information about data collection procedures. For example, the report did not indicate who collected the data, how self-report instruments were administered (orally or in writing), and where follow-up data were collected (i.e., in the participants' homes, in clinics, and so on).

Most of the outcome measures selected by the researchers appear to have been thoughtful choices that were adequately described in the report. Table 1, which outlined the timing and frequency of administering the various measures, provided an excellent summary. Most of the instruments and methods seemed to be appropriate measures of the outcome variables in which the researchers were interested, and for most the researchers provided some information about the measure's quality. For example, the measure for shoulder function was a scale with adequate internal consistency and test-retest reliability. The report did not provide evidence relating to the validity of the measures, but for the most part their measures had high face validity, such as the measures of pain and range of motion.

It appears that the range of motion measurements were made by several different research assistants, which the authors themselves described as a study limitation. However, the problem is not so much that there were multiple data collectors as that there is no information about the reliability of these measurements. The researchers should have described how these data collectors were trained, and also should have required high inter-rater reliability during training before allowing them to collect the data.

Although the measures used in this study generally seemed appropriate, there was no discussion of why a measure of family stress and strengths (the Family Stressor Inventory) was included. This outcome was not mentioned in the hypotheses, nor was there a discussion of how it might be affected by the intervention. One further thought is that the researchers did not collect any information from the significant others, who were the true recipients of the researchers' teaching intervention. The researchers could have measured a number of outcomes with the significant others (e.g., their well-being, their sense of efficacy, their feeling of closeness to the women, etc.) and could also have obtained valuable qualitative information from those in the E group about their experiences (e.g., was the training clear? did it motivate them to perform the massage? what improvements to the intervention could be made? why did they perform the number of massages they did? and so on.)

The researchers apparently *did* collect qualitative data from the women in the E group regarding their perceptions of the treatment, i.e., for the results described in the subsection "Feedback from the Intervention Group." However, there is no information in the report about how or when these data were collected, how many women were questioned, what exactly was asked, or how it was recorded and analyzed.

ETHICAL ASPECTS

The authors did not provide much information about human subjects considerations—

which does *not* mean that there were ethical transgressions. No mention was made of having the study approved by a human subjects committee (an IRB or Research Ethics Board), for example. The only information in the report was a notation in the "Inclusion Criteria" subsection that both the women and their significant other had to consent to participate and had to be able to give informed consent. There is no indication in the report that the subjects were harmed, deceived, or mistreated in any way.

■ Results

The results section addressed each of the study hypotheses, and also included an analysis of the qualitative feedback regarding reactions to the intervention from women in the treatment group. It would have been useful to learn more about how these data were gathered, as just noted, but the information was valuable and offered some suggestions about how the intervention might be improved (e.g., longer massages).

The statistical analyses focused on group differences on the outcome variables, that is, whether the E-C groups differed significantly in terms of pain, perceptions of pain control, swelling, range of motion, shoulder function, family stress and strengths, use of health care services, and health care costs. It would have also been possible to present statistical information about changes over time for most of these outcomes (e.g., how family stress changed from baseline to 4 months after surgery), but the researchers chose to focus on tests of their hypotheses.

One notable absence in the Results section, as previously mentioned, was a table summarizing E-C group characteristics at the outset. The text provides a description of the overall sample, but it is important for readers to understand whether the two groups were similar with respect to demographic characteristics and baseline measures of the outcomes—that is, whether randomization was successful in equating the groups with regard to key attributes.

The researchers used *t*-tests to compare group means on the outcomes. This statistical test is technically appropriate for comparing group means, but it is not necessarily the best analytic method—especially when there is evidence that the groups were not equivalent at the outset. It is not clear why the researchers chose not to use analysis of covariance, using baseline measures of the outcome variable as the covariate. This analytic strategy would have added precision and strengthened the internal validity of the study, because it would have statistically adjusted for any initial group differences. ANCOVA might have even changed some of the conclusions, but further speculation is constrained because the researchers did not share much descriptive information—for example, what the range of motion scores for the two groups were at baseline and at the two follow-up points when this variable was measured.

The findings indicated that the women in the E group reported lower pain and greater pain control than women in the C group in the first few days post-surgery. There were also favorable and significant group differences with regard to shoulder function 10–14 days after surgery. Thus, even with a small sample size and the absence of statistical controls, there were significant and encouraging group differences in the predicted direction for these outcomes. However, contrary to prediction, there appeared to be significantly more swelling in the E than in the C group (Table 4). The authors attribute this group differences to the effect of a single outlier, meaning that one woman in the E group had extremely high measurements. When the outlier was removed from the analysis, the group difference was no longer significant (although it narrowly missed significance, and a difference of that magnitude would have been significant with a larger sample). The legitimacy of removing the outlier is not clear, but the researchers should have also used statistical controls (ANCOVA) for this analysis, in particular. With or without the outlier, the hypothesis regarding swelling being lower in the E group was not supported. The findings with regard to family stress and strengths were erratic, sometimes favoring the E group and sometimes favoring the C group. With regard to health care costs and utilization, there were no significant group differences, although one difference relating to social costs approached significance. Overall, given some of the design and analytic problems already mentioned, the pattern of findings is not easily interpreted, but some of the positive results are nevertheless encouraging.

Discussion

Forchuk and her colleagues began their discussion with a review of some of the study's limitations. They made note of the biggest problem (small sample size), but failed to note other important ones (lack of blinding, selection bias). The researchers also noted that the study's generalizability was limited by the fact that only women who had a significant other could be included in the study.

The discussion and interpretation of the findings focused exclusively on the positive results. Similarly, the implications for nursing practice were developed with the positive findings in mind. A more balanced analysis of the study, factoring in the study limitations and the nonsignificant or contrary results, would have been desirable. On the other hand, it would appear that there is merit in the researchers' assertion that "teaching the significant other the simple massage technique may provide a tangible helping role that has traditionally has not existed." The authors would have done well to urge replications and extensions of the study so that the evidence regarding the effectiveness of a massage for women with lymph node dissection could be strengthened.

Presentational Issues

This report was well written and well organized, but would have benefited from the inclusion of some additional details. The results section had a nice mixture of text and tables, although the tables could have been organized somewhat better and had more information. For example, a table with E-C differences for all major outcomes (including baseline and follow-up means and SDs) would have been useful. A particularly regrettable presentational lapse is the absence of sufficient information for computing effect sizes, which would be needed to include this study in a meta-analysis. One last issue is that there appear to be some errors in the tables (which could be the fault of the publisher and not the authors). For example, the pain scores were described as ratings from 0 to 10, and yet the means in Table 2 were double-digit numbers, for example, 83.18 for the experimental group on Day 1. Moreover, the row label indicates "Mean (%)", so it is not clear what information is being provided—means or percentages.

Response from Cheryl Forchuk

Thanks for the critique. Overall the comments are accurate with regards to what is in the report.

It is mentioned that we did not specify which outcome measure was used for the sample size calculation—in fact all outcome measures were used and the results reflected the largest sample size required by any measure (in this case costs).

The research assistants were blinded until the last data collection period. They then opened an envelope (after all other measures were collected) so that they would know whether or not to ask the additional questions about feedback related to the intervention.

Ethics approval was through both the university and hospital.

All these points were of course in earlier drafts (including much more on the data collection procedure, etc.) and had to be removed to meet the page limitations. I think your critique will be useful to students—but they also need to know about page limitations of journals.

APPENDIX H

Beliefs and Rituals in Traditional Birth Attendant Practice in Guatemala

Linda V. Walsh

▶ Childbearing women and infants in developing countries continue to experience unacceptably high rates of mortality and morbidity in spite of targeted initiatives to address the problem. The aim of this study was to identify the beliefs and rituals of traditional birth attendants (TBAs) in one indigenous Guatemalan community to better understand the cultural influences on perinatal care practices. Ethnographic methods were used to increase understanding of the practice of 10 Mayan TBAs. Three themes were constructed: sacred calling, sacred knowledge and sacred ritual.

▶ ***Key Words:*** midwifery · pregnancy · birth · rituals · spirituality · clinical area—maternal/child

Childbearing women and infants in developing countries continue to experience unacceptably high rates of mortality and morbidity in spite of targeted initiatives to address the problem. It is estimated that the average maternal mortality rate in developing countries is approximately 20 times that experienced in developed countries (World Health Organization [WHO], 2000). Approximately one half of all births in developing countries are attended by traditional birth attendants (TBAs), and it has been suggested that in rural areas, as many as 95% of women are attended by TBAs (Kruske & Barclay, 2004). For example, it is estimated that 59% of births in Guatemala are attended by TBAs or unskilled family members or friends; in rural areas, this proportion is undoubtedly higher (Pan American Health Organization [PAHO], 1998). The most common attendant at birth in Guatemala, particularly in the indigenous communities, is the *comadrona*, a traditional birth attendant who may or may not have formal training for her role. Comadronas are typically women who have been recognized by community members as trusted, wise women who have accepted the calling to midwifery.

However, because of their lack of education, their gender, and their ethnicity, they are commonly devalued by those in the formal health care system, and comadronas are often the scapegoat for the high mortality rates in the country.

For the past 30 years, international health groups have called for the training of TBAs as a means to decrease maternal and perinatal mortality and morbidity. In 1987, a group of international agencies founded the Safe Motherhood Inter-Agency Group with the goal of halving the maternal mortality rate in developing countries by the year 2000 (Kruske & Barclay, 2004). Despite attention to TBA training and community education, by 2001 there was little change in the mortality rates (Anderson & Johnson, 2001). In response to the lack of improvement of health indicators for childbearing women, the WHO has suggested that ensuring that all women having access to a skilled birth attendant (physician, midwife, or nurse professionally prepared for the provision of perinatal care) will decrease

Reprinted with permission from *Journal of Transcultural Nursing* 2006; 17[2]:148–154. Copyright © Sage Publications.

the high number of preventable deaths. This statement reflects a Western medicine worldview held by members of the WHO that is that birth attendants with more skills will decrease the perinatal mortality and morbidity. The primary ritual associated with that belief is medically directed prenatal and perinatal care. However, it has been suggested that poverty, low levels of literacy, and the poor social and economic status of women may have a far stronger influence on pregnancy outcome than previously acknowledged, and that the training programs that were initiated were ineffective in part because of the lack of attention to community belief systems.

In addition to differences in belief systems and explanatory models for poor perinatal health indicators, there are practical concerns as well. Although the WHO has set a target of increasing the proportion of births attended by a skilled attendant to 90% by 2015, it appears that developing countries will have a difficult time recruiting and training a significant body of practitioners in that time frame. To solve this problem, Kruske and Barclay (2004) argued that rather than continuing to develop interventions grounded in a Western medicine worldview of health care delivery, we need instead to develop programs that are inclusive of healers who reflect the sociocultural beliefs of the community. To accomplish this, it is imperative that we increase our knowledge and understanding of the beliefs held and rituals valued by community members in developing countries. The aim of the current study was to describe the beliefs and rituals identified as central to the birth experience by comadronas serving a primarily indigenous Mayan population in Guatemala. This is an important target population because the traditional Mayan communities experience a disproportionately high rate of maternal and infant mortality and morbidity in the country.

■ Method

A poststructuralist approach was used to understand the lives of the comadronas and the researchers, namely, "The world as it is known is constructed through acts of representation and interpretation" (Denzin & Lincoln, 2000, p. 1055). Ethnographic methods were chosen because the purpose of the current study was to obtain in-depth information about the behaviors and beliefs of people in naturally occurring social settings (Atkinson & Hammersley, 1998). In the current study, observation, participation, and key informant interviewing were used to identify the beliefs and practices of Mayan TBAs. In addition, artifacts identified and used by these native healers were observed and entered into the analysis.

Traditional methods of participant observation with their goal of "emotional involvement and objective detachment" were not employed in this study (Tedlock, 2000, p. 465). Rather "observation of participation" was used to explore the comadronas world. This view acknowledges the engagement of the researcher in the social, political, and cultural web of a community. In this context, participation is "a context in which researchers who define themselves as members of those social settings interact in dialogic fashion with other members of those settings" (Angrosino & Mays de Perez, 2000, p. 690). Observation in the homes of pregnant women and, in some cases, small community health centers, provided the opportunity to develop an understanding of the resources available and the process of care offered by the comadronas. Observation in the homes of the comadronas provided the opportunity to view areas in which the comadronas kept materials used during their provision of care. A few of the comadronas also shared artifacts that included rocks and candles used for creating sacred spaces in their homes and the homes of pregnant women.

Participation included the provision of prenatal examinations with the comadronas, as well as interaction during monthly reunions, meetings in which there were trainings and time for social interaction. The principal investigator (PI) additionally participated in prenatal care and attendance at births in the small clinic in San Lucas

Toliman, often with a comadrona also in attendance. Ethnographic research typically requires a significant immersion in a site to allow the investigator to comprehend the life-ways of the community members. Depending on the research question, this period of time can range from 1 month to years (Foster, 2004; Speziale, 2003). The PI has been a participant and an observer in the practice of midwifery for more than 25 years and has been working with community birth attendants and health promoters in San Lucas Toliman, Guatemala, for 4 to 6 weeks per year during the past 5 years.

Key informant interviews were done primarily in the comadronas' homes, although at two comadronas' request, they were done in the bed of the pickup truck used for transportation to provide increased privacy. All interviews were audiotaped, and they were 60 to 80 minutes in length. In addition, the PI wrote field notes that included observations of the participant's actions, the physical environment, and artifacts associated with the practice rituals. Each participant was *interviewed once* and was assigned an identifying number that was used in all taping and notes to maintain confidentiality.

■ Setting

San Lucas Toliman is located on the southeast shore of Lake Atitlan in the highlands of Guatemala and is the commercial center for about 28 surrounding rural remote communities. About 82% of the inhabitants are indigenous Mayans. The remainder of the population is "Ladino," or mixed indigenous and Spanish race. The primary languages in the communities surrounding San Lucas Toliman are Spanish and Kakchiquel, one of the traditional Mayan dialects. It is estimated that 91% of the indigenous population lives in extreme poverty (PAHO, 1998). Families with one wage earner, usually the father who does agricultural work, must survive on the minimum wage of 14 quetzales per day (approximately US$2).

Almost all of the births in this rural part of the country are attended by comadronas. Each community typically has one or two practicing comadronas, and it is unusual for comadronas to attend births outside their own communities. There have been past efforts to offer government-sponsored training for birth attendants and isolated training programs offered by nongovernmental organizations [Unfortunately, there has been no coordinated effort to ensure basic minimal competencies for comadronas attending births.]

■ Sample

There are approximately 40 comadronas in the communities surrounding San Lucas Toliman, although many comadronas have limited practices with few births each year. Ten comadronas maintain busy practices, attending at least five births per month. Each of these comadronas was asked to participate, and all agreed to be interviewed. Their ages ranged from 37 years to 74 years, and their length of practice was 4 to 45 years. Nine reported marriage or "unida," which means living in a committed relationship without formal church or civil certification. They had personally experienced 4 to 11 pregnancies. All had started work as comadronas when there were still dependent children in the household. Only two comadronas were able to read and write. Most comadronas provided only pregnancy-related care, primarily assistance at birth and during the immediate postpartum period. A few also provided counseling and care for other medical problems using traditional interventions and herbs. One comadrona in the sample also served as a health promoter (community health worker) in her community.

■ Consent Procedure

The health promoter employed by La Parroquia San Lucas Toliman (the Roman on being sick.... Now as a midwife I'm not sick anymore."

The dreams and the struggle with making the decision to do the work sometimes presented in frightening ways. One comadrona described,

> I started [dreaming] at a very young age, I was 10 yours [sic] old, before my own menstruation, and I started to dream that I was seeing puddles of blood. I was bathing children, and things like that. Then at 28 years of age I started to get sick. I was sick a lot. The doctors from the church started to realize I was sick. I had high blood pressure at 29, very very high. When I was pregnant, I went around seven times to Guatemala City. There they ran tests on me and told me that there was nothing wrong with me, that I had no disease.

This comadrona experienced often incapacitating physical and mental illnesses during the course of several years until she decided not to reject the calling any more. Once she began the work as a comadrona, she regained her health.

Mayan spiritual beliefs include a strong integration of nature and the spiritual world. The sacred calling described by the comadronas often included symbols and objects linked to nature. One comadrona described walking down a path and finding a small stone with the shape of a face. This meant to her that she would start the work of a midwife. Another related, "I picked up a little doll made of stone in the form of a child. This was my first sign that I was to be a midwife."

One of the very experienced comadronas expanded her discussion of sacred rocks while showing her basket of rocks to the PI. She started simply. "I picked up some little stones... they represented being a midwife." She then went on to explain that she had had a dream directing her to walk on a particular trail where she would find the stone that would signify her calling into midwifery. She followed the directions and found the first of what would become a basketful of sacred rocks. One stone appears to have a face carved on it; however, she believes it was not carved by man but rather sent from the spiritual world as the sign of her calling to midwifery.

Among the Mayans, inanimate natural objects like the stones often are given sacred powers. As she talked about her sacred stones, the comadrona told a story. She left one of her stones in the cooking area of her house. She forgot about the stone and did not return it to the basket of sacred rocks. One of the pregnant women under her care came to her door and said to her, "How is it possible that you are burning me a lot?" She looked around the kitchen and saw that her daughter had put the stone under a pan to steady it, and the stone was hot and full of smoke. When she removed the stone from the hearth, the pregnant woman no longer felt like someone was burning her.

In Mayan tradition, birds are also seen as connecting the physical and the spiritual. While describing her early work as a comadrona, one participant said,

> I was called to see a pregnant woman in [village]. And I was walking when I saw up in the sky something that looked like a swallow or a bird flying... it came in front of me and dropped something and I picked it up and it was like a little paper and there was a little bit of dust in it. I saw it as a sign for my work.

While telling the story, this comadrona took a piece of paper, dropped some soil from the ground on it, and folded it. She then dropped it to the ground as a way to demonstrate how the paper fell in front of her.

When the work of the comadrona was begun, participants believed that they were doing God's work. One said, "I dreamt of being a midwife. But now, thank God, I already have become a midwife." Another comadrona shared that she "fears God very much and knows that God was the one that granted me that work, and if I don't do it, I think that God can take away my life."

SACRED KNOWLEDGE

All of the comadronas began their work caring for pregnant women without any formal training or apprenticeship. Many described learning the work through dreams or visions and they expressed the belief that the dreams were direct communication from God. One related,

> Nobody taught me how to do an examination, no one told me how, but I dreamed how to do this type of examination on women... how to measure them with a finger [points to knuckle on her finger that she uses to assess station of the presenting part] and when it gets smaller up here, that's a sign that they are going to give birth.

Another explained, "God is beautiful because He teaches everything, when the babies are coming feet first, buttocks first or sideways one has the practice to examine them. God gave me this gift. He gave me the vision to help people, to help the community."

One shared,

> And if God, if it is my fate to leave it [the work of being a midwife] to the Lord, I take it with all my heart, and I tell my patients I do my best for them so the children are born properly, that I deliver them with affection.

The comadronas also described dreams that foretold births. One explained that she

> dreams before going to take care of the delivery, [dreams that] people often arrive and ask that she go with them. Sometimes men come to tell me, to express in the dream "be very careful because that delivery brings complications."

Another explained that she receives messages through dreams:

> Sometimes you dream that you are out in the market buying only things for the kitchen, pots and baskets and that's the month that more girls are born. And there are some months that you dream of buying a machete, hatchet and all that stuff... and sometimes that's when boys are born.

Comadronas also describe receiving somatic signs that they interpret as messages from God. "When my right eye or right arm twitch[es], it will be a normal delivery. If it's the left side, there will be complications." Another comadrona explained that when her arm twitches, she'll then dream of a birth, and the next day she'll hear a knock on the door, and someone will call her to attend a birth. Yet another described a "tingling" in her arms that she feels, and the veins in her arms become more prominent shortly before being called for a birth. Because knowledge acquisition and the somatic signs are seen as communication from God, the knowledge gained in this way was believed to be sacred.

SACRED RITUAL

All of the comadronas described similar preparation for attending a birth. When called to attend a birth, the comadronas first pray before leaving their own homes. One explained that "always before I leave, I burn some incense at home and pray first before leaving the house." Similarly, one describes going to church and lighting a candle in front of the Holy Virgin and praying for a safe delivery. On arriving at the home of the laboring woman, the comadronas describe praying before entering the home. "I always pray before going in with the patient, before entering with the patient. I haven't touched, still haven't seen anything about the patient so what I do is pray." "The first thing [at my home] is to ask God, ask God that everything will be all right, and when I arrive at the house of the person too." Yet another explained, "When I first get there, I don't touch the patient. No, first I have to pray for half an hour."

"[From the time I leave my house to go to a birth] I am always asking God for wisdom. When I get to the house, always, and when I kneel in the, in the bed with the patient, I pray always to God." Often the laboring women themselves participate in the spiritual rituals. "I kneel with the woman and ask God to help in this."

The comadronas also spoke of using candles, incense, and other religious artifacts to create sacred space in the homes of the laboring woman. One described purchasing special candles for the births and "burning the candle and incense for any work I am going to do." Another noted, "I light a candle, a special candle and pray for the lives of the woman and the baby." The comadronas also described creation of sacred space by the families themselves. "Some people have religious pictures and light candles around them. They light the candles so God will help the women

What is your purpose as a midwife?

Are there any particular rituals or practices that you use when you attend a birth?

Were you taught anything to ensure that the birth goes well?

Are there physical rituals (like washing your hands) or spiritual rituals (like saying a prayer) that you do while you are with a woman in labor or birth?

Please tell me about a birth that was very special to you.

Do you think birth is sacred? Why?

Do you think that midwives have any special purposes in addition to "receiving" the baby?

Author's Note: The author wishes to thank Jesus Antonio Perez Aguilar for his assistance in recruitment and translation.

REFERENCES

Anderson, F., & Johnson, T. R. B. (2001). Commentary: Maternal mortality in developing countries. *Journal of Midwifery and Women's Health, 46*, 90.

Angrosino, M. V., & Mays de Perez, K. A. (2000). Rethinking observation: From method to context. In N. Denzin & Y. Lincoln (Eds.), *Handbook of qualitative research* (pp. 673-702). Thousand Oaks, CA: Sage.

Atkinson, P., & Hammersley, M. (1998). Ethnography and participant observation. In N. Denzin & Y. Lincoln (Eds.), *Handbook of qualitative research* (pp. 110-136). Thousand Oaks, CA: Sage.

Denzin, N., & Lincoln, Y. (2000). *Handbook of qualitative research*. Thousand Oaks, CA: Sage.

Foster, J. (2004). Fatherhood and the meaning of children: An ethnographic study among Puerto Rican partners of adolescent mothers. *Journal of Midwifery and Women's Health, 49*, 118-125.

Halifax, J. (1979). *Shamanic voices—A survey of visionary narratives*. New York: Penguin Books.

Hammersley, M. (1992). *What's wrong with ethnography? Methodological explorations*. London: Routledge.

Hammersley, M., & Atkinson, P. (1995). *Ethnography: Principals and practice*. New York: Tavistock Arkana.

Kruske, S., & Barclay, L. (2004). Effect of shifting policies on traditional birth attendant training. *Journal of Midwifery and Women's Health, 49*, 306–311.

Pan American Health Organization. (1998). *Health in the Americas* (Vol. 2). Washington, DC: Author.

Paul, L., & Paul, B. (1975). The Mayan midwife as sacred specialist: A Guatemalan case. *American Anthropologist, 2*, 707–725.

Prechtel, M. (1998). *Secrets of the talking jaguar—Memoirs from the living heart of a Mayan village*. New York: Jeremy P. Tarcher/Putnam.

Rist, R. (2000). Influencing the policy process with qualitative research. In N. Denzin & Y. Lincoln (Eds.), *Handbook of qualitative research* (pp. 1001-1017). Thousand Oaks, CA: Sage.

Ryan, G. W., & Bernard, H. R. (2000). Data management and analysis methods. In N. Denzin & Y. Lincoln (Eds.), *Handbook of qualitative research* (pp. 769-802). Thousand Oaks, CA: Sage.

Speziale, H. J. S. (2003). Ethnography as method. In H. J. S. Speziale & D. R. Carpenter (Eds.), *Qualitative research in nursing* (pp. 153-180). Philadelphia: Lippincott, Williams & Wilkins.

Tedlock, B. (2000). Ethnography and ethnographic representation. In N. Denzin & Y. Lincoln (Eds.), *Handbook of qualitative research* (pp. 455-486). Thousand Oaks, CA: Sage.

Woods, C. M. (1968). *Medicine and culture change in San Lucas Toliman: A highland Guatemala community*. Unpublished doctoral dissertation, Stanford University, Stanford, CA.

World Health Organization. (2000). *Safe motherhood: A newsletter of world-wide activity* (Vol. 28). Geneva, Switzerland: Author.

CRITIQUE OF WALSH'S ETHNOGRAPHIC STUDY, "BELIEFS AND RITUALS IN TRADITIONAL BIRTH ATTENDANT PRACTICE IN GUATEMALA"

■ Overall Summary

Walsh's ethnographic study of traditional birth attendant practices in rural Guatemalan communities provided a rich description of how cultural beliefs affect the delivery of maternal and child care in a part of the world where mortality relating to childbearing is high and the incorporation of current medical knowledge is low. Walsh, who had spent many months in the communities under study, collected a rich array of data via participation, observation, and in-depth interviews with 10 women who worked as *comadronas*, or traditional birth attendants. Although Walsh made efforts to enhance the integrity of her research, additional actions could have been taken to strengthen trustworthiness. Nevertheless, the report provides a rich and compelling picture of birthing practices in a remote area of a developing country.

■ Title

The title of the study conveyed the central focus of the study, namely the beliefs and rituals in traditional birth attendant practices in Guatemala. The title, although perfectly acceptable, lacks "grab." It also fails to convey information about the key themes or findings, as titles for qualitative reports often do. A more appealing and informative title might be, "The sacred work of comadronas: Traditional birth attendant practice in Guatemala."

■ Abstract

The abstract was brief but communicated some important information. The abstract began with a brief problem statement, followed by the study purpose. The abstract then indicated that the study was an ethnography. Some information about the sample was provided (e.g., that data were collected from 10 Mayan traditional birth attendants). However, details about specific ethnographic methods used (e.g., participant observation) and the amount of time spent in the field were not mentioned in the abstract. The abstract concluded by mentioning the three primary themes that emerged in the analysis. The abstract did not summarize any conclusions or implications for nursing practice. Overall, then, a bit more detail about the study would have been desirable, but the journal in which this paper was published may have imposed word limits for abstracts that constrained Walsh's ability to provide more information.

■ Introduction

STATEMENT OF THE PROBLEM

The problem that this research addressed was articulated in the first paragraph of the paper, and Walsh made a persuasive argument about its significance. In developing countries such as Guatemala, childbearing women and their infants have high mortality and morbidity rates, despite initiatives to address the problem. Even after training and community education have been provided to traditional birth attendants (TBAs), there has been little change in mortality rates. Walsh argued that, instead of continuing to develop interventions based on a Western medical view of health care, programs need to be sensitive to local sociocultural beliefs.

The central phenomena of interest were clearly stated in the introduction, namely the beliefs and rituals relating to the birth experience by comadronas serving the Mayan women in Guatemala. Walsh did not specifically address the significance of the problem for nursing. However, community education and training of indigenous healers and TBAs (the *comradonas*) undoubtedly involve health care teams that include nurses.

REVIEW OF THE LITERATURE

Literature relating to the phenomena of interest was not described in the introduction—although several relevant studies on traditional Mayan birth practices were briefly described in the discussion. The citations in the introduction highlighted the significance of the problem, but did not summarize prior research on the central topic of this research. For example, the statement, "It is estimated that the average maternal rate in developing countries is approximately 20 times that experienced in developing countries (World Health Organization [WHO], 2000)" supports the need for the study, but does not summarize what is already known. It is not unusual for qualitative reports to forego a detailed literature review in the introduction. Nevertheless, it might have been useful to provide readers with a context by noting that previous studies on this topic had been done decades earlier and therefore little was known about current practices.

CONCEPTUAL UNDERPINNINGS

Walsh did not describe any theoretical or conceptual basis for her study.

RESEARCH QUESTION

Walsh did not explicitly state a research question, but she did articulate the specific aim of her study, namely "to describe the beliefs and rituals identified as central to the birth experiences by comadronas serving a primarily indigenous Mayan population in Guatemala." The congruence between the research purpose and the paradigm and methods used was excellent. Walsh chose a naturalistic paradigm for her study so that the voices and interpretations of the comadronas could yield insights regarding birth rituals.

■ Method

RESEARCH DESIGN

An ethnographic approach was appropriate in this research, given the aim to understand the beliefs and rituals of the comadronas and members of the communities they served. Because ethnographies typically involve a large investment of time in the field, the methods associated with ethnography are particularly well suited for gaining in-depth knowledge about the beliefs and lifeways of a culture.

Walsh cited Hammersley and Atkinson (1995) as the reference for her ethnographic methods. Ideally, Walsh should have described this particular approach to ethnography in greater detail, but journal constraints may have made such elaboration impossible.

A strength of this ethnography was the prolonged time that Walsh spent in the field prior to starting her study. Walsh reported that she had worked with the community birth attendants and health promoters in the rural highlands of Guatamala (near the commercial center of San Lucas Toliman) for 4–6 weeks per year for the previous 5 years. Walsh did not, however, provide information about the time spent in the field for the actual collection of her data.

Given Walsh's argument about the need to "develop programs that are inclusive of healers who reflect the sociocultural beliefs of the community," this study might well have adopted a *critical* ethnographic approach. However, her aim was not so much to use ethnography to promote local change as to develop insights that could be useful in developing sensitive higher-level policies and programs.

SAMPLE AND SETTING

Walsh provided a fair amount of important detail about the study setting, which was in rural remote communities near San Lucas Toliman. She described the area's geographic location, the ethnicity and languages of the inhabitants, and the high level of poverty of the area's families. One important piece of information that was missing, however, concerned religion. Given the prominence of religion and spirituality in the study findings, it would have been useful to know what percentage of the population was Roman Catholic, and more about how Catholicism and indigenous religions were intertwined.

The primary sample for this study included 10 comadronas who served as Walsh's key informants. Walsh reported that there were about 40 comadronas who served the communities around San Lucas Toliman, but only 10 of them maintained busy practices (i.e., attended 5 or more births per months). Walsh opted to recruit only these 10 women, and all 10 of them agreed to participate. It might have been useful to interview 2 or 3 of the comadronas with less busy practices, as a means of validating understandings and searching for some disconfirming evidence for her thematic analysis. This might have yielded important insights about why some women chose "full-time" practices, while most TBAs opted for less intensive work.

Walsh provided basic demographic information about her 10 key informants. She recruited comadronas representing a range of characteristics. Comadronas' ages ranged from 37 to 74 years and their length of practice ranged from 4 to 45 years. Only 2 of the comadronas in her sample were able to read and write.

The report indicated that a health promoter who was employed by the Roman Catholic Parish helped Walsh recruit comadronas for her study. This health promoter played a vital role in recruitment, data collection, and translation in this study. Walsh could have helped readers to better understand the sociopolitical context of the study by providing more information about the health promoter's characteristics, background, and role in the community.

ETHICAL CONSIDERATIONS

Walsh took multiple, appropriate steps to ensure informed consent was obtained. The health promoter employed by the Roman Catholic Parish obtained verbal consent in the comadronas' primary language because most TBAs did not read or write. One of the traditional Mayan dialects is Kakchiquel. The health promoter translated for the TBAs who spoke this dialect. Back translation was used to make sure the translated informed consent from English to Spanish was equivalent. The consent form was read to each comadrona in Spanish or Kakchiquel. The two TBAs who could read and write signed the informed consent. The remaining eight comodronas consented by drawing a line on the form. An American research assistant, who served as translator from English into Spanish, was the witness for all the informed consents.

With regard to confidentiality, the informants were given a choice of where the interviews would take place, and some (perhaps to maintain privacy) opted not to be interviewed in their homes. The report indicated that informants were assigned an identification number that was used "in all taping and notes to maintain confidentiality." No names were used in presenting the results.

DATA COLLECTION

Walsh used a variety of data collection approaches that are congruent with the ethnographic research tradition—namely observation, participation, key informant interviewing, and analysis of artifacts.

Interviews were conducted with key informants, the comadronas, mostly in their homes. Each of the 10 key informants was interviewed once, in interviews that lasted between 60 and 80 minutes. All the interviews were audiotaped, and a professional transcription service transcribed all the interviews in Spanish and English for subsequent analysis. The actual process of interviewing was not described in the report, however. Presumably Walsh asked the questions in English, and then had questions translated into Spanish (by the research assistant) or by the health promoter (in Kakchiquel), but greater clarity about the process would have been helpful to understand the dynamics of the interviewing situation.

Walsh used a topic guide to structure her semi-structured interviews with the key informants. In the interviews, Walsh asked the TBAs to tell their stories about their journeys to becoming comadronas, and to describe the manner in which they practiced. Walsh also asked them to describe a recent birth that moved them. Laudably, Walsh included the topic guide as an appendix to her report. The questions were generally broad and appeared appropriate for the study aims. At least one question, however, might be considered leading, in that it could have influenced the data the comadronas provided and the researcher's interpretations of the data: "Do you think birth is sacred?"

The researcher made observations in the homes of pregnant women, in small community health centers, and in the homes of the comadronas. Some of the comadronas shared artifacts, such as rocks and candles that were used to create sacred spaces in homes. Walsh also participated in providing prenatal care with the comadronas and she also interacted with others at monthly reunions and training meetings. Walsh attended births in a small clinic in San Lucas Toliman. Walsh did not indicate the amount of time spent in such observations, nor how many of each type of observation were made.

An essential component of data collection in ethnography is writing field notes. Walsh stated that she wrote field notes about the observations, participations, the physical environment, and artifacts that the comadronas used in practice rituals. Her field notes recorded not only her various observations, but also her personal reflections.

ENHANCEMENT OF STUDY INTEGRITY

Commendably, Walsh used multiple strategies to enhance the trustworthiness of her data. She used three criteria identified by Hammersley (1992): Plausibility, credibility, and relevance. To address plausibility she reviewed her findings with community members and compared her findings with other published information. With regard to credibility, Walsh used member checking by sharing a draft of her findings with the two comadronas who could read. Relevance was achieved when the researcher, on a subsequent visit to San Lucas Toliman, shared the results with community members to make certain the findings represented the comadronas' experiences.

Another critical strategy that Walsh used to strengthen the integrity of her study was *triangulation*. Her insights about the beliefs and rituals of the comadronas were enhanced by her use of multiple sources and types of data. She also used triangulation in her analysis, by having another nurse researcher immerse herself in the texts and assist in coding the transcripts. Subsequent discussions about coding decisions continued until consensus was achieved.

Additional methods Walsh used to enhance the rigor of her findings included audiotaping all the interviews and checking the accuracy of the translations of the interviews with the health promoter and several participants. Walsh also wrote her reflections as the researcher in her field notes. Her immersion in the site of San Lucas Toliman for 4–6 weeks per year for the previous 5 years was extremely valuable in enhancing the trustworthiness of the findings.

There are some hints in the report, however, that further steps could have been taken to enhance readers' confidence in the integrity of the data collection and analysis. For example, Walsh did not indicate that saturation had been achieved, and so it is not possible to know whether additional interviews would have altered the interpretations. It is also not clear whether one interview was sufficient to get the full story from each comadrona about her experiences and practices in delivering babies. And, as previously noted, Walsh did not collect potentially disconfirming evidence from "part-time" comadronas. The inclusion of a direct question on the topic guide about the sacredness of births suggests a pre-existing inclination on Walsh's part to interpret the comadronas' experiences and responses in terms of themes of sacredness. Although Walsh provided certain information about her background, which enhanced the credibility of the study (e.g., she had 25 years of practice in midwifery), it might be illuminating to know more about her religious and spiritual orientation.

DATA ANALYSIS

Walsh's description of her data analysis was quite general, and a stronger description of her analytic methods would have been useful (although, again, journal page constraints likely contributed to this problem). Walsh stated that she and another nurse researcher skilled in qualitative methods developed codes from the texts until consensus was achieved. Then "from these codes, categories were developed from the texts through interpretive analysis," resulting in six categories. From these categories, the three overarching themes were developed. Walsh did not provide any references for the specific ethnographic data analysis method she used, nor did she explain what she meant by "interpretive analysis." A table or figure providing an illustration of how categories and themes were related might have proved helpful.

FINDINGS

From Walsh's interpretive analysis three themes emerged: sacred calling, sacred knowledge, and sacred ritual. Walsh summarized the findings succinctly and chose good excerpts to bring alive the themes for the readers, providing "thick description" about the lives and experiences of the comadronas. The results suggest a thoughtful presentation of the beliefs and values of the comadronas in Guatemala.

■ Discussion

Walsh presented a fairly well-constructed discussion of the findings. Walsh compared her results with previous research on Mayan midwives. Three studies from the 1970s and 1980s were used to help interpret the findings. Walsh concluded that even though over 50 years had past since Paul and Paul's (1975) study of Mayan midwives in another Lake Atitlan village, their results and those of Walsh's current study were very similar. In both, the comadronas' birthing practices were firmly grounded in spirituality.

Walsh also discussed her findings within an appropriate cultural context. According to

Walsh, current formal health care practices in Guatemala mirror the dominant medical view and do not take traditional cultural values and beliefs into account. Even though there has been a dramatic increase in technological knowledge in villages in Guatemala, traditional healers still adhere to spiritual beliefs and practices for childbirth.

Walsh listed only one limitation of her study, namely that with her small sample of comadronas, the findings might not be representative of TBAs in other communities. Walsh could perhaps have been a bit more insightful in considering other study limitations.

She made a suggestion for future research. Walsh suggested that research is needed to determine the effect of training programs and delivery of interventions that incorporate the TBA's strong spiritual beliefs as a strategy for improving maternal and child outcomes.

Implications for clinical practice in international health were also noted. Walsh called for creative strategies that incorporate the cultural beliefs and rituals of traditional healers. She provided an excellent example of how comadronas changed their clinical practices to incorporate new knowledge from monthly training sessions within the context of their cultural views and spiritual beliefs. Indeed, this finding, presented in a late paragraph of the discussion rather than in the results section, is intriguing and merits fuller elaboration.

■ Presentational Issues

Walsh's report was well written, well organized, and in sufficient detail for critical analysis. The results were rich and vivid. One concern is that there were several instances of editorializing, or inserting personal opinions within the text of the report. For example, Walsh's assertion in the introduction that "comadronas are often the scapegoat for the high mortality rates in the country" is not supported with citations.

APPENDIX I

Development of the Purposeful Action Medication-Taking Questionnaire

Mary Jayne Johnson • Sandra Rogers

► This three-phase study describes the development and psychometric properties of the Medication-Taking Questionnaire (MTQ) to measure the purposeful action domain (reasons individuals decide to accept medication treatment) in the medication adherence model for hypertension. During Phase I, items were evaluated for content validity and clarity. Item analysis, internal consistency, and exploratory factor analysis were preformed during Phase II to finalize the MTQ: Purposeful Action as 12 items and 2 subscales (treatment benefits and medication safety). Phase III evaluated the MTQ: Purposeful Action for temporal stability and construct validity. The final version MTQ: Purposeful Action demonstrated good internal consistency, temporal stability, and construct validity. The MTQ: Purposeful Action appears to have good psychometric characteristics that represent the decision-making process for adherence in medication treatment for hypertension.

► ***Keywords:*** hypertension; medication adherence; health attitudes; compliance; beliefs

Hypertension is a prevalent health problem that affects an estimated 63 million people or 24% of the U.S. population, with the prevalence increasing to 60% in individuals reaching the ninth decade of life (Burt et al., 1995; Ionita et al., 2005). Nonadherence is a major reason for inadequate control of high blood pressure and has been identified as the principle clinical problem in the management of hypertension (Haynes, McDonald, Garg, & Montague, 2001; Joint National Committee VI, 1997). This article describes the development and validity testing of a questionnaire to assess whether an individual will cognitively choose to take medications.

▪ The Medication-Taking Process

Forty years of adherence research has demonstrated that adherence is a multifactor phenomenon with more than 250 factors contributing to non-adherent or adherent behaviors (Haynes, 1979; Haynes et al., 2001). Medication taking for chronic illness is complicated requiring continual decision making and lifestyle changes to become adherent with prescribed treatment. Original adherence theories were developed to address the cognitive components of health behaviors in response to perceived health threats (Leventhal, Leventhal, & Contrada, 1998; Rosenstock, 1974). Leventhal et al. (1998) expanded on existing frameworks by addressing the feedback process individuals encounter during dynamic changes in health. Many chronic diseases are asymptomatic, exerting a seemingly nonthreatening silent impact on health. Applying current adherence theories to the context of medication-taking for chronic disease, consequently, has been mostly ineffective. Non-adherence continues to be a major reason for treatment failure (Haynes et al., 2001; Jayne & Rankin, 2001).

Several instruments exist to measure health beliefs about medication taking. The limitations of existing measures include the use of items unrelated to medication-taking behaviors, items that demonstrate potential response bias, failure of items to focus on reasons to take medications, or limited items addressing issues associated with long-term medication taking (Hamilton et al., 1993; Hill & Berk, 1995; Morrell, Park, Kidder, & Martin, 1997; Streiner & Norman, 1995). Most adherence scales measuring individual perceptions use five or fewer response options, potentially increasing the possibility of ceiling effect, which is common in individuals self-reporting adherence (Craig, 1985; Haynes et al., 2001; Streiner & Norman, 1995).

The medication adherence model (MAM) was conceptualized to meet the need for a framework that addressed medication taking in low-threat situations and was user friendly in the clinical setting (Johnson, 2002a, 2002b; Johnson, Williams, & Marshall, 1999). Two types of nonadherence drove the development of the MAM: the intentional decision to take or miss medications and the unintentional interruptions that cause medications not to be taken (Hughes, 2004; Johnson et al., 1999; Kingsnorth & Wilkinson, 1996; Wroe, 2002). The MAM identifies three concepts (purposeful action, patterned behavior, and feedback) that are responsible for long-term adherence to prescribed hypertension medications. The model suggests that patients must first make deliberate decisions, termed purposeful action, to use medications for the control of blood pressure. Patients then develop patterned behaviors to take medications regularly through regular access, routines, and techniques to facilitate remembering. Feedback, such as blood pressure readings, reinforces the purposeful intent to take medications and guides the patient's capacity to maintain medication routines. The MAM outlines the dynamic process of initiating and maintaining adherence to medications. A detailed discussion of the MAM and its relationship to existing adherence theories can be found in Johnson (2002a, 2002b).

Successful treatment of hypertension is first dependent on an individual's perceptions of the efficacy of medications. The concept of purposeful action parallels other constructs that address individual health beliefs and also captures the salient factors influencing an individual's decision to take medications. The subdomains for purposeful action included: perceived need (need), which assesses an individual's perception that medications are needed to control blood pressure to maintain and promote health and well-being; perceived effectiveness (effectiveness), which evaluates an individual's perception that medications are effective in controlling blood pressure and in preventing health problems; and perceived as safe (safe), which assesses an individual's perception that medications are generally safe and do not pose serious health problems. Because no measure of purposeful action exists, an instrument that reflects prevention and health promotion with relation to the MAM needs to be developed.

■ Purpose

The purpose of this study was to develop a psychometrically sound questionnaire to assess the purposeful action domain, or the decision to take medications.

■ Design

A methodological study was conducted in three phases to establish initial reliability and validity estimates for the Medication-Taking Questionnaire (MTQ): Purposeful Action.

Content validity was undertaken during Phase I. Phase II consisted of finalizing the factor structure of the MTQ: Purposeful Action through item analysis, internal consistency analysis, and exploratory factor analysis (EFA). Phase III evaluated test-retest reliability and construct validity. A confirmatory factor analysis (CFA) and multitrait-multimethod (MT-MM) analysis were used to examine construct validity of the finalized MTQ: Purposeful Action.

■ Sample

Institutional review board approval was obtained from participating facilities ($N = 7$). Content validity testing was conducted in a sample of five hypertensive patients and five health care professionals who examined the MTQ: Purposeful Action for clarity and content relevance (Imle & Atwood, 1988; Lynn, 1986). Professionals were invited to participate in the study based on their known experience with antihypertensive treatment and included two family physicians, a cardiology nurse practitioner, a nurse working with a statewide cardiovascular disease program, and a nurse researcher who had published articles on adherence. All professionals were Anglo American and were nearly equally divided with regard to gender.

Participants for the content validity phase who had been prescribed antihypertensive medications and lived in a situation in which they managed their own medications were recruited through healthy aging clinics, work-site wellness programs, hospital outpatient clinics, and hospital emergency departments in the intermountain west. The five hypertensive participants were Anglo American, had at least a high school education, and ranged in age from 48 to 90 years ($M = 62.0 \pm 16.4$).

A sample of 229 individuals enrolled from the same sites and meeting the same enrollment criteria for content validity was recruited for Phases II and III. The mean age of the participants was 61.5 years (range = 24–94; $SD = 15$). Participants were invited to participate in the study by employees of the participating facilities and then referred to the principal investigator. Fewer than 10 individuals refused to participate when the principal investigator explained the study to them. Most of the participants were female ($n = 147$; 64.9%), Anglo American ($n = 218$; 96%), and married ($n = 167$; 72%) and had a high school education or higher ($n = 234$; 93%). Length of diagnosis with hypertension ranged from less than 6 months to longer than 10 years, with 60% ($n = 138$) having the diagnosis longer than 5 years. Approximately 66% of individuals ($n = 151$) indicated they had medication insurance coverage. Individuals were asked to rate their health on a 5-point, Likert-type scale (1 = *poor*, 5 = *excellent*); 75% of individuals ($n = 171$) indicated they had good health or better.

The number of blood pressure pills taken ranged from 0 to 7, with most participants taking one pill per day ($M = 1.5 \pm 1.1$; $Mdn = 1.0$). Individuals were asked to rate how well they were able to take their medication for a given week on a 10-point adherence visual analog scale (1 = *not at all able to take my medications, 10 = never miss my medications*). Most participants rated themselves as generally adherent ($n = 179$; $M = 8.5$; $SD = 2.3$). A small number of participants ($n = 14$; 6%) indicated they had low adherence (a rating of 1-3) in taking their antihypertensive medications; however, only 50% of participants stated they took their medications 100% of the time.

■ Method

PHASE I: INITIAL INSTRUMENT DEVELOPMENT AND CONTENT VALIDITY TESTING

A total of 20 items (need, $n = 8$; effectiveness, $n = 6$; and safe, $n = 6$) were initially developed to tap the three underlying dimensions of purposeful action based on the statements given by participants in a qualitative study (Johnson, 2002a; Johnson et al., 1999). The method for item construction was guided by the principles outlined in DeVellis (1991) and Streiner and Norman (1995). Items were worded at approximately a sixth-grade reading level, evaluated by using the Flesch-Kincaid grade-level assessment program in Microsoft Word 2000 (Rasin, 1997). Items ranged from a 1.0 to 6.2 grade level, with a 3.5 grade level readability score for the overall questionnaire. After the items were constructed, psychometric testing was formally conducted.

Content validity testing was undertaken to determine clarity and relevance of content. Participants and experts were given verbal instructions and a packet consisting of a consent form, written instructions, clarity instrument, content validity instrument, and demographic questionnaire. The clarity instrument asked participants to rate items as clear or unclear (Imle & Atwood, 1988). Participants were given a definition of each subscale and asked to rate each item's relevancy using a 4-point scale from 1 (*irrelevant*) to 4 (*extremely relevant*; Lynn, 1986). Space was provided to make comments after each rating procedure.

PHASE II: FINALIZING ITEMS AND SUBSCALES

The MTQ: Purposeful Action was subjected to further psychometric testing after revisions were made based on the clarity and content validity analysis in a separate sample of individuals prescribed hypertensive medications. After the study purpose was explained and the consent was signed, participants were asked to complete a demographic questionnaire and the revised MTQ: Purposeful Action.

The MTQ: Purposeful Action items were arranged in a 7-point, Likert-type format describing responses based on agreement (7 = *always agree*, 6 = *very frequently agree*, 5 = *usually agree*, 4 = *occasionally agree*, 3 = *rarely agree*, 2 = *almost never agree*, 1 = *never agree*). The 7-response option was used in an attempt to obtain optimal variance while discouraging a ceiling effect (Streiner & Norman, 1995). Higher scores for the MTQ: Purposeful Action indicated greater intent to take medications based on perceived need, effectiveness, and safety.

PHASE III: STABILITY AND CONSTRUCT VALIDITY

At the time of Phase II enrollment, individuals were randomized into two groups to participate in the Phase III analyses (temporal stability or construct validity testing). Three Phase II participants declined to participate in Phase III. The MTQ: Purposeful Action was readministered 1 week after first completing the questionnaire to evaluate temporal stability ($n = 116$) because medication adherence was thought to change even within a 1-week period.

Participants ($n = 111$) randomized to the construct validity testing, in addition to completing the MTQ: Purposeful Action, were asked to complete the Hamilton Health Belief Model Hypertension Scale (HBM scale) and Lifestyle Busyness Questionnaire (LBQ) and to keep a Blood Pressure Feedback Log (FB Log) daily for 1 week.

The HBM scale (Hamilton, 1982) is an 18-item, 5-choice, self-report scale (1 = *not at all*, 5 = *a lot*) developed to measure patients' perceptions of hypertension and their health, which was hypothesized to be similar to the purposeful action domain. This instrument has four subscales: (a) Susceptibility, (b) Severity, (c) Benefits, and (d) Barriers. The HBM scale overall coefficient alpha for this sample was .86, with subscale coefficient alphas of .79 for HBM-Susceptibility, .43 for HBM-Severity, .86 for HBM-Benefits, and .36 for HBM-Barriers.

The LBQ is a 13-item scale developed to assess patients' consistency in keeping general daily routines (routines) and level of general busyness (busyness), which was hypothesized to be related to the behavioral component of medication adherence and be dissimilar to purposeful action (Park et al., 1999). The LBQ's overall coefficient alpha for this sample was .70, with a Busyness subscale alpha of .90 and a Routine subscale alpha of .71.

The FB Log was developed specifically for this study to capture the actual appraisal process of taking antihypertensive medications, which was hypothesized to represent feedback frequency and be dissimilar to an individual's belief structure characterized as purposeful action (Burman, 1995; Johnson, 2002a, 2002b). Study participants were asked to check items (concrete and intuitive) that reflected influences on adherence for 7 days. There were two 8-item sections. The first section listed reasons why participants did not take their medications (FB Log: Nonadherent). The second section listed reasons why participants took their medications (FB Log: Adherent). Log scores were counted based on the frequency of events checked by the participant.

■ Data Analysis

Data were analyzed using SPSS (Version 13.0), except the CFA was analyzed using AMOS 5.0. Descriptive statistics were used to summarize demographic data. Items met the clarity criterion if 70% of participants rated the item as clear and the content validity criterion if 80% of participants rated the item as 3 or 4 (Imle & Atwood, 1988; Lynn, 1986). The comments from the clarity and content validity criterion were used to revise the MTQ: Purposeful Action items and subscales.

The Phase II sample data were used to conduct item analyses, internal consistency analyses, and EFA. Item analysis was used to evaluate the individual performance of each item in relation to the overall instrument (Ferketich, 1991). Internal consistency estimates (coefficient α) reflected the average correlation among items within the instrument and indicated how well items clustered together or represented a single construct. Factor analysis is a grouping technique that allows for evaluation of the dimensionality of scales (Munro, 2001; Nunnally & Bernstein. 1994). A principal axis factoring solution with an oblimen rotation, considered the best analysis for achieving a theoretical solution uncontaminated by unique and random error variability, was undertaken (Nunnally & Bernstein, 1994; Tabachnick & Fidell, 1996).

The choice of subscale construction and item retention was guided by the desire to achieve a balance in the following criteria: (a) item variability with standard deviations > 1.0, (b) no ceiling effect ($M < 6.5$), (c) factor eigenvalues > 1 (amount of variance in all the items explained by a given factor), (d) item-to-factor loadings $> .40$ (the correlation between the item and the factor), (e) no cross-loading of an item on more than two factors of $< .20$ between factors to ensure the item was unique to its factor, (f) maximized total explained variance of the factor solution, (g) maximized coefficient alphas with at least $\geq .70$ for each subscale and total MTQ, and (h) keeping in mind subscales need to make theoretical sense (DeVellis, 1991: Nunnally & Bernstein, 1994; Pett, Lackey, & Sullivan, 2003; Streiner & Norman, 1995).

Temporal stability was calculated in two ways: (a) by undertaking correlations between Time 1 and Time 2 (traditional test-retest, t_{rr}, estimate) and (b) by calculating an intraclass coefficient (ICC; Berk, 1975; Meek, 1998). ICC is able to partition random from systematic error (Crocker & Algina, 1986).

A CFA using the Phase II data and MT-MM analyses using the Phase III data were conducted to examine initial construct validity. CFA examined model fit of the items and latent variables for the finalized MTQ: Purposeful Action. The following fit statistics were considered: relative chi-square, normative fit index (NFI), comparative fit index (CFI), and the root mean squared error of approximation (RMSEA; Bryne, 2001; Kline, 1998). The relative chi-square is an informal measure examining chi-square to the degrees of freedom. A value of > 3.0 is generally preferred for indication of good model fit. The NFI is an indicator of the proportion of the overall fit of the hypothesized model with the null model, though it has a tendency to underestimate fit with small sample sizes. The CFI is a revised version of the NFI that accounts for sample size. Good estimates of model fit will demonstrate values of $> .90$, with CFI values best in the .95 range. The RMSEA is a hypothetical comparison of the covariance matrix between the participants under study and the general population in terms of error of approximation. An RMSEA value of $\leq .08$ represents reasonable errors of approximation in the target population with a p value of $< .05$ (Bryne, 2001; Munro, 2001).

The MT-MM analysis for the overall MTQ: Purposeful Action and subscales was evaluated by comparing them with measures hypothesized to have similar constructs (convergent coefficients) and dissimilar constructs (discriminate coefficients). The MTQ: Purposeful Action should have higher Pearson correlations with related constructs than with differing constructs. The MTQ: Purposeful Action was hypothesized to have convergent correlations with Hamilton's (1982) HBM scale because they represent the cognitive aspect of the medication-taking process. The LBQ and FB Log were hypothesized to demonstrate discriminant correlations because they were believed to represent patterns of behavior and the feedback process, respectively.

■ Results

CLARITY AND CONTENT VALIDITY

Of the 20 MTQ: Purposeful Action items, 19 achieved clarity and content validity agreement. The 1 item that had an unacceptable clarity agreement was eventually eliminated from the questionnaire. Professionals expressed a concern about the lack of specificity in the questions, but that was not an issue for the hypertensive participants. For example, one professional indicated that the item, "Blood pressure pills keep me from having problems," lacked specificity. Because the purpose of this questionnaire was to establish a general screening tool for individuals who potentially may choose not to take their medications rather than to create a diagnostic tool, the participants' scores were given priority. Of the 20 items, 12 underwent minor grammatical revisions guided by the comments of both the participants and professionals. For example, items were made specific to blood pressure and the term *medication* was changed to *pills*. Several items were reworded, or the tense of a verb was changed.

ITEM ANALYSIS, INTERNAL CONSISTENCY, AND EFA

A total of 236 persons were enrolled in Phase II of the study, with 229 completing the questionnaires. Seven participants were dropped from the study because they did not cooperate in completing the study or did not meet the inclusion criteria. The sample exceeded the recommended 200 for undertaking a reliability analysis and 10 participants per item for the factor analysis (Nunnally & Bernstein, 1994).

Prior to undertaking the EFA, two items were eliminated because of ceiling effect or redundancy with other items (the original items and their statistics can be seen in Table 1). An EFA using principal axis factoring with an oblimen rotation ($\Delta = 0$) was undertaken to determine the underlying dimensions of the MTQ: Purposeful Action. The EFA yielded two interpretable factors (see Table 2), which eliminated six additional items because of factor loadings $< .40$. The first factor merged the need and effectiveness items along with one item from the Safe subscale. This factor was renamed treatment benefits (benefits). The second factor, renamed medication safety (safety), was reduced to three of the original safe subscale items.

The Benefits subscale retained nine items that focused on the actual perceived benefits of treatment, such as preventing a stroke, controlling blood pressure, preventing further health problems, and feeling better when taking medications, which indicated a desire to control blood pressure to maintain and promote health and well-being. The subscale had an eigenvalue of 5.5 and a total item variance explained by the factor of 46%. Pattern factor loadings ranged from .54 to .84. The internal consistency estimate was strong ($\alpha = .90$). The item means ranged from 5.4 to 6.4. The standard deviations ranged from 1.3 to 1.8. The alpha for items if deleted from the scale ranged from .88 to .90, and interitem correlations ranged

Table 1. Medication-Taking Questionnaire: Purposeful Action Initial 20 Items Statistics

	M	*SD*	Item-Total Correlation	Mann-Whitney Adherence *p* Values[a]
Perceived need				
My blood pressure pills keep me from having a stroke.	5.8	1.5	.58	.08
I need to take my blood pressure pills.	6.4	1.4	.77	.01
I take my blood pressure pills for my health.	6.5	1.3	.75	.01
Blood pressure pills keep me from having health-related problems.	5.7	1.5	.63	.17
I could have health problems if I do not take my blood pressure pills.	6.1	1.3	.74	.13
It's not a problem if I miss my blood pressure pills.[b]	5.1	2.0	.30	.02
I would rather treat my blood pressure without pills.[b]	4.1	2.3	.37	.26
I am OK if I do not take my blood pressure pills.[b]	5.6	1.8	.64	.012
Perceived effectiveness				
My blood pressure will come down enough without pills.[b]	5.4	1.8	.40	.10
I will have problems if I don't take my blood pressure pills.	6.1	1.4	.63	.001
My blood pressure pills control my blood pressure.	6.0	1.4	.66	.46
Blood pressure pills benefit my health.	6.1	1.4	.74	.01
I feel better when I take my blood pressure pills.	5.4	1.8	.56	.01
I have problems finding pills that will control my blood pressure.[b]	5.7	1.8	.09	.059
Perceived as safe				
The side effects from my blood pressure pills are a problem.[b]	5.2	1.9	.40	.10
The side effects from my blood pressure pills are harmful.[b]	5.6	1.8	.63	.27
My blood pressure pills are safe.	5.8	1.4	.66	.47
Taking my blood pressure pills is not a problem because they benefit my health.	6.0	1.4	.74	.02
My blood pressure pills cause other health problems.[b]	5.4	1.8	.56	.35
I will become dependent on my blood pressure pills.[b]	3.9	2.3	−.05	.20

a. Difference between low (scored 1–3) versus high (scored 7–10) adherence.
b. Reverse coded.

Table 2. Principal Axis Factor Analysis With Oblimen Rotation Pattern (and Structure in Parentheses) Coefficients for the MTQ: Purposeful Action Two Factor Solution

	Factor Loadings			Eigenvalue	% Variance Explained	Coefficient α
	1	2	h^2			
Treatment benefits				5.5	45.9	.90
I need to take my blood pressure pills.	.84 (.85)	(.34)	.73			
Taking my blood pressure pills is not a problem because they benefit my health.	.82 (.84)	(.35)	.72			
I could have problems if I do not take my blood pressure pills.	.81 (.84)	(.21)	.70			
Blood pressure pills keep me from having health-related problems.	.81 (.79)	(.16)	.63			
My blood pressure pills keep me from having a stroke.	.75 (.75)	(.23)	.55			
I feel better when I take my blood pressure pills.	.74 (.74)	(.21)	.55			
My blood pressure pills control my blood pressure	.74 (.74)	(.26)	.55			
I am OK if I do not take my blood pressure pills.[a]	.72 (.71)		.52			
My blood pressure will come down enough without pills.[a]	.54 (.48)		.30			
Medication safety				1.9	15.6	.80
The side effects from my blood pressure pills are harmful.[a]	(.19)	.87 (.86)	.74			
The side effects from my blood pressure pills are a problem.[a]	(.27)	.84 (.84)	.71			
My blood pressure pills cause other health problems.[a]	(.29)	.82 (.83)	.70			
Total				7.4	61.5	.88

Note. $n = 229$.
a. Item required reverse coding. Factor loadings in parenthesis represent structure coefficients. If patterned or structure coefficient is not listed the value was $< .15$.

from .25 to .72, with one interitem correlation less than .30. This subscale's mean score was 52.0 (range 9.0–63.0), with a *SD* of 10.3.

The Safety subscale (three items) focused on side effects of medications. This subscale had an eigenvalue of 1.9 and a total item variance explained by the factor of 16%. Pattern factor loadings ranged from .82 to .87. The internal consistency estimate was good for a newly developed instrument (α = .80). The item means ranged from 5.2 to 5.6. The item standard deviations were good, ranging from 1.8 to 1.9. The interitem correlations ranged from .57 to .58. The coefficient alpha for items if deleted from the scale ranged from .59 to .80. The Safety subscale had a mean of 16 (range 3–21) and a *SD* of 4.7. Together, the two factor solution had a coefficient alpha of .87 and an explained variance of 62%. The overall MTQ: Purposeful Action mean was 68.6 (range 15.0–84.0) with a *SD* of 12.7.

PHASE III: STABILITY AND CONSTRUCT VALIDITY

The test-retest correlation and ICCs were good (MTQ: Purposeful Action t_{rr} = .80, ICC = .86; Benefits subscale t_{rr} = .81, ICC = .80; Safe subscale t_{rr} = .80, ICC = .79). The test-retest and intraclass correlation for the overall MTQ: Purposeful Action suggested that approximately 14% to 21% of the variance was attributed to random time sampling error with little systematic error (Crocker & Algina, 1986).

A first order model with two latent factors, treatment benefit and medication safety, was judged to have good model fit. The relative chi-square value was 2.09. The NFI (.92) and the CFI (.96) indicated that the overall model fit was very good. The RMSEA was .07 (Cl .05–.087) with a *p* value of .042, indicating reasonable errors of approximation in the population.

Construct validity attempts to establish what underlying constructs an instrument is actually measuring (Nunnally & Bernstein, 1994). The MT-MM results appears to support the hypothesized relationship with the HBM scale, indicating that the perceptions of medication benefit and safety had a moderately positive association with perceptions of hypertension and individual health, especially between purposeful action and Benefits subscale and between HBM and Benefits subscale (r = .63; see Table 3). Very low correlation was seen, as expected, between the LBQ and MTQ: Purposeful Action. The intentional decision to take medications (MTQ: Purposeful Action) had a moderately positive correlation with reasons participants did take their medications (FB: Adherent, r = .53) and the intentional decision to take medications (MTQ: Purposeful Action) had a moderately negative correlation with reasons individuals did not take their medications (FB: Nonadherent, r = −.60), which were hypothesized to have little if any correlations.

■ Discussion

The inductively generated MTQ: Purposeful Action demonstrated good psychometric characteristics. The clarity results identified potentially problematic areas that were corrected based on participants' comments. The content analysis provided a formal opportunity to seek outside review, thus affording a cost-effective and efficient way to establish fundamental validity, reliability, and contemporary relevance of MTQ: Purposeful Action (Cronbach, 1988; Lynn, 1986; Messick, 1988; Nunnally & Bernstein, 1994).

The originally hypothesized factor structure for the MTQ: Purposeful Action was supported (considering that the Benefits subscale is a merger of the Perceived Need and Perceived Effectiveness subscales as a result of the EFA). The newly defined Benefit subscale contributed to a more parsimonious interpretation of the cognitive factors contributing to long-term medication taking.

The problem with measuring temporal stability in relation to medication adherence is determining when to readminister the instrument so that memory effect is not a factor, yet true change has not occurred (Waltz, Strickland, & Lenz, 1991). A 1-week retest

Table 3. Validity Correlation Coefficients for the MTQ: Purposeful Action and Subscales

	MTQ: Purposeful Action	MTQ Benefit Subscale	MTQ Safe Subscale
Hamilton HBM Scale[a]	.30**	.43**	−.12
HBM: Susceptibility subscale	.36**	.41**	.01
HBM: Severity subscale	.00	.12	−.27**
HBM: Benefits subscale	.58**	.63**	.19
HBM: Barriers subscale	−.49**	−.42**	−.41**
Lifestyle Busyness Questionnaire[b]	.08	.11	−.02
Busyness subscale	.10	.13	.01
Routine subscale	−.07	−.06	−.06
Blood Pressure Feedback Log[c]			
Adherent	.53**	.54**	.25*
Nonadherent	−.60**	−.50**	−.53**

Note. HBM is Health Belief Model Hypertension Scale.
a. $n = 107$.
b. $n = 104$.
c. $n = 102$.
*$P < .05$. two-tailed. **$p < .01$, two-tailed.

period was selected because of the hypothesis that adherence behavior may be volatile and that no information concerning stability has been reported in the literature. With the retest period of 1 week, however, the estimates may be deceptively high. A test-retest reliability study at various lengths of time would be needed to assess the dynamic nature of the cognitive component of adherence (Nunnally & Bernstein, 1994).

The CFA supported the hypothesis that benefits and safety underlie the cognitive component of medication taking in hypertensive medications. MT-MM estimates supported the hypothesis that the MTQ: Purposeful Action measures the decision component rather than the behavioral component of medication taking. The relationship between the MTQ: Purposeful Action and the FB Log was much stronger than expected. Because the FB Log represents the frequency of events that occur that reinforce medication benefits and safety, results may implicate that feedback may be more likely to influence intention to take medications rather than establishing routines.

The intended purpose for developing this questionnaire was to generate a valid measure of purposeful action that would be predictive of health beliefs important to taking antihypertensive medications. The reliability and construct validity estimates indicate this measure could be used for individual assessment of factors influencing a patient's decision to take antihypertensive medication (Perrin et al., 1997). Adequate assessment of an individual's actual health beliefs regarding medication taking may help health care providers determine medical and educational interventions that will assist patients with making informed decisions regarding taking antihypertensive medications during the long term.

There were several limitations with this study. The first was finding participants who would admit to low and moderate adherence behavior. Although a nonparametric analysis of levels of adherence indicated that some of the items could differentiate between individuals who self-reported high and low levels of adherence to medications, further investigation using more reliable measures of adherence would be required to confirm these results. The second limitation is the inability to generalize the results to ethnic groups other than Anglo Americans, to those in low-income situations, and to those with low literacy levels. Ethnically diverse groups were under-sampled because of the limitation of enrolling only individuals who could read English and the population demographics of the location of the study. Further testing is required to see if the underlying construct of purposeful action is generalizable to other groups.

The quality of MT-MM coefficients is dependent on the finding of reliable instruments that measure similar traits (Streiner & Norman, 1995). Low coefficients were obtained between some of the MTQ: Purposeful Action and its subscale and the HBM Severity and Susceptibility subscales. Possible contributing factors in obtaining low correlations could either be because of the low alpha coefficients for the HBM Severity and Susceptibility subscales and/or that these subscales have little association with the benefits and safety of medication treatment.

The MTQ: Purposeful Action appears, given its apparent limitations, to be representative of the purposeful action construct (the intentional decision to take medication) in the MAM. The MTQ: Purposeful Action provides a new instrument to further study the aspects of intentional medication taking in relationship to behavior and individual feedback with regard to hypertension and actual adherence. The sample was of sufficient size and variance to generalize the results to moderately and highly adherent individuals. This instrument may best be used to identify individuals' perceptions of the benefits and safety of antihypertensive treatment; however, further testing is needed to determine its responsiveness. Additional psychometric testing is needed to determine the predictive, discriminate, and responsive characteristics of the MTQ: Purposeful Action in a more diverse population.

***Mary Jayne Johnson**, PhD, APRN, is assistant professor at the College of Nursing, Brigham Young University.*

***Sandra Rogers**, DNSc, RN, is associate professor, and international vice president at Brigham Young University.*

REFERENCES

Berk, R. A. (1975). Utility of analysis of variance with repeated measures programs for estimating reliability. *Perceptual and Motor Skills, 41,* 441–442.

Bryne, B. M. (2001). *Structural equation modeling with AMOS: Basic concepts, applications, and programming.* Mahwah, NJ: Lawrence Erlbaum.

Burman, M. E. (1995). Health diaries in nursing research and practice. *Image: Journal of Nursing Scholarship, 27,* 147–152.

Burt, V. L., Whelton, P., Roccella, E.J., Brown. C., Cutler, J. A., Higgins, M., et al. (1995). Prevalence of hypertension in the U.S. adult population: Results from the Third National Health and Nutrition Survey. 1988–1991. *Hypertension, 25,* 305–313.

Craig, H. M. (1985). Accuracy of indirect measures of medication in hypertension. *Research in Nursing and Health,* 8, 61–66.

Crocker, L., & Algina, J. (1986). *Introduction to classical and modern test theory.* Fort Worth TX: Harcourt Brace Jovanovich College.

Cronbach, L. J. (1988). Five perspectives on validity argument. In H. Wainer & H. Braum (Eds.), *Test validity* (pp. 3–17). Hillsdale, NJ: Lawrence Erlbaum.

DeVellis, R. F. (1991). *Scale development: Theory and applications.* Newbury Park, CA: Sage.

Ferketich. S. (1991). Focus on psychometrics: Aspects of item analysis. *Research in Nursing and Health 14.* 165–168.

Hamilton, G. A. (1982). A *multivariate approach to compliance in hypertension.* Unpublished doctoral dissentation. Boston University.

Hamilton. G. A., Roberts. S. J., Johnson, J. M., Tropp, J. R., Anthony-Odgren. D., & Johnson. B. F. (1993). Increasing adherence in patients with primary hypertension: An intervention. *Health Values: Achieving High Level Wellness. 17,* 3–11.

Haynes, R. B. (1979). Introduction. In R. B. Haynes, D. W. Taylor, & D. L. Sackett (Eds.). *Compliance in health care* (pp. 1–7). Baltimore: Johns Hopkins University Press.

Haynes. R. B., McDonald, H., Garg, A. X., & Montague. P. (2001). Interventions for helping patients to follow prescriptions for medications

Additionally, reduction in blood pressure,[3,20] and improvement in aerobic capacity[2] in patients with heart disease have been reported. Tai Chi requires no special facility or expensive equipment and can be performed either individually or in groups. Tai Chi movements are suited for persons of all ages, regardless of previous exercise experience and aerobic capacity.[14,21] Tai Chi is a low impact, low to moderate intensity exercise incorporating elements of balance, strength, flexibility, relaxation, and body alignment. Features of Tai Chi exercise include weight-shifting between right and left legs, knee flexion, straight and extended head and trunk, rotation, and asymmetrical diagonal arm and leg movements with bent knees.[22,23] The exercise intensity of Tai Chi is variable and can be adjusted by the height of the postures, duration of the practice session, and training style.[22,23] Tai Chi is performed in a semisquat position. A high-squat posture and short-training session are well suited for deconditioned persons, including those with heart disease and older adults.[22,23] The exercise intensity of Tai Chi, height of the postures, and duration are all likely to affect overall improvements in aerobic capacity. However, there is a paucity of literature on the aerobic benefits of Tai Chi exercise.

Lan and colleagues[22] reported the exercise intensity during performance of the classical Yang style among experienced Tai Chi practitioners to be at 55% of the subjects' peak oxygen uptake. Zhuo and colleagues[24] reported the estimated energy costs of performing the classical Yang style of Tai Chi to be 4.1 metabolic equivalents (METs), with work intensity not exceeding 50% of an individual's maximum oxygen uptake. Schneider and Leung[25] reported that the exercise intensity of performing Tai Chi was 4.6 METs. Zhuo and colleagues[24] have also reported that the energy cost for performing a simplified form of Tai Chi requires an average of 2.9 METs with a maximum oxygen uptake at less than 40%. Energy requirements for Tai Chi Chih, a simplified form of Tai Chi, were reported by Fontana[26] to range from 1.5 to 2.6 METs,[26] depending on whether the subject was sitting or standing. There seems to be a wide range of exercise intensities associated with Tai Chi performance, ranging from 1.5 to 4.6 METs.

Maximum oxygen consumption ($\dot{V}O_2$ max) is considered the best measure of aerobic capacity and provides important information about cardiorespiratory function.[27,28] $\dot{V}O_2$ max is the greatest amount of oxygen a person can take in from inspired air while performing dynamic exercise involving a large part of total muscle mass.[27] $\dot{V}O_2$ max is considered the gold standard for determining aerobic capacity,[27,28] though not feasible or appropriate for some patient populations. Aerobic capacity is derived from gas exchange during exercise testing and is difficult to obtain in older populations and those with compromised cardiopulmonary functioning. In high risk or diseased populations, it may be more appropriate to obtain $\dot{V}O_2$ peak if symptoms such as angina, deconditioning or other factors prevent subjects from achieving maximum oxygen consumption levels.[27,28] Oxygen consumption derived from $\dot{V}O_2$ peak during exercise testing is most accurate when measured directly from expired gases.[27,28] Another term to express oxygen consumption is *metabolic equivalents*.[27,28] One metabolic equivalent (MET) is a unit of resting oxygen uptake (~3.5 mL of O_2 per kilogram of body weight per minute [$mL \cdot kg^{-1} \cdot min^{-1}$]).[29] In this meta-analysis, $\dot{V}O_2$ peak in $mL \cdot kg^{-1} \cdot min^{-1}$ is used as the measure of aerobic capacity.

The effect of Tai Chi exercise on aerobic capacity is important to know if clinicians want to recommend Tai Chi as an alternative form of aerobic exercise. The majority of the published studies examining cardiorespiratory responses to Tai Chi exercise by measuring aerobic capacity have small sample sizes. A meta-analysis involves the integration of several studies with small or large sample sizes, enabling the investigator to summarize the research results into useful clinical information. Therefore, the purpose of this meta-analysis was to estimate the extent to which Tai Chi exercise affects aerobic capacity.

■ Methods

LITERATURE SEARCH AND STUDY SELECTION

A computerized search of 7 databases (PubMed, CINAHL, Current Contents, Cochrane Library, Digital Dissertations, PsychINFO, and SocAbstracts) was done using key words for the various English language spellings of Tai Chi (eg, Tai Chi, Tai Chi Chuan, Tai Chi Quan, Tai Ji, and Tai Ji Quan). All languages were accepted. A total of 441 citations were obtained. Abstracts of all research studies were reviewed using a study selection form to determine whether subjects were randomly assigned to a Tai Chi exercise intervention or whether a Tai Chi exercise group was compared with another group; and if aerobic capacity was an outcome measure. The following types of articles were rejected: review, commentary, case report, research methodology paper, a reanalysis of data, a meta-analysis, an overview, qualitative research not related to the meta-analysis topic, or if aerobic capacity was not included as an outcome variable. Several articles appeared in more than one database.

Following initial selection criteria, 14 studies and 1 doctoral dissertation were examined in depth to determine whether they met the selection criteria. A total of 8 studies investigated Tai Chi and aerobic capacity and met the inclusion criteria. Four of the articles were experimental studies (2 randomized clinical trials,[19,20] 2 quasi-experimental[2,4]), 3 were cross-sectional studies,[5,25,30] and 1 was a prospective cohort study.[6] In the cross-sectional studies, 2 groups of different subjects were matched on age, gender, and body composition, allowing for adequate group comparisons. The prospective cohort study examined age-related deterioration in aerobic capacity and how Tai Chi may slow progressive decline. Subjects in the Tai Chi exercise and control groups in the prospective cohort study had statistically significant different baseline $\dot{V}O_2$ scores. Thus, group comparisons at the end of the study were not feasible,[6] and the study was not included in this meta-analysis. Characteristics of the subjects in these studies can be found in Table 1 (experimental) and Table 2 (cross-sectional).

DEVELOPMENT OF STUDY QUALITY SCORING TOOL

A study quality scoring tool was developed on the basis of previous work from Chan and Bartlett.[31] A total of 16 study elements were critically appraised to determine a study quality score. Elements reviewed included study design, sample selection, description of the independent variable (Tai Chi), description of the outcome measure (aerobic capacity), data analyses, and results. The highest possible study quality score was 32; each item had a possible score of 0 to 2 (0 = absent, 1 = partially defined, 2 = clearly defined), with possible scores ranging from 0 to 32. The methodological quality of both experimental and cross-sectional studies could be assessed using this tool. Any study with a quality score below 67% (<21) of the total possible score[31] was eliminated from this analysis.

MEASUREMENTS OF EFFECTS OF TAI CHI EXERCISE ASSESSED

In order to measure the benefits of exercise, the frequency, intensity, duration, type, and preference of exercise need consideration.[27,28] Current recommendations by the American College of Sport Medicine[27,28] include exercise frequency of 3 to 5 days per week, an intensity of either 65% to 90% of maximum heart rate or 50% to 85% of maximal oxygen uptake, duration of 20 to 60 minutes per session, aerobic type activity, and participation in an enjoyable aerobic activity. In very unfit individuals, the exercise intensity based on 55% to 64% of an individual's predicted maximum heart rate may be most suitable.[27,28] Aerobic capacity is influenced by age, weight, gender, exercise habits, genetic factors, and cardiovascular clinical status. Effects of Tai Chi exercise on aerobic capacity in this meta-analysis included study design, gender, physical activity habits, style of Tai

Table 1. Experimental Studies

Author/ Year	Study Design	Size	Gender	Mean Age in Years (SD)	Tai Chi Style	Length of Intervention	Group	Baseline Mean $\dot{V}O_2$ Peak, $mL \cdot kg^{-1} \cdot min^{-1}$ (SD)	Follow-up Mean $\dot{V}O_2$ peak, $mL \cdot kg^{-1} \cdot min^{-1}$ (SD)	Effect Size	LBCI	UBCI
Brown et al 1995	RCT	11	Male	50.4 (6.7)	Not specified	16 wk	Tai Chi	31.7 (5.1)	30.8 (4.1)	−0.3580	−1.154	+0.4379
		14	Male	50.5 (7.4)			Control (sedentary)	31.9 (5.4)	32.7 (5.8)			
		7	Female	51.5 (8.3)		16 wk	Tai Chi	25.0 (4.4)	23.8 (4.7)	−0.3101	−1.1857	+0.5830
		17	Female	53.6 (9.4)			Control (sedentary)	26.7 (6.0)	25.2 (4.4)			
Lan et al 1998	Quasi-exper	9	Male	65.2 (4.2)	Yang, 108 postures	52 wk	Tai Chi	24.2 (5.2)	28.1 (5.4)	+0.8176	−0.1442	+1.779
		9	Male	66.6 (3.9)			Control (sedentary)	24.0 (4.8)	23.6 (5.0)			
		11	Female	64.9 (4.7)		52 wk	Tai Chi	16.0 (2.5)	19.4 (2.8)	+1.334	+0.3609	+2.307
		9	Female	65.4 (3.8)			Control (sedentary)	15.8 (2.5)	15.6 (2.6)			
Lan et al 1999	Quasi-exper	9	Male	55.7 (7.1)	Yang, 108 postures	52 wk	Tai Chi	26.2 (4.4)	28.9 (5.0)	+0.6572	−0.2469	+1.561
		11	Male	57.2 (7.6)			Control (walking program)	26.0 (3.9)	25.6 (4.6)			
Young et al 1999	RCT	27	Not specified	Not specified	Yang, 13 movements	12 wk	Tai Chi	Not specified	0.97* (4.1)	−0.1598	−0.7105	+0.3909
		24	Not specified	Not specified			Control (aerobic exercise)	Not specified	1.64* (4.1)			

Note. RCT denotes randomized clinical trial; Quasi-exper, quasi-experimental study; WK, week; LBCI, lower bound confidence interval; and UBCI, upper bound confidence interval. Effect size is not significant if 0 is included in the confidence interval.
*Mean change in aerobic capacity.

Table 2. Cross-Sectional Studies*

Author/Year	Study Design	Size	Gender	Mean Age in Years (SD)	Group	Tai Chi Style	Mean $\dot{V}o_2$ Peak, $mL \cdot kg^{-1} \cdot min^{-1}$ (SD)	Effect Size	LBCI	UBCI
Schneider et al 1991	Cross-sectional	10	Male	35.5 (3.9)	Tai Chi	Not specified	44.3 (6.6)	+0.1571	−0.7208	+1.035
		10	Male	30.0 (5.0)	Wing Chun	. . .	43.4 (4.0)			
Lai et al 1993	Cross-sectional	21	Male	58.7 (3.9)	Tai Chi	Yang, 108 postures	33.9 (6.3)	+1.3836	+0.7252	+2.0421
		23	Male	59.1 (4.0)	Sedentary	. . .	26.3 (4.4)			
		20	Female	58.3 (4.8)	Tai Chi	Yang, 108 postures	21.8 (2.2)	+0.8943	+0.2834	+1.5052
		26	Female	57.5 (4.7)	Sedentary	. . .	19.0 (3.6)			
Lan et al 1996	Cross-sectional	22	Male	70.4 (4.1)	Tai Chi	Yang, 108 postures	26.9 (4.7)	+1.2289	+0.5503	+1.9076
		18	Male	69.5 (4.2)	Sedentary	. . .	21.8 (3.1)			
		19	Female	66.9 (2.7)	Tai Chi	Yang,108 postures	20.1 (2.9)	+1.3965	+0.6670	+2.1260
		17	Female	67.1 (2.8)	Sedentary	. . .	16.5 (2.0)			

Note. LBCI denotes lower bound confidence interval; UBCI denotes upper bound confidence interval. Effect size is not significant if 0 is included in the confidence interval.
*Matched on gender, age, and body composition.

Chi exercise, and the duration of the Tai Chi exercise intervention-training period.

DATA ABSTRACTION AND CALCULATION OF EFFECT SIZE

Using the data abstraction form developed for this meta-analysis, information from the 7 studies was abstracted (by Ruth Taylor-Piliae) to record study sample characteristics, the independent variable (Tai Chi), the outcome variable (aerobic capacity, expressed as $\dot{V}O_2$ peak in $mL \cdot kg^{-1} \cdot min^{-1}$), results, and statistical methods. Effect sizes were calculated from the standardized mean differences using means and standard deviations reported on the outcome measure (aerobic capacity).

The standardized mean difference effect size (ES_{sm}), also called d, is a scale-free measure that can contrast results for 2 groups, with continuous underlying distributions.[32,33] Effect sizes are important for power calculations when designing research studies and help clinicians and researchers understand the magnitude and direction of a relationship.[33,34]

The following formula[34] was used:

$$ES_{sm} = \frac{Mean_{Rx} - Mean_{c}}{S_{pool}}$$

Where Rx denotes Tai Chi exercise group, C denotes control or comparison group, and

$$S_{pool} = \sqrt{\frac{(n_1 - 1)s_1^2 + (n_2 - 1)s_2^2}{n_1 + n_2 - 2}}$$

where n = sample size and s = standard deviation.

D-STAT* software was used to calculate the ES_{sm} and the 95% confidence intervals. The ES_{sm} for each study was weighted by the sample size and pooled variance. The postintervention mean aerobic capacity ($\dot{V}O_2$ peak) was used to contrast the experimental and control group in the experimental studies, as there was no difference in the baseline mean scores in these studies. The ES_{sm} for 1 of the experimental studies[20] was calculated by D-STAT using the mean change in aerobic capacity, because of incomplete descriptive data. The ES_{sm} in the cross-sectional studies were derived from group contrasts between the Tai Chi exercise and the comparison groups. All relevant data derived from the studies were coded and entered into SPSS (10.0)[35] for analysis.

INTERPRETATION OF EFFECT SIZES

Cohen[33] has previously presented guidelines for assessing effect sizes. An effect size (ES) of 0.20 is judged to be a small effect, 0.50 as a medium effect, and 0.80 as a large effect.[33] In addition, a proportion of variance (η^2) can be calculated. Analysis of variance is a t-test statistic for means greater than 2. The analysis of variance ES is called f; and $f = d/2$. Using the formula $\eta^2 = [d^2/(d^2 + 4)]$, the percentage of variance between 2 groups can be calculated.[33] Finally, interpretation of the ES can be expanded by transforming the ES into a percentile. The percentile is obtained by referring to a normal distribution table and identifying the area under the curve associated with the ES, referred to as the measure of nonoverlap, (U_3).[33] U_3 is the percentage of the control distribution exceeded by the upper 50% of the treatment population.[36] U_3 readily provides the clinician with information regarding the success or failure of a treatment or intervention. For example, if the ES = 0.85, then 80% of the control group is below the average person in the treatment group. Also, it is important to note that when 50% of the control group is below the average person in the treatment group, then the ES = 0 (eg, no nonoverlap).[32,33,36]

■ Results

DESCRIPTIVE DATA FROM STUDIES IN META-ANALYSIS

Quality scores ranged from 22 to 28 (mean = 25.1, SD = 2.0) and no studies were excluded on the basis of their quality. The purpose of

*Johnson, BT D-STAT: Software for the Meta-Analytic Review of Research Literature. Lawrence Erlbaum Associates, Inc; 1989.

each study was clearly defined in all of the studies included in the meta-analysis. All but 1 of the studies had a complete and comprehensive description of subject characteristics. All of the studies had the dependent variable (aerobic capacity) clearly defined. However, only 1 of the 7 studies had the rater blinded to group assignment when collecting the data on aerobic capacity.

Within these studies, a total of 344 subjects participated; 166 subjects were in Tai Chi exercise groups. There were 82 males and 57 females, and no gender was specified for the remaining 27 subjects practicing Tai Chi. There were 178 subjects in either control or comparison groups. Sample sizes ranged from 7 to 27 subjects per group. Mainly, healthy older adults participated in these studies (n = 6). In the Tai Chi exercise groups, on average men were 56.0 years old (SD = 12.3) and women were 60.4 years old (SD = 7.0). Control/comparison groups were similar with regard to age and health status (men = 55.5 years, SD = 14.2; women = 60.9 years, SD = 6.4).

Four of the 7 studies had subjects perform the classical Yang style of Tai Chi, which constitutes 108 postures. One study had a modified 13-movement Yang style of Tai Chi, while Tai Chi styles were unspecified in 2 of the studies. In the 2 experimental studies, the duration of the Tai Chi exercise sessions ranged from 45 to 60 minutes, 3 to 5 times per week. The length of the Tai Chi intervention-training period ranged from 12 to 52 weeks. The workload of the outcome variable, aerobic capacity, was provided either by treadmill or cycle ergometer in all of the studies.

In 6 of the studies,[2,4,5,19,25,30] aerobic capacity was derived from $\dot{V}O_2$ peak through estimations obtained from subjects' expired air. One study[20] used predicted maximal workload using published equations by plotting heart rate and estimating workload at the predicted maximal heart rate. Thus $\dot{V}O_2$ max is not likely to have been achieved in these studies. Though use of $\dot{V}O_2$ peak and established equations for estimating oxygen consumption during exercise testing is common, aerobic capacity may have been overestimated due to wide variance inherent with multistage testing.[27,28]

■ Effects of Tai Chi on Aerobic Capacity

The effect size and the 95% confidence interval were calculated for each study, weighted by the sample size and pooled variance. Effects of Tai Chi exercise on aerobic capacity in this meta-analysis also included study design, gender, physical activity habits, style of Tai Chi exercise, and the length of the Tai Chi exercise intervention-training period. The percent of variance between groups (η^2) and the measure of nonoverlap (U_3), was only calculated for effects found to be statistically significant (Table 3).

The average effect size for the cross-sectional studies was large (ES_{sm} = 1.01; CI = +0.37, +1.66) (Fig 1), while in the experimental studies the average effect size was small (ES_{sm} = 0.33; CI = −0.41, +1.07) (Fig 2). In the cross-sectional studies, approximately 20% (η^2 = 0.20) of the variance in aerobic capacity could be explained by group. Aerobic capacity for the average subject in a Tai Chi exercise group was higher than 84% of the subjects in the comparison groups in the cross-sectional studies.

Six of the 7 studies[2,4,5,19,25,30] reported gender-specific descriptive statistics and enabled gender-specific effects to be calculated. Effect sizes of aerobic capacity in women (ES_{sm} = 0.83; CI = −0.43, +2.09) were somewhat higher than those for men (ES_{sm} = 0.65; CI = −0.04, +1.34), though not statistically significant.

Effect sizes examining aerobic capacity based on the physical activity habits of subjects in the control and comparison groups were also calculated. Four of the studies[4,5,19,30] had sedentary subjects as comparisons, while the other 3 studies[2,20,25] involved subjects doing other exercise, such as walking. Approximately 14% (η^2 = 0.14) of the variance in aerobic capacity could be explained

Table 3. Aerobic Capacity Effects Sizes and 95% Confidence Intervals ($n = 344$)

Selected Group for Analysis	n	ES	LBCI	UBCI	η^2	U_3
Study Design						
Cross-sectional	186	1.01*	+0.37	+1.66	0.20	0.84
Experimental	158	0.33	−0.41	+1.07		
Gender†						
Women	126	0.83	−0.43	+2.09		
Men	167	0.65	−0.04	+1.34		
Physical Activity Level						
Sedentary comparisons	253	0.80*	+0.19	+1.41	0.14	0.79
Other exercise	91	0.22	−0.81	+1.24		
Style of Tai Chi						
Classical Yang style	224	1.10*	+0.82	+1.38	0.23	0.86
Modified or unspecified	120	−0.17	−0.54	+0.20		
Length of Tai Chi Intervention‡						
52 weeks	58	0.94*	+0.06	+1.81	0.18	0.83
12 or 16 weeks§	100	−0.28*	−0.53	−0.02	0.02	0.61

Note. n denotes sample size; ES, effect size; LBCI, lower bound confidence interval; UBCI, upper bound confidence interval; η^2 = percent of explained variance between groups (η^2) and U_3 = percentage of the treatment group above the control group mean. The effect size is not significant if 0 is included in the confidence interval; η^2 and U_3 are reported only for significant ES.
*significant ES.
†51 subjects not included due incomplete descriptive data.
‡Sample of 158 subjects.
§Control group better than 61% of the subjects in treatment group.

by physical activity habits. Aerobic capacity for the subjects in a Tai Chi exercise group was higher than 79% of the sedentary subjects (average ES_{sm} = 0.80; CI = +0.19, +1.41).

Dose-treatment effects of Tai Chi exercise were calculated by the style of Tai Chi exercise performed. Four of the 7 studies[2,4,5,30] utilized the longest form of the Yang style of Tai Chi with 108 postures. The other 3 studies had subjects perform a simplified Yang style form (13 movements)[20] or the style of Tai Chi was not specified in 2 of the studies.[19,25] Approximately 23% (η^2 = 0.23) of the variance in aerobic capacity could be explained by style of Tai Chi exercise. Aerobic capacity for the average subject performing the classical Yang style form of Tai Chi exercise was higher than 86% of the subjects in the control or comparison groups (average ES_{sm} = 1.10; CI = +0.82, +1.38).

In the 4 experimental studies,[2,4,19,20] Tai Chi exercise session ranged from 45 to 60 minutes (mean = 56 minutes, SD = 7.5), 3 to 5 times per week (mean = 4 times per week, SD = 0.8). The length of Tai Chi intervention training period ranged from 12 to 52 weeks (mean = 33 weeks, SD = 22). Only effect sizes examining aerobic capacity based on length of the Tai Chi intervention were calculated. Approximately 18% (η^2 =

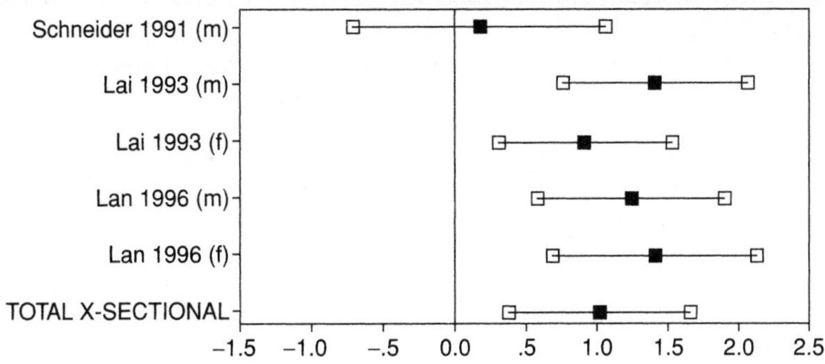

Figure 1. Cross-sectional studies, *n* = 3.

0.18) of the variance in aerobic capacity could be explained by length of the Tai Chi exercise-training period. Aerobic capacity for the average subject participating in a 52-week Tai Chi exercise group was higher than 83% of the subjects in the control group (average ES_{sm} = 0.94; CI = +0.06, +1.18). On the other hand, the improvement in aerobic capacity for the average subject in the 12-week or 16-week control group was better than 61% of the subjects in the Tai Chi exercise group (average ES_{sm} = −0.28, CI = −0.53, −0.02). However, this result is not likely to be clinically relevant, only 2% (η^2 = 0.02) of the variance in aerobic capacity could be explained by the number of weeks subjects remained in the control condition.

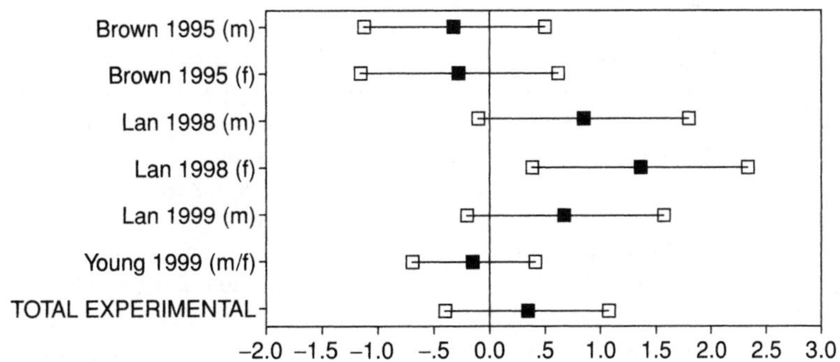

Figure 2. Experimental studies, *n* = 4.

■ Discussion

Given the limited number of studies pertaining to the effects of Tai Chi exercise on aerobic capacity in women (n = 126), these results need to be interpreted with caution. However, this early review appears to indicate potential gender differences in the effectiveness of Tai Chi exercise on aerobic capacity. Effect sizes of Tai Chi exercise on aerobic capacity in women were greater than those for men, though not statistically significant. This finding suggests that it may be important to consider, and future studies could clarify if there are gender differences by designing stratified randomization (based on gender). The development of alternative exercise programs for women including Tai Chi exercise could be of value, as previous research has reported that women desired exercise options other than using the treadmill or cycle.[37] Further, 1 of the experimental studies[20] did not provide gender information for the subjects completing the study. It is unknown if an effect based on gender would have resulted in different findings.

The degree of improvement in aerobic capacity depends on the exercise intensity, duration, and frequency, as well as the subject's initial level of physical activity. Persons who were sedentary before beginning Tai Chi exercise made greater gains with a more favorable effect. This finding is consistent with the traditional western exercise literature wherein the most sedentary persons demonstrate the greatest benefit when they initiate a regular program of exercise.[38] However, consideration needs to be given to possible selection bias, as Tai Chi masters were compared with sedentary subjects (>5 years), matched on age and gender, in 2 of the cross-sectional studies.[5,30] This selection of subjects with distinctly different exercise proficiencies is likely to influence the large effect sizes obtained. Further, the extent to which diet and other lifestyle practices influenced the results was not measured.

Tai Chi exercise styles varied among the studies reviewed. The classical Yang style comprises 108 postures and is more difficult to learn.[5,30] Simpler forms have fewer postures and exclude some of the more strenuous movements, such as deep squatting or vigorous kicking. While the simplified forms of Tai Chi are shorter and easier to learn, they may have a reduced training benefit. The 4 studies[2,4,5,30] that utilized the classical Yang style of Tai Chi had larger effect sizes. The findings are likely due to the inclusion of more strenuous movements and the longer time needed to complete the entire set of postures.

In the 4 experimental studies, the Tai Chi exercise intervention ranged from 45 to 60 minutes, 3 to 5 times per week, and is consistent with the current recommendations for western-style exercise.[27,28] However, the length of the Tai Chi intervention training period varied, ranging from 12 to 52 weeks. Subjects in 2 of the 4 experimental studies[2,4] had longer intervention times (52 weeks) than the other 2 experimental studies (12 or 16 weeks).[19,20] The largest effect was seen in the studies with the 52-week intervention time. However, the improvement in aerobic capacity for the average subject in the 12-week or 16-week control group was significantly better than subjects in the Tai Chi exercise groups. This finding may partially be attributed to a threshold effect when performing Tai Chi exercise or a dropout effect.

Subjects in the 12-week or 16-week Tai Chi exercise groups participated in either a simplified or unspecified form of Tai Chi and may have had a reduced training benefit. In the study by Young and colleagues,[20] moderate-intensity aerobic exercise, instead of sedentary controls, may partially explain why the improvement in aerobic capacity for the average 12-week control subject was greater than the average subject in the Tai Chi exercise group. Further, the mean change in aerobic capacity within and between the 12-week or 16-week control and Tai Chi exercise groups was small in these 2 studies.

Finally, the dropout rate for subjects participating in a 52-week intervention was approximately 26.5%, while the 12-week and 16-week intervention studies reported dropout rates of 17% and 8% respectively. Future research could help explain these findings by examining dose-response effects of Tai Chi exercise.

■ Conclusion

The findings of this meta-analysis fill a gap in the literature and highlight a potential benefit in aerobic capacity when performing Tai Chi. This meta-analysis included a total of 7 studies, only 4 of which used an experimental design. It is likely that the small samples in these studies had insufficient power for the researchers to detect significant differences between groups, assuming that $\alpha = .05$ and power = 0.80 were utilized.

Tai Chi may be an additional form of aerobic exercise, suitable for sedentary older adults and those with heart disease.[2,3,20] The slow and graceful movements of Tai Chi have several advantages over other forms of exercise, as Tai Chi does not require any special clothing or equipment, making Tai Chi a cost-effective and affordable form of exercise. Tai Chi may also foster adherence due to its practical utility (may be performed any time and at any place). Moreover, Tai Chi might be an enjoyable and preferred form of exercise for some.[1]

Future research studies examining the effect the Tai Chi on aerobic capacity should consider using the same frequency, duration, and intensity of Tai Chi exercise as that recommended by the American College of Sports Medicine.[27,28] This is necessary in order to have valid comparisons of the effect of Tai Chi exercise to traditional forms of exercise, such as walking. Further, it is recommended that an established style of Tai Chi be used, such as the classical Yang style, rather than unspecified or modified forms, so as to provide a comparison to published findings. Research among diverse populations, including persons with chronic diseases, would help to expand current knowledge about the effect of Tai Chi on aerobic capacity. However, aerobic capacity is only 1 potential outcome, and improvements in balance,[7-9] muscular strength,[10-12] flexibility,[5,13,14] relaxation[15,16] and mood state[15,17-19] may be additional benefits of doing Tai Chi.

Ruth E. Taylor-Piliae, *RN, CNS, MN*
Doctoral Candidate, Department of Physiological Nursing, School of Nursing, University of California, San Francisco, Calif.
Erika S. Froelicher, *RN, MPH, PhD, FAAN*
Professor, Department of Physiological Nursing, School of Nursing, University of California, San Francisco, Calif.

This research project was supported by grant 1 F31 NR08180-01 from the National Center for Complementary and Alternative Medicine and the National Institutes of Health, US Department of Health and Human Services and a Graduate Opportunity Fellowship from the University of California, San Francisco, awarded to Ruth Taylor-Piliae.
The authors thank Dr Kathryn A. Lee for her advice and helpful comments on previous drafts of this article and Dr Steven M. Paul for his assistance with the statistical analyses.
Corresponding author
Ruth E. Taylor-Piliae, RN, CNS, MN, Department of Physiological Nursing, School of Nursing, 2 Koret Way, Box 0610, San Francisco, CA 94143 (e-mail: rtaylor@itsa.uscf.edu).

REFERENCES

1. Kutner NG, Barnhart H, Wolf SL, McNeely E, Xu T. Self-report benefits of Tai Chi practice by older adults. *J Gerontol B Psychol Sci Soc Sci. 1997; 52*:P242–P246.
2. Lan C, Chen SY, Lai JS, Wong MK. The effect of Tai Chi on cardiorespiratory function in patients with coronary artery bypass surgery. *Med Sci Sports Exerc*. 1999;31:634–638.
3. Channer KS, Barrow D, Barrow R, Osborne M, Ives G. Changes in haemodynamic parameters following Tai Chi Chuan and aerobic exercise in patients recovering from acute myocardial infarction. *Postgrad Med J*. 1996;72:349–351.
4. Lan C, Lai JS, Chen SY, Wong MK. 12-month Tai Chi training in the elderly: its effect on health fitness. *Med Sci Sports Exerc*. 1998;30:345–351.
5. Lan C, Lai JS, Wong MK, Yu ML. Cardiorespiratory function, flexibility, and body composition among geriatric Tai Chi Chuan practitioners. *Arch Phys Med Rehabil*. 1996;77:612–616.
6. Lai JS, Lan C, Wong MK, Teng SH. Two-year trends in cardiorespiratory function among older Tai Chi Chuan practitioners and sedentary subjects. *J Am Geriatr Soc*. 1995;43:1222–1227.

7. Wolf SL, Coogler C, Xu T. Exploring the basis for Tai Chi Chuan as a therapeutic exercise approach. *Arch Phys Med Rehabil.* 1997;78:886–892.
8. Yan JH. Tai Chi practice improves senior citizens' balance and arm movement control. *J Aging Phys Activity.* 1998;6:271–284.
9. Hain TC, Fuller L, Weil L, Kotsias J. Effects of T'ai Chi on balance. *Arch Otolaryngol Head Neck Surg.* 1999;125:1191–1195.
10. Parker MG, Hocking K, Katus J, Stockert E, Gruby R. The effects of a three-week Tai Chi exercise program on isometric muscle strength and balance in community- dwelling older adults: a pilot study. *Issues Aging.* 2000;23:9–13.
11. Wolfson L, Whipple R, Derby C, et al. Balance and strength training in older adults: intervention gains and Tai Chi maintenance. *J Am Geriat Soc.* 1996;44:498–506.
12. Lan C, Lai JS, Chen SY, Wong MK. Tai Chi Chuan to improve muscular strength and endurance in elderly individuals: a pilot study. *Arch Phys Med Rehabil.* 2000;81:604–607.
13. Hugel K, Sciandra T. The effects of a 12-week Tai Chi program on thoracolumbar, hip and knee flexion in adults 50 years and older. *Issues Aging.* 2000;23: 15–18.
14. Hong Y, Li JX, Robinson PD. Balance control, flexibility, and cardiorespiratory fitness among older Tai Chi practitioners. *Br J Sports Med.* 2000;34:29–34.
15. Jin P. Efficacy of Tai Chi, brisk walking, meditation, and reading in reducing mental and emotional stress. *J Psychosom Res.* 1992;36:361–370.
16. Sun WY, Dosch M, Gilmore GD, Pemberton W, Scarseth T. Effects of a Tai Chi Chuan program on Hmong American older adults. *Educ Gerontol.* 1996;22:161–167.
17. Ross MC, Bohannon AS, Davis DC, Gurchiek L. The effects of a short-term exercise program on movement, pain, and mood in the elderly. Results of a pilot study. *J Holist Nurs.* 1999;17:139–147.
18. Jin P. Changes in heart rate, noradrenaline, cortisol and mood during Tai Chi. *J Psychosom Res.* 1989;33: 197–206.
19. Brown DR, Wang Y, Ward A, et al. Chronic psychological effects of exercise and exercise plus cognitive strategies. *Med Sci Sports Exerc.* 1995;27:765–775.
20. Young DR, Appel LJ, Jee S, Miller ER III. The effects of aerobic exercise and T'ai Chi on blood pressure in older people: results of a randomized trial. *J Am Geriatr Soc.* 1999;47:277–284.
21. Taylor-Piliae RE. Tai Chi as an adjunct to cardiac rehabilitation exercise training. *J Cardiopulm Rehabil.* 2003;23:90–96.
22. Lan C, Chen SY, Lai JS, Wong MK. Heart rate responses and oxygen consumption during Tai Chi Chuan practice. *Am J Chin Med.* 2001;29: 403–410.
23. Lan C, Lai JS, Chen SY. Tai Chi Chuan: an ancient wisdom on exercise and health promotion. *Sports Med.* 2002;32:217–224.
24. Zhuo D, Shephard RJ, Plyley MJ, Davis GM. Cardiorespiratory and metabolic responses during Tai Chi Chuan exercise. *Can J Appl Sport Sci.* 1984;9:7–10.
25. Schneider D, Leung R. Metabolic and cardiorespiratory responses to the performance of Wing Chun and T'ai Chi Chuan exercise. *Int J Sports Med.* 1991;12:319–323.
26. Fontana JA. The energy costs of a modified form of T'ai Chi exercise. *Nurs Res.* 2000;49:91–96.
27. American College of Sports Medicine (ACSM). *ACSM's Resource Manual for Guidelines for Prescription Testing and Prescription.* Philadelphia: Lippincott Williams & Wilkins; 2001.
28. American College of Sports Medicine (ACSM). *ACSM's Guidelines for Exercise Testing and Prescription.* Philadelphia: Lippincott Williams & Wilkins; 2000.
29. Fletcher GF, Balady GJ, Amsterdam EA, et al. Exercise standards for testing and training: a statement for healthcare professionals from the American Heart Association. *Circulation.* 2001;104: 1694–1740.
30. Lai JS, Wong MK, Lan C, Chong CK, Lien IN. Cardiorespiratory responses of Tai Chi Chuan practitioners and sedentary subjects during cycle ergometry. *J Formos Med Assoc.* 1993;92: 894–899.
31. Chan WW, Bartlett DJ. Effectiveness of Tai Chi as therapeutic exercise in improving balance and postural control. *Phys Occup Ther Geriatr.* 2000; 17:1–22.
32. Lee KA. Meta-analysis: a third alternative for student research experience. *Nurse Educ.* 1988;13: 30–33.
33. Cohen J. *Statistical Power Analysis for the Behavioral Sciences.* Hillsdale, NJ: Lawerence Erlbaum; 1988.
34. Lipsey MW, Wilson DB. *Practical Meta-Analysis.* Thousand Oaks, Calif: Sage; 2001.
35. Norusis MJ. *SPSS 10.0: Guide to Data Analysis.* Upper Saddle River, NJ: Prentice-Hall; 2000.
36. Lipsey MW. *Design Sensitivity: Statistical Power for Experimental Research.* Newbury Park, Calif: Sage; 1990.
37. Moore SM. Women's views of cardiac rehabilitation programs. *J Cardiopulm Rehabil.* 1996;16:123–129.
38. Haskell WL. JB Wolffe Memorial Lecture. Health consequences of physical activity: understanding and challenges regarding dose-response. *Med Sci Sports Exerc.* 1994;26:649–660.

APPENDIX K

Parenting Preterm Infants

A Meta-Synthesis

Martha K. Swartz

- ***Purpose:*** To synthesize the findings of qualitative studies on parenting preterm infants and present a framework that will enable clinical nurses to provide better care.
- ***Study Design and Methods:*** A meta-ethnographic approach was used to synthesize the findings of 10 qualitative research studies that focused on parenting the preterm infant upon hospital discharge and on into the toddler years.
- ***Results:*** Five themes of parenting preterm infants emerged: adapting to risk, protecting fragility, preserving the family, compensating for the past, and cautiously affirming the future.
- ***Clinical Implications:*** Nurses provide expert care, anticipatory guidance, and education for NICU babies and families, but should also foster the inclusion of all family members in the NICU setting, provide opportunities for parental peer support, establish effective systems of continuity of care, and advocate for parents of preterms in policy-making arenas.

- ***Key Words:*** Infant, premature · Parenting · Qualitative research

The incidence of preterm birth has steadily increased in the United States over the past several decades, and now 12.1% of all infants are born before 37 weeks of gestation (Martin et al., 2003). Significant improvements in the survival rates of small, preterm infants have occurred as well. However, compared with term infants, follow-up studies of preterm infants indicate a higher rate of medical complications and neurodevelopmental impairments in these children (Escobar, Littenberg, & Petitti, 1991).

While steady progress has occurred in the field of neonatal intensive care, it is important to consider what strides have been made in caring for the parents of these vulnerable infants. In examining studies from previous decades, nurses have shown that mothers of preterm infants experience more severe levels of psychological distress, notably anxiety and depression, in the neonatal period than mothers of term infants (Brooten, Gennaro, & Brown, 1988). Moreover, maternal depression has been linked to negative effects on the child's cognitive, emotional, and behavioral development (Field, 1995; Walker, Ortiz-Valdes, & Newbrough, 1989). Even as the prematurely born child approaches the toddler stage, mothers remain concerned about the child's health, development, and behavioral management; their strong maternal feelings of protection may interfere with their ability to set appropriate limits and encourage independence (Miles, Holditch-Davis, & Shepherd, 1998). It has also been noted that the prematurity might compromise the quality of interactions between the preterm infant and the mother, which may lead to poorer outcomes in subsequent development of the infant (Barnard et al., 1989; Sumner & Spietz, 1996).

What are the unique concerns expressed by parents of preterm infants? What generalizations can be obtained from qualitative studies

Reprinted with permission from *The American Journal of Maternal Child Nursing* 2005; 30[2]:115–120.

on parenting preterm infants that would enable nurses in newborn special care and primary care sites to provide better care? How would this information not only provide the basis for more effective clinical care, but also inform larger policy issues of creating systems that would provide for optimal parent-child outcomes? To address these questions, a meta-synthesis was conducted examining the results of qualitative research findings concerning the parenting of preterm infants.

■ Study Design and Methods

WHAT IS META-SYNTHESIS?

One of the goals of meta-synthesis is to translate findings from several qualitative studies and place them within a larger interpretive context to derive implications for practice and policy. (Sandelowski, Docherty, & Emden, 1997). Ideally, the result of a meta-synthesis will protect the particulars of each individual qualitative study but achieve a higher analytical goal and add to nursing knowledge by building a "grand narrative" (a generalization from all the studies). In this way the interpretive possibilities of the findings in the sample studies are further expanded.

PROCEDURE

The meta-ethnographic approach of Noblit and Hare (1988) involves a systematic comparison of studies in which the findings of qualitative studies are translated into one another. This comparison and translation is accomplished through the following phases:

- *Getting started.* To get started, the researcher identifies an area of interest or a topic that qualitative research might inform.
- *Deciding what is relevant to the initial interest.* At this phase, the researcher develops a list of studies that might be included in the review and decides on what studies should be included according to his or her interest and the audience.
- *Reading the studies.* The studies are read and re-read with particular attention to the participant findings reported in each study, so as not to be limited by the metaphors or concepts used by the authors.
- *Determining how the studies are related.* Across studies, participant accounts may either be directly comparable (reciprocal), stand in opposition to each other (refutational), or represent a more interpretive line of argument.
- *Translating the studies into one another.* Translations are comparisons of the themes of one study with the themes of the other studies included in the meta-synthesis in such a way that the particulars of the participant accounts are protected.
- *Synthesizing translations.* In the synthesis of the multiple accounts or studies, reciprocal translation or overarching themes emerge.
- *Expressing the synthesis.* The synthesis is driven by a concern to inform other practitioners. After assessing the audience, the results of the synthesis should be communicated in an appropriate format.

SAMPLE

For this review, the following computer library databases were searched for publications between 1990 and 2003: the Cumulative Index to Nursing and Allied Health Literature (CINAHL), MedLine, PsycInfo, SilverPlatter, and Dissertation Abstracts. The combined search delimiters used were "infant premature" and "parenting." Also, in CINAHL, the search term "qualitative research" was used, limited to the infant age group. The search yielded 68 studies, of which 10 were chosen for the meta-synthesis because they were qualitative research studies aimed at understanding the phenomenon of parenting a preterm infant (Table 1). Four of the research studies utilized content analysis as a methodology, three studies used grounded theory as the analytic approach, and three studies (including one doctoral dissertation) were phenomenologic research projects.

Table 1. Qualitative Studies on Parenting Preterm Infants

Study	Sample	Qualitative Design/Method
Casteel (1990)	18 mother/father parents of preterms were interviewed before and after discharge of their preterm infants	Content analysis
Gennaro et al. (1990)	65 mothers of babies born <37 weeks gestation and hospitalized <16 weeks	Content analysis
McCain (1990)	20 mothers, 4 fathers with babies ages 24–48 months who were born weighing <1500 g	Content analysis
Murphy (1990)	20 mothers and 20 fathers interviewed at home 1 month after the discharge of their preterm infant	Constant comparative method
Miles & Holditch-Davis (1995)	27 primary caretakers of infants born <1500 g were interviewed before and after hospital discharge	Constant comparative method
Vazquez (1995)	14 parents of very-low-brithweight (<1500 g) infants interviewed at 1, 3, and 5 months after hosptial discharge	Constant comparative method
Findlay (1997)	9 parents whose preterm infants were at least 4 weeks old were interviewed	Interpretive phenomenology
Miles et al. (1998)	30 mothers and 4 grandmothers with legal custody were interviewed when their pretern infants reached the age of 3	Content analysis
Bissell & Long (2003)	10 sets of parents of infants born at <37 weeks gestation; interviewed 1 week before and 6 weeks after discharge	Descriptive phenomenology
Jackson et al. (2003)	7 sets of parents of infants born at ≤34 weeks at 1–2 weeks after the infants birth, and at 2, 6 and 18 months of age	Descriptive phenomenology

■ Results

In this meta-synthesis, the metaphors or themes of each study were directly compared with one another and then translated into one another through a process of reciprocal connection. Five reciprocal translations concerning the process of parenting preterm infants emerged: (1) adapting to risk, (2) protecting fragility, (3) preserving the family, (4) compensating for the past, and (5) cautiously affirming the future.

ADAPTING TO RISK

Overwhelming concerns of the parents about their baby's health and development were pervasive. In the immediate period after birth, parents confronted and coped with known risks and the interventions necessary to sustain the infant's life. This was a time when parents would gather personal and environmental resources to be as informed as possible about the baby's care and to provide the best possible nurturing that they could. Gennaro et al. (1990) identified parental concerns regarding infant health, weight, and development as paramount. A parent interviewed by Bissell and Long (2003) stated that "*I was completely obsessed by her medical state, and I never thought beyond that, really. I was worried all the time.*" These concerns were expanded upon in the research by McCain (1990), which indicated that parents held onto the perception that these infants are at risk for future physical and behavioral problems. Vasquez (1995) described this early stage as a time of gathering resources to provide sustenance. The notion of risk remained even as the babies became toddlers, as parents kept in mind the potential physical, emotional, or mental disabilities that might ensue as a result of the premature birth. This sense of risk particularly emerged in the interviews conducted by Findlay (1997): "*They're saying that her hearing and vision more than likely will correct itself in time. And surgery for her eyes, and her ears, and legs. There's a whole bundle of things that could go wrong*" (Findlay, 1997, p. 97). As several other mothers described. "It's hard for me to cope with it when she gets sick 'cause I don't know what's going to happen next"... "I'm terrified of her getting sick. When she does get sick I panic"... "I was wondering when it was going to stop—-you know, that he was going to able to just live normal and we won't have to run back and forth to the doctor every two weeks or every month" (Miles et al., 1998, p. 73).

PROTECTING FRAGILITY

The parental feelings of vulnerability were closely tied with the process of providing protection, which clearly emerged across five of the studies reviewed (Casteel, 1990; Miles & Holditch-Davis, 1995; Miles et al., 1998; Vasquez, 1995). Parents described a sense of vulnerability and reported feeling especially protective when the baby came home from the hospital; "*At first, to me he was like if you had a glass and you drop it and it might break, so I was real protective of him. I might have been a little too protective*" (Miles et al., 1998). From another parent: "*It takes time to get attached to him.... I'm afraid of losing him even though he's come home. He's so small and fragile. He's not like a normal baby. Every time I see him I can't believe he's alive and doing fine*" (Jackson et al., 2003, p. 125). These heightened feelings of protection permeated the parents' everyday lives: "*Really, what I do in my life now is dedicated to him. Every meal I dedicate it to him in prayer, before I go to sleep, I dedicate it to him. He will probably be an only child and I just want to concentrate on him*" (Findlay, 1997, p. 100).

Parents were also especially careful to shield the infant from potential hazards and exposure to germs from family members: "*When people come over...mostly relatives ... I did tell them that they couldn't touch the baby. I felt so bad*" (Vasquez, 1995, p. 621). As another mother put it: "*I'm still protective of him. I believe I always will be like that, I just think it has to do with the way he was born. He's just my little miracle baby. I'm always going to have a sense of protection with him, more so than with the other kids*" (Miles et al., 1998, p. 73).

PRESERVING THE FAMILY

With the birth of a preterm infant, parents and the family unit were faced with stresses that challenged their coping resources and brought about changes in role relationships. As one father described: "*It was like you were both in the ocean and drowning. You're both drowning together. One of you has got to be strong enough to try and save both of you*" (Murphy, 1990, p. 35). For some parents, this was accompanied by a sense that they were under surveillance by healthcare providers as well as family members, which placed the young family at risk for disunity. They would turn inward to continue to shield and protect the infant while also mobilizing internal family resources. As one parent stated about those outside the immediate family: "*They're afraid of him. Some people are afraid to touch him... he's so small. I'm talking about relatives, the people that I expect to love him. They love him... but don't show it. They haven't celebrated his birth yet. It's been seven months*" (Vasquez, 1995, p. 622).

For some, family finances related to health-care costs was also a major source of stress: *"Our long financial struggle since then has been very hard on all of us...we were forced to file bankruptcy on all our outstanding medical and doctor bills to get us out of debt. We have no credit and no bank will loan us money for a home, which is still very much a part of our dreams. I don't wish to have any more children only because I can't give them a home to grow up in"* (McCain, 1990, p. 469).

In order to cope, many parents realized that a higher level of communication between them was necessary. According to one father: *"I think it is important to share. It is important to talk about things. If you have concerns, if you have fears, even, talk about them, in order to help each other out"* (Murphy, 1990, p. 39).

COMPENSATING FOR THE PAST

Closely aligned with the theme of protecting fragility was the process of compensating for the babies' past experience in the newborn intensive care unit (NICU), especially as the children became toddlers. Miles and Holditch-Davis (1995) identified a core concept of compensatory parenting, which evolved out of two paradoxical views the mothers had of their preterm children as being both normal and special. As one mother described: *"I have always had to make myself look back to the [NICU] when I got ready to discipline Katie. That she went through as much as she did and fought as hard as she did to be here. I always have to give her that little bit of leniency in discipline"* (Miles & Holditch-Davis, 1995, p. 247).

This alteration in parenting style was also evident in the transcripts of the interviews conducted by Findlay (1997). One participant stated: *"I can tell you, I'm going to be much more lenient than I'd ever planned on doing. I won't be able to punish him in any way because he's had such a hard time"* (Findlay, 1997, p. 98). Another parent said: *"After going through what he's been through... the suffering and the turmoil and the pain, I feel like there should be nothing in the world that I couldn't give him if he ask for it... due to the fact that his life already has been harder than my life will probably ever be... or the average kid that he will be along side of"* (Findlay, 1997, p. 98).

CAUTIOUSLY AFFIRMING THE FUTURE

As the parents emerged from the initial stages of adapting to risk, protecting fragility, and preserving the family, they tended to reaffirm their family unit and reconnect with extended family members and friends. For some families, the premature infant's actual age was a difficult concept to grasp: *"Just the other day we were talking about celebrating her birthday. When she turns one... will she really be one? Developmentally, she will be a little behind. We'll just do it on her real birthday, the day she should have been born"* (Vasquez, 1995, p. 623). Although thoughts of potential long-term difficulties resurfaced, for most families, this was a time when parents began to engage in more reciprocal interactions with the infant and finally achieve some reinforcement from that process. *"Once he starts smiling and listening to your voice, you're getting something back... It's been really hard"* (Vasquez, 1995, p. 622).

▪ Clinical Implications

The results of this meta-synthesis illustrate the paths that parents and families of preterm infants may move through prior to hospital discharge and then into the child's toddler years. The findings indicate the need for clinical nursing interventions targeted at the concerns that the families revealed.

As parents adapt to risk and focus on protecting their fragile infant, the concerns about the infant's health and development become paramount. Nurses should be prepared to provide expert, evidence-based clinical care and to offer anticipatory guidance and education that will enable the parents and family to cope with an infant at risk. Helping parents to build on their intuitive strengths and empowering them in caring for their infant are two other important aspects of nursing care for these families. Creative models of providing support to vulnerable parents while the infant is hospitalized should also be explored and implemented. For example, in their study of a parent "buddy" system, Preyde and Ardal (2003) found that when other mothers whose infants had previously been in the NICU provided telephone support to the parents, the mothers of the hospitalized infants experienced less anxiety, less depression, and greater perceived social support.

As the parents of preterm infants struggle to preserve their family, nurses should offer their teaching and recommendations based on a thorough understanding of the unique needs and values of the family unit, encouraging family members to visit the infant as much as possible. Current guidelines state that parents should be allowed unrestricted visits to the NICU, and that flexible and liberal visiting policies for all family members should be encouraged (American Academy of Pediatrics & American College of Obstetricians and Gynecologists, 2002). Sibling visitation should also be encouraged for children who are prepared in advance, who are supervised by an adult, who carefully wash their hands, and who show no signs or symptoms of acute illness or communicable disease. Nurses should assess for any barriers that may hinder family involvement (such as lack of transportation, changes in employment status, and day care needs) and work with an interdisciplinary team to help the family address those needs.

Families may also encounter significant financial stress if parents are losing time from work or if there are needs for additional equipment and home health services upon discharge. One parent stated that she needed a "corporate voice" to be empowered when negotiating with insurance companies (Swartz, personal communication, 2000). Every effort should be made to enable the family to effectively coordinate with insurance and community providers so that the transition home is as seamless as possible. In so doing, it is less likely that parents will be burdened with the role of case manager and thus will have greater resources to devote to the well-being of their baby and family.

Continuity of care remains important upon the infant's discharge and transfer to a primary care site or newborn follow-up clinic. For infants who were hospitalized for an extended period of time, it may be advisable to create a system whereby NICU nurses rotate through the newborn follow-up clinic, or even provide home care consultation, to facilitate continuity of care after discharge (Gennaro, Zukowsky, Brooten, Lowell, & Visco, 1990).

After discharge, a mechanism for peer support as described above may continue to be an important resource for parents. Interestingly, group prenatal care has been shown to be an effective intervention (Ickovics et al., 2003; Klima, 2003), and in one study resulted in higher birth-weights for infants of women receiving group versus individual prenatal care (Ickovics et al., 2003). This concept could be extended to newborn follow-up care and may provide a continuing source of social support for parents.

The infant's behavior and quality of the parent-child interactions should be continually assessed and provide the framework for further intervention both in the practice setting as well as in the home. The repetitiveness of child care routines and the lack of reinforcement that may accompany parenting a preterm infant who is not easily readable, predictable, or responsive can become a source of parental frustration. As Barnard et al. (1989) have noted, mothers may become intrusive or "aggressive" with the infant to compensate for perceived developmental and behavioral delays. As the child develops, the parenting issues of compensation, stimulation, overprotection, and discipline should be considered within the larger family context.

Finally, the work of policy makers and legislators in healthcare financing arenas is of considerable consequence for these families and children. The allocation of resources for this population is an ethically complex and emotionally charged issue. By attending to the eloquent voices of parents who are living the day-to-day experience of caring for high-risk, preterm infants, nurses can empower policy makers to make conscientious decisions that will improve the quality of life for these families.

Martha K. Swartz is an Associate Professor and Assistant Dean for Academic Affairs, Yale University School of Nursing, New Haven, CT. She can be reached via e-mail at martha.swartz@yale.edu.

REFERENCES

American Academy of Pediatrics & American College of Obstetricians and Gynecologists. (2002). *Guidelines for perinatal care* (5th ed.) Washington, DC: Author.

Barnard, K., Hammond, M., Booth, C., Bee, H., Mitchell, S., & Speiker, S. (1989). Measurement and meaning of mother child interaction. In F. Morrison & C. Lee (Eds.), *Applied developmental psychology* (pp. 39–80). San Diego: Academic Press.

Brooten, D., Gennaro, S., & Brown, L. (1988). Anxiety, depression and hostility in mothers of preterm infants. *Nursing Research, 37*, 213–216.

Casteel, J. (1990). Affects and cognitions of mothers and fathers of preterm infants. *Maternal Child Nursing Journal, 19*(3), 211–220.

Escobar, G., Littenberg, B., & Petitti, D. (1991). Outcomes among surviving very low birth weight infants: A meta-analysis. *Archives of Disease in Childhood, 66*, 204–211.

Field, T. (1995). Infants of depressed mothers. *Infant Behavior and Development, 18*, 1–13.

Gennaro, S., Zukowsky, K., Brooten, D., Lowell, L., & Visco, A. (1990). Concerns of mothers of low birth weight infants. *Pediatric Nursing, 16*(5), 459–462.

Ickovics, J. R., Kershaw, T. S., Westdahl, C., Rising, S. S., Klima, C., Reynolds, H., et al. (2003). Group prenatal care and preterm birth weight: results from a matched cohort study at public clinics. *Obstetrics and Gynecology, 102*(5 Pt 1), 1051–1057.

Klima, C. S. (2003). Centering pregnancy: A model for pregnant adolescents. *Journal of Midwifery and Women's Health, 48*(3), 220–225.

Martin, J. A., Hamilton, B. E., Sutton, P. D., Ventura, S. J., Menacker, F., & Munson, M. L. (2003). Births: final data for 2002. *National Vital Statistics Report, 52*(10), 1–114.

Miles, M., & Holditch-Davis, D. (1995). Compensatory parenting. How mothers describe parenting their 3-year-old prematurely born children. *Journal of Pediatric Nursing, 10*(4), 243–253.

Miles, M. Holditch-Davis, D., & Shepherd, H. (1998). Maternal concerns about parenting prematurely born children. *MCN: The American Journal of Maternal Child Nursing, 23*(2), 70–75.

Noblit, G., & Hare, R. (1988). *Meta-ethnography Synthesizing qualitative studies*, Newbury Park, CA: Sage Publications.

Preyde, M., & Ardal, F. (2003). Effectiveness of a parent "buddy" program for mothers of very preterm infants in a neonatal intensive care unit. *Canadian Medical Association Journal, 168*(8), 969–973.

Sandelowski, M., Docherty, S., & Emden, C. (1997). Qualitative meta-synthesis: Issues and techniques. *Research in Nursing and Health, 20*, 365–371.

Singer, L., Salvatore, A., Guo, S., Collin, M., Lilien, L., & Bailey, J. (1999). Maternal psychological distress and parenting stress after the birth of a very low-birth-weight infant. *Journal of the American Medical Association, 281*(9), 799–805.

Sumner, G., & Spletz, A. (1996). *NCAST caregiver/parent-child teaching manual.* Seattle: University of Washington NCAST publications.

Vasquez, E. (1995). Creating paths: Living with a very-low-birth-weight infant. *Journal of Obstetric, Gynecologic and Neonatal Nursing, 24*(7), 619–624.

Vohr, B., Wright, L., Dusick, A., Mele, L., Verter, J., Steichen, J., et al. (2000). Neurodevelopmental and functional outcomes of extremely low birth weight infants in the National Institute of Child Health and Human Development Neonatal Research Network, 1993–1994. *Pediatrics, 105*(6), 1216–1226.

Walker, L. S., Ortiz-Valdes, J. A., & Newbrough, J. R. (1989). The role of maternal employment and depression in the psychological adjustment of chronically ill, mentally retarded and well children. *Journal of Pediatric Psychology, 14*(3), 357–370.

APPENDIX L

Older Adults' Response to Health Care Practitioner Pain Communication

Grant Application to NINR, Summary Sheet, and Letter of Response to Reviewer Comments

Deborah Dillon McDonald

Form Approved Through 09/30/2007 OMB No. 0925-0001

Department of Health and Human Services Public Health Services **Grant Application** *Do not exceed character length restrictions indicated.*	**LEAVE BLANK—FOR PHS USE ONLY.** Type / Activity / Number Review Group / Formerly Council/Board (Month, Year) / Date Received

1. TITLE OF PROJECT *(Do not exceed 81 characters, including spaces and punctuation.)*
Older Adults' Response to Health Care Practitioner Pain Communication

2. RESPONSE TO SPECIFIC REQUEST FOR APPLICATIONS OR PROGRAM ANNOUNCEMENT OR SOLICITATION ☐ NO ☒ YES
(If "Yes," state number and title)
Number: PA-03-152 Title: Biobehavioral Pain Research

3. PRINCIPAL INVESTIGATOR/PROGRAM DIRECTOR	**New Investigator** ☐ **No** ☒ **Yes**	
3a. NAME (Last, first, middle) McDonald, Deborah Dillon	3b. DEGREE(S) BS MS PhD	3h. eRA Commons User Name
3c. POSITION TITLE Associate Professor	3d. MAILING ADDRESS *(Street, city, state, zip code)* The University of Connecticut School of Nursing 231 Glenbrook Road, Unit 2026 Storrs, CT 06269-2026	
3e. DEPARTMENT, SERVICE, LABORATORY, OR EQUIVALENT School of Nursing		
3f. MAJOR SUBDIVISION N/A		
3g. TELEPHONE AND FAX *(Area code, number and extension)* TEL: 860-486-3714 FAX: 860-486-0001	E-MAIL ADDRESS: deborah.mcdonald@uconn.edu	

4. HUMAN SUBJECTS RESEARCH ☐ No ☒ Yes	4b. Human Subjects Assurance No. FWA00007125		5. VERTEBRATE ANIMALS ☒ No ☐ Yes	
	4c. Clinical Trial ☒ No ☐ Yes	4d. NIH-defined Phase III Clinical Trial ☒ No ☐ Yes	5a. If "Yes," IACUC approval Date	5b. Animal welfare assurance no. A3124-01
4a. Research Exempt ☒ No ☐ Yes	If "Yes," Exemption No.			

6. DATES OF PROPOSED PERIOD OF SUPPORT *(month, day, year—MM/DD/YY)*		7. COSTS REQUESTED FOR INITIAL BUDGET PERIOD		8. COSTS REQUESTED FOR PROPOSED PERIOD OF SUPPORT	
From	Through	7a. Direct Costs ($)	7b. Total Costs ($)	8a. Direct Costs ($)	8b. Total Costs ($)
5/01/06	4/30/08	$100,000	$148,000	$175,000	$259,000

9. APPLICANT ORGANIZATION	10. TYPE OF ORGANIZATION
Name University of Connecticut Address Office for Sponsored Programs 438 Whitney Road Ext., Unit 1133 Storrs, CT 06269-1133 Telephone: 860-486-3622 Fax: 860-486-3726; Email: osp@uconn.edu	Public: ☐ Federal ☒ State ☐ Local Private: ☐ Private Nonprofit For-profit: ☐ General ☐ Small Business ☐ Woman-owned ☐ Socially and Economically Disadvantaged 11. ENTITY IDENTIFICATION NUMBER 06-0772160 DUNS NO. 614209054 Cong. District Second

12. ADMINISTRATIVE OFFICIAL TO BE NOTIFIED IF AWARD IS MADE	13. OFFICIAL SIGNING FOR APPLICANT ORGANIZATION
Name Carol Welt, PhD Title Executive Director & Assist. V. Prov. Research Address Office of Sponsored Programs 438 Whitney Road Ext., Unit 1133 Storrs, CT 06269-1133 Tel: 860-486-8704 FAX: 860-486-3726 E-Mail: carol.welt@uconn.edu	Name Carol Welt, PhD Title Executive Director & Assist. V. Prov. Research Address Office of Sponsored Programs 438 Whitney Road Ext., Unit 1133 Storrs, CT 06269-1133 Tel: 860-486-8704 FAX: 860-486-3726 E-Mail: carol.welt@uconn.edu

14. PRINCIPAL INVESTIGATOR/PROGRAM DIRECTOR ASSURANCE: I certify that the statements herein are true, complete and accurate to the best of my knowledge. I am aware that any false, fictitious, or fraudulent statements or claims may subject me to criminal, civil, or administrative penalties. I agree to accept responsibility for the scientific conduct of the project and to provide the required progress reports if a grant is awarded as a result of this application.	SIGNATURE OF PI/PD NAMED IN 3a. *(In ink. "Per" signature not acceptable.)*	DATE
15. APPLICANT ORGANIZATION CERTIFICATION AND ACCEPTANCE: I certify that the statements herein are true, complete and accurate to the best of my knowledge, and accept the obligation to comply with Public Health Services terms and conditions if a grant is awarded as a result of this application. I am aware that any false, fictitious, or fraudulent statements or claims may subject me to criminal, civil, or administrative penalties.	SIGNATURE OF OFFICIAL NAMED IN 13. *(In ink. "Per" signature not acceptable.)*	DATE

PHS 398 (Rev. 09/04) Face Page **Form Page 1**

Principal Investigator/Program Director (Last, First, Middle): McDonald, Deborah Dillon

DESCRIPTION: See instructions. State the application's broad, long-term objectives and specific aims, making reference to the health relatedness of the project (i.e., relevance to the **mission of the agency**). Describe concisely the research design and methods for achieving these goals. Describe the rationale and techniques you will use to pursue these goals.

In addition, in two or three sentences, describe in plain, lay language the relevance of this research to **public** health. If the application is funded, this description, as is, will become public information. Therefore, do not include proprietary/confidential information. **DO NOT EXCEED THE SPACE PROVIDED.**

How practitioners communicate with patients about their pain has been overlooked as a factor contributing to effective pain management. Eliciting important pain information from patients enables practitioners to prescribe more specific pain treatments, and significantly decrease pain. The aim of our study is to test the effect of practitioners asking patients an open-ended question about pain that does not encourage a socially desirable response. A posttest only double blind experiment will test how the phrasing of health care practitioners' pain questions, open-ended and without social desirability bias; closed-ended and without social desirability bias; or open-ended and with social desirability bias, affects the pain information provided by people with chronic pain. Three hundred community dwelling older adults with chronic osteoarthritis pain will be randomly assigned to one of the three practitioner pain communication conditions. Older adults will watch and verbally respond to a videotape clip of a practitioner asking the patient about their pain. The clips will be identical except for the pain question asked by the practitioner. After responding to the pain question, all of the older adults will respond to a second videotape clip of the practitioner asking if there is anything further they want to communicate. The older adults will then respond to a third videotape clip asking if there is anything further they want to communicate about their pain. Responses to the three videotape clips will be audiotaped. To control for pain differences between participants, the Brief Pain Inventory Short Form will be administered to measure present pain intensity and pain interference with functional activities. Participants' audiotaped responses will be transcribed and content analyzed using a priori criteria from national guidelines to identify communicated pain information and omitted pain information important for osteoarthritis pain management. The three groups will be compared for the communicated pain information and omitted pain information while controlling for present pain intensity and pain interference with activities. The goal is to identify practitioner pain communication strategies that allow patients to describe pain information important for guiding effective pain management, and to substantiate what pain information is missed when practitioners use less effective pain communication. The results will provide empirically tested communication strategies that can be used in practitioner and patient pain communication.

PERFORMANCE SITE(S) (organization, city, state)

University of Connecticut School of Nursing, Storrs, CT
P.C. Smith Towers, Hartford, CT
Betty Knox Apartments, Hartford, CT
Capitol Towers, Hartford, CT
Fireside Apartments, Bridgeport, CT
Harborview Towers, Bridgeport, CT
Park Ridge I and II, New Haven, CT
Tower One/Tower East, New Haven, CT

Principal Investigator/Program Director (Last, First, Middle): McDonald, Deborah Dillon

KEY PERSONNEL. See instructions. *Use continuation pages as needed* to provide the required information in the format shown below.
Start with Principal Investigator. List all other key personnel in alphabetical order, last name first.

Name	eRA Commons User Name	Organization	Role on Project
McDonald Deborah Dillon		University of Connecticut	PI
Katz, Leonard		University of Connecticut	Statistical Consultant
Rosiene, Joel		Eastern CT State Univ.	Computer Consultant
Maura Shea		University of Connecticut	Graduate Assistant
Leonie Rose		University of Connecticut	Graduate Assistant

OTHER SIGNIFICANT CONTRIBUTORS

Name	Organization	Role on Project
N/A		

Human Embryonic Stem Cells ☒ **No** ☐ **Yes**

If the proposed project involves human embryonic stem cells, list below the registration number of the specific cell line(s) from the following list: http://stemcells.nih.gov/registry/index.asp. *Use continuation pages as needed.*

If a specific line cannot be referenced at this time, include a statement that one from the Registry will be used.

Cell Line

Disclosure Permission Statement. Applicable to SBIR/STTR Only. See SBIR/STTR instructions. ☐ Yes ☐ No

Number the *following* pages consecutively throughout the application. Do not use suffixes such as 4a, 4b.

Principal Investigator/Program Director (Last, First, Middle): McDonald, Deborah Dillon

The name of the principal investigator/program director must be provided at the top of each printed page and each continuation page.

RESEARCH GRANT

TABLE OF CONTENTS

Appendix (*Five collated sets. No page numbering necessary for Appendix.*)

Appendices NOT PERMITTED for Phase I SBIR/STTR unless specifically solicited. ☒ Check if Appendix is Included

Number of publications and manuscripts accepted for publication (*not to exceed 10*) 5

Other items (list):

Brief Pain Inventory Short Form

Demographic Form

Principal Investigator/Program Director (Last, First, Middle): McDonald, Deborah Dillon

BUDGET JUSTIFICATION PAGE
MODULAR RESEARCH GRANT APPLICATION

	Initial Period	2nd	3rd	4th	5th	Sum Total (For Entire Project Period)
DC less Consortium F&A	100,000 *(Item 7a, Face Page)*	75,000				175,000 *(Item 8a, Face Page)*
Consortium F&A						
Total Direct Costs	100,000	75,000				$ 175,000

Personnel
Deborah Dillon McDonald, RN, PhD, Principal Investigator (Y1-20% & 50% summer; Y2-20% & 50% summer) will be responsible for the overall administration and completion of the project. She will collaborate with the videotape production company to produce the health care practitioner videotape clips. She will consult with Dr. Rosiene to program the laptop computer with touch screen. She will train and supervise the GA. She will prepare the sites for data collection and maintain contact with sites throughout the study. She will conduct the content analysis with the GA, statistically analyze the data in consultation with Dr. Katz, write, and submit manuscripts reporting the findings.

Leonard Katz, PhD, Consultant (Y2-1% effort) will advise the PI regarding statistical analyses.

Joel Rosiene, PhD, Consultant (Y1-5% effort) will program the laptop computer with the SuperLab 3.0 software and insert the health care practitioner videotape clips as the experimental manipulation. He will test the program and resolve any programming issues. He will remain available for consultation in the event of future programming problems.

TBA, Graduate Assistant (Y1-8 mos., 20 hrs/wk; Y2-4 mos., 20 hrs/wk; Y2-4 mos., 10 hrs/wk) will recruit eligible older adults, provide informed consent, data collect, debrief, and compensate the older adults. The GA will also transcribe the audiotaped responses. The GA will content analyze the data with the PI, enter the data into a SPSS data base, and clean the data to remove input errors.

Explanation for Budget Deviation
The increased budget by $25,000 during year one is due to the cost of video development and the need for the 20 hour per week GA during eight months.

Consortium

N/A

Fee (SBIR/STTR Only)
N/A

Principal Investigator/Program Director (Last, First, Middle): McDonald, Deborah Dillon

BIOGRAPHICAL SKETCH

Provide the following information for the key personnel and other significant contributors in the order listed on Form Page 2.
Follow this format for each person. **DO NOT EXCEED FOUR PAGES.**

NAME Deborah Dillon McDonald	POSITION TITLE Associate Professor
eRA COMMONS USER NAME	

EDUCATION/TRAINING *(Begin with baccalaureate or other initial professional education, such as nursing, and include postdoctoral training.)*

INSTITUTION AND LOCATION	DEGREE *(if applicable)*	YEAR(s)	FIELD OF STUDY
Marycrest College, Davenport, IA	BSN	1975	Nursing
University of Connecticut, Storrs, CT	MS	1981	Nursing
Columbia University, New York, NY	PhD	1990	Social Psychology

A. Positions and Honors

1975-1978	Navy Regional Medical Center, Long Beach, CA; Lieutenant in Nurse Corps
1978-1979	Hartford Hospital, Hartford, CT; Staff
1981-1983	Elms College, Chicopee, MA; Assistant Professor of Nursing
1983-1986	University of Connecticut, Storrs, CT; Assistant Professor of Nursing
1988-1990	National Center for Nursing Research Pre-doctoral Fellowship at Columbia University, New York, NY; Pre-doctoral Fellow
1990-present	University of Connecticut, Storrs, CT; Associate Professor

B. Selected Peer-Reviewed Publications

McDonald, D. (1993). Postoperative narcotic analgesic administration: A pilot study. *Applied Nursing Research. 6*, 106-110.

McDonald, D. (1994). Gender and ethnic stereotyping and narcotic analgesic administration. *Research in Nursing & Health, 17*, 45-49.

McDonald, D. (1996). Nurses' memory of patient's pain. *International Journal of Nursing Studies. 23*, 487-494.

McDonald, D., & Sterling, R. (1998). Acute pain reduction strategies used by well older adults. *International Journal of Nursing Studies, 35*, 265-70.

Wessman, A., & McDonald, D. (1999). Nurses' personal pain experiences and their pain management knowledge. *Journal of Continuing Education in Nursing, 30*, 152-157.

McDonald, D. (1999). Postoperative pain after hospital discharge. *Clinical Nursing Research, 8*, 347-359.

McDonald, D., McNulty, J., Erickson, K., & Weiskopf, C. (2000). Communicating pain and pain management needs after surgery. *Applied Nursing Research, 13*, 70-75.

McDonald, D., Freeland, M., Thomas, G., & Moore, J. (2001). Testing a preoperative pain management intervention for elders. *Research in Nursing & Health, 24*, 402-409.

McDonald, D. & Weiskopf, C. (2001). Adult patients' postoperative pain descriptions and responses to the Short-Form McGill Pain Questionnaire. *Clinical Nursing Research, 10*, 442-452.

Tafas, C., Patiraki, E., McDonald, D. & Lemonidou, C. (2002). Testing an instrument measuring Greek nurses' knowledge and attitudes regarding pain. *Cancer Nursing, 25* (1), 1 – 7.

McDonald, D., Pourier, S., Gonzalez, T., Brace, J., Lakhani, K., Landry, S. & Wrigley, P. (2002). Pain problems in young adults and pain reduction strategies. *Pain Management Nursing, 3*(3), 81-86.

McDonald, D. & Molony, S. (2004). Postoperative pain communication skills for older adults. *Western Journal of Nursing Research, 26*, 836 – 852, 858 - 859.

Patiraki - Kourbani , E., Tafas , C., McDonald , D., Papathanassoglou , E., Katsaragakis , S. & Lemonidou , C. (2004). Greek nurses' personal and professional pain experiences. *International Journal of Nursing Studies, 41*, 345-54.

McDonald, D., Thomas, G., Livingston, K. & Severson, J. (2005). Assisting older adults to communicate their postoperative pain. *Clinical Nursing Research, 14,* 109-126.

McDonald, D., LaPorta, M., & Meadows-Oliver, M. (2006). Nurses' response to pain communication from patients: A post-test experimental Study. *International Journal of Nursing Studies.*

C. Research Support

National Institute of Nursing Research, 1R21NR009848-01, 3/16/06 – 3/15/08, McDonald PI
Older Adults' Response to Health Care Practitioner Pain Communication
The aim of our study is to test the effect of practitioners asking patients an open-ended question about pain that does not encourage a socially desirable response.

Donaghue Foundation, 10/1/01 – 10/1/02; McDonald PI
Assisting Elders to Communicate their Pain After Surgery
The goal of the study was to refine our videotape intervention teaching older adults about postoperative pain communication and pain management, and test the effects of the videotape intervention on the pain outcomes of older adults after major surgery.

National Institute of Nursing Research, 1 R15 NR04876-03, 5/1/99 – 10/1/01; McDonald PI
Postoperative Pain Communication Skills for Older Adults
The goal of the study was to develop a videotape intervention teaching older adults about postoperative pain communication and pain management, and test the effects of the videotape intervention on the pain outcomes of older adults after major surgery.

University of Athens, Athens, Greece, 11/98 – 1/03; McDonald Co-Investigator
Nurses' Knowledge Regarding Pain and Cancer Patients' Reports of Pain Control
The goal of the study was to test the construct validity, test-retest reliability, and internal consistency of the Greek version of the Nurses' Knowledge and Attitudes Survey Regarding Pain (NKASRP) with Greek nurses, as phase I in a series of studies examining how to improve pain outcomes for cancer patients in Greece.

Principal Investigator/Program Director (Last, First, Middle): McDonald, Deborah Dillon

Resources

Clinical: We will recruit and conduct the study at seven independent living elder housing sites throughout Connecticut. The urban sites in Bridgeport, New Haven and, Hartford, CT increase the opportunity to include Black or African Americans, Hispanic and Asian elders. The sites include P.C. Smith Towers, Capitol Towers, and the Betty Knox Apartments in Hartford, CT; Park Ridge I and II and Tower One/Tower East in New Haven, CT; and Fireside Apartments and Harborview Towers in Bridgeport, CT. The sites contain from 193 to 248 housing units each, insuring a large group of older adults for our study.

Computer: The PI has a Dell Pentium 4 computer 2.4 GHz with 256 MB RAM, loaded with SPSS-13.0 and Word 2000 professional operating system; and a Hewlett Packard LaserJet5 printer in her university office. Additional computer resources are available through the Center for Nursing Research (CNR) in the School of Nursing at the University of Connecticut. Fourteen new Dell computers each with Intel Pentium 4 processor 520's are available. There are two HP LaserJet IV printers, one HP LaserJet III printer, one HP LaserJet 1200, one HP LaserJet 5L printer, one Laser Jet 1100 printer, and an HP Office jet 5110 all-in-one copier, scanner, and printer. All computers have direct access to the university mainframe computer, the university library system, and the Internet. Software programs available on the PCs in the CNR relevant for our study include: Power and Precision, QRS N6 (NUD*IST), and SPSS 12.0.

Office: The PI has a private university office, telephone, and four locked filing cabinets. Various support personnel are available through the Center for Nursing Research at the School of Nursing. Work-study students, graduate assistants, and secretaries are available for assisting with all aspects of a research project. In addition, a program for doctoral study in the School of Nursing offers a pool of well-qualified graduate nursing students from which to select a research assistant for the study.

Other: The Seven Seas Film Company located in Madison, CT will produce the three videotape clips of the health care practitioner asking the older adults about their pain, the two follow up videotape clips, and the test videotape that will be used to adjust the audibility of the videotapes for each participant. Seven Seas produced our 15-minute documentary style pain communication videotape tested with older adults and reported in McDonald, et al., (2005). Seven Seas has produced films for the Public Broadcasting Service (PBS) and major universities.

MAJOR EQUIPMENT: List the most important equipment items already available for this project, noting the location and pertinent capabilities of each.
The University of Connecticut School of Nursing offers access to additional equipment. There are multiple copiers (i.e. Cannon IR3300, Savin 4060 SP, all with sorter and stapler, a color scanner (HP Office jet 9130), a color printer (Hewlett Packard color laser jet 5550hdn) and two independent fax lines. In addition to readily available equipment, there is ample conference meeting space and facilities for use in research projects.

Principal Investigator/Program Director (Last, First, Middle): McDonald, Deborah Dillon

A. Specific Aims

Management of patients' pain is one of the most enduring challenges facing all health care practitioners. Assessment of pain is now an assumed standard of practice required by the Joint Commission for Accreditation of Health Care Organizations. Pain communication between patients and practitioners provides a critical link for the assessment and management of pain.

Inadequate pain communication between patients and health care practitioners[1-3] can result in sustained or increased pain for patients.[4] Researchers have shown that pain remained undiagnosed for 53% of patients with moderate pain and 30% with severe pain during their primary care outpatient visit,[5] indicating that pain was not addressed despite a pressing need to talk about pain. Nearly half of the people reported moderate levels of acute[6] or chronic pain[7] in two recent surveys. Communicating about pain involves more than use of pain assessment measures. Hospitalized patients did not consider responding to a numerical pain intensity scale equivalent to communicating about pain.[2] Effective pain communication involves talking with patients in ways that permit patients to more fully discuss salient aspects of their pain experience. Research is needed to test communication strategies that enhance patient and practitioner communication about pain.

The aim of this study is to test how practitioners' pain communication affects the pain information provided by older adults. The study will specifically test the effect of asking an open-ended question about pain that does not direct a socially desirable response. We suspect that a question about pain presented in what might be perceived as a social exchange ("How are you feeling?") might not be sufficient to elicit clinically meaningful and important information if patients perceive a social, rather than a clinical, source of the question.

Hypothesis

Older adults asked about their pain with an open-ended question without social desirability bias will describe more important pain information and omit less information than older adults asked about their pain with a closed-ended question without social desirability or an open-ended question with social desirability bias.

To test the hypothesis, three videos will be developed that portray a health care practitioner asking participants about their pain in one of three different ways: open-ended without social desirability, closed-ended without social desirability, and open-ended with social desirability. Older adults with chronic osteoarthritis pain will be randomly assigned to watch and respond to one of the three videos. The second and third parts of the videos, after the first part of questioning, will be the same. All participants will next watch and respond to the second part of the video with the practitioner asking if there is anything further participants want to communicate in general, and then the third part with the practitioner asking if there is anything further they want to communicate about their pain. Participants' audio taped responses will be content analyzed for important included and omitted pain information.

Older adults with chronic pain due to osteoarthritis will be randomly assigned to one of the three practitioner pain communication conditions. Present pain will be measured with the counterbalanced Brief Pain Inventory Short Form (BPI-SF) to statistically control for pain differences between participants evident after random assignment while controlling for the timing of the BPI-SF. Participants' audio taped responses will be content analyzed using a priori criteria from the American Pain Society[8] guidelines for the management of pain in osteoarthritis to identify pain communication content important for osteoarthritis pain management, and important omitted pain information. The three groups will be compared for the included and omitted pain information while controlling for pre-existing, current pain intensity and pain interference with activities. The immediate goal is to identify practitioner pain communication strategies that allow patients to describe important pain information that can more effectively guide pain management, and significantly reduce or eliminate pain. The long-term goal is to incorporate empirically tested, theory driven pain communication strategies into health practitioner curricula and patient education.

Principal Investigator/Program Director (Last, First, Middle): McDonald, Deborah Dillon

B. Background and Significance

Communication About Pain Management

Effective pain communication involves more than practitioners encouraging patients to identify when patients have pain. An intervention that encouraged terminally ill patients to talk with their physicians about their pain showed that 43.4% of patients continued to have a pain problem at hospital discharge, and less than half received a pain intervention.[9] Interventions that only encourage patients to talk about their pain might be inadequate for promoting pain communication. Increased communication between patients and practitioners was not associated with increased pain relief, perhaps because communication was restricted to discussing pain treatments, and asking the patient to alert practitioners when pain occurred.[10] Clinical contexts where routine pain communication should be part of standard practice continue to demonstrate deficiencies in pain communication. Physicians discussed pain during only 72% of the outpatient palliative care visits, and initiated the pain topic only half of the time.[11] Cancer patients and family caregivers have clearly identified the need for improved communication with their health care practitioners.[12] Patients and practitioners need research-based support to help them communicate about pain in ways that lead to greater pain relief for patients.

Reasons for the inadequate pain communication might be directly attributable to the way that practitioners speak with patients. Constructing pain assessment questions in the form of social conversation (i.e. "How are you today?") encourages patients to respond in a socially desirable manner by suppressing their pain concerns.[3,13] These types of approaches might be seen as directing social exchange rather than soliciting important clinical assessment data. Giving little attention to patients' reports of pain, and controlling pain communication by interrupting patients, minimizing or dismissing the reports of pain, and curtailing patient responses to yes/no responses were techniques observed to be used by physicians in a descriptive study of oncology patients consulting with their physicians.[13] Again, these methods to ask for pain information are more directing in soliciting a response than merely asking a patient, "tell me about your pain." Physicians challenged and attempted to disconfirm biological explanations for the pain, insisting on psychological explanations when talking with chronic pain patients who had no apparent medical reason for their pain.[14] When subjected to practitioner statements suggesting where the pain might be felt, patients reported significantly more referred pain, and more intense pain.[15] The preceding communication techniques thwart complete and accurate pain discussions between patients and practitioners. Randomized controlled clinical trials are needed to link specific pain communication strategies to patient outcomes.

Patient factors impact pain communication. Patient factors include low expectations for pain relief,[16-17] reluctance to bother busy staff,[3,12,18] concern about repercussions from staff if patients complain about pain,[4] fear of addiction to opioids,[17,19-20] fear of unpleasant opioid side effects,[3,19-21] belief that health care providers innately know best how to manage their pain;[17] and general lack of information about pain management, and difficulty articulating pain management needs.[4] Hospitalized patients reporting more intense pain communicated about their pain more often, but were less satisfied with the information communicated by the nurse. Older adults communicated less about their pain, but voiced greater satisfaction with the information provided by nurses.[2] When given the opportunity, many patients clearly describe their pain (e.g. "my leg is going to burst," "someone turning a knife under my skin."[22] Patients have the ability to clearly communicate their pain, but multiple barriers continue to restrain patients from communicating about pain with practitioners.

Pain Communication Interventions

Promising interventions to assist patients to describe their pain have been tested, such as individual coaching prior to an office visit,[23] and combinations of written scripts and individual coaching.[24] Both interventions resulted in a significant decrease in pain. These findings suggest that patients can be assisted to effectively communicate their pain and receive interventions that significantly reduce their pain. The cost of the individual coaching interventions might limit the widespread use of coaching interventions. Both studies involved patients with cancer pain. Individual coaching interventions for patients with different pain etiologies might not be as effective in eliciting more responsive pain management from practitioners.

Practitioner Influence in Health Care Communication

Health care communication research, conducted mainly in psychology and medicine, provides insight about pain management communication. The Bayer Institute for Health Care Communication literature review on health care practitioner and patient communication identified only six medical studies that examined eliciting patients' agenda.[25] All six were limited to descriptive medical studies. Primary care physicians interrupted opening statements by their patients during 77% of the visits, and patients completed only 1 out of 52 interrupted statements.[26] Physician communication remained virtually unchanged 12 years later when physicians again interrupted 72% of the opening statements.[27] Physicians using problem defining communication skills, which included starting off with an open-ended question to delineate the patient's problem, identified significantly more patients with emotional distress than physicians not taught problem defining skills. Six months later patient distress remained significantly reduced for patients of physicians using problem defining communication skills.[28] Female physicians use more positive statements, more psychosocial information giving, more active partnership behaviors, but also more closed-ended questions during office visits.[29] The ability to gather or omit potentially important information from patients is influenced by how health care practitioners communicate with patients.

Patient Influence in Health Care Communication

Descriptive and intervention studies have examined patients' contribution to their health care interaction. During a family practice office visit, younger, more educated, and more anxious patients who asked more questions received more diagnostic health information. Patients who asked more questions and expressed more concern received more treatment information from their physicians.[30] Similarly, parents of pediatric patients received more information when they asked more questions and expressed more affect.[31] Patients communicated more and provided more biomedical and psychosocial information, promoted more partnership building, and talked more positively with female physicians.[32] Patients trained via a booklet and coaching to talk with their family practice physicians asked more questions about medically related topics, elicited more information from the physician, and provided more information about their medical problems than untrained patients.[33] Women either prompted to think about their questions prior to seeing their women's health physician or informed that the physician was open to questions were significantly more likely to ask all of the questions that they wanted compared to women in a control group.[34] Participants who watched a video with a patient either asking questions or making disclosures communicated more than participants who watched a video without patient interaction. [35] Patients who prior to their office visit were instructed to think about the instructions the physician gave them during the visit, imagine carrying out the instructions, and to ask the physician questions about problems that they anticipated, communicated significantly more than patients not given any additional instructions, or patients instructed that the physician was open to answering questions.[36] Preliminary evaluation of a community based intervention teaching people how to communicate with their physician by teaching them communication skills and helping them practice the skills was associated with a moderate increase in patient confidence for communicating with the physician.[37] The variety of successful communication interventions indicates that people can successfully communicate with their health care practitioners when supported to do so.

Linking increased practitioner and patient communication with improved health outcomes substantiates the impact of communication during health care interactions. Patients with diabetes, hypertension, ulcer disease, and breast cancer were tested during three randomized controlled trials and a nonequivalent control trial respectively for the effect of an intervention to improve communication by patients during health care visits.[38] The intervention for each study consisted of providing each patient with individualized information about their medical care, and coaching about actively communicating during the visit. The communication techniques included more effective ways to ask questions, keeping focused on the medical care, and negotiating skills. Improved hemoglobin A1c and lowered diastolic blood pressure resulted from more patient control, less physician control, more negative affect expressed by both, more information seeking by patients, and more patient communication. How patients with chronic health problems communicate with practitioners during their health care visits can directly impact their health outcomes. The success of the individualized coaching intervention demonstrates that patients with different chronic health problems can be assisted to communicate more effectively and impact their health outcomes. The resource intensity of the intervention remains a drawback.

Pain Communication and Health Practitioner Curricula

Practitioner pain management education has been the major means for improving pain outcomes, but medical and nursing curricula have generally not included education about pain communication beyond pain assessment (e.g. Giamberardino[39]), even though experts have identified pain communication skills as an essential component of training in medical education.[40] The benefit of increased education in pain communication was provided by a recent study with pediatric residents.[41] An 18-hour educational intervention teaching physicians a more patient centered approach when communicating about pain problems with patients with fibromyalgia found that patients felt that they were allowed to fully discuss their pain,[42] perhaps because of a Hawthorne effect for the physicians, or low expectations by patients. This resource intensive intervention supported increased pain communication between patients and practitioners, but the specific communication strategies that promoted the full discussion remain unclear, and the effect on patient pain outcomes was not measured. Further research is needed to test specific pain communication strategies essential for practitioner pain management education.

Communication Theory Attuning Strategies

Communication Accommodation Theory (CAT) has been used to guide causal research about communication behaviors with older adults.[43] CAT describes the motivations and behaviors of people as they adjust their communication in response to their own needs and the perceived behavior of the other person.[44-45] Paying attention to the other person when communicating provides useful information that can enhance communication. This attention has been termed attuning strategies.[46] Attuning strategies include discourse management and interpersonal control strategies. Discourse management strategies involve evaluating the social aspects of the communication interaction, such as selecting and sharing a topic. Interpersonal control strategies pertain to identifying the relationship between the communicators.

Within the context of pain management communication CAT provides strategies that practitioners can use to enhance communication with patients. For example, practitioners could use a topic sharing discourse management strategy by using an open-ended question to inquire about pain

Principal Investigator/Program Director (Last, First, Middle): McDonald, Deborah Dillon

to allow patients more freedom to respond in the way they feel most helpful in communicating their pain. An interpersonal control strategy by practitioners would be to avoid phrasing questions about pain in a socially desirable way, clarifying that the pain communication is taking place within a health care rather than a social context. Testing how different strategies affect pain communication between practitioners and patients can lead to more effective use of the communication strategies to decrease pain.

Summary the Literature Review

Pain communication has emerged as an important, but poorly understood aspect of pain management. Descriptive studies document problems with pain communication and patient related barriers to pain communication. Clinical trials have demonstrated the benefits of resource intensive coaching interventions for patients prior to office visits. An extensive pain communication education intervention with physicians did not clarify if pain was adequately discussed, or how individual communication strategies affected pain communication. Our study addresses gaps in pain communication research by using theory based pain communication strategies in a rigorously designed study to test how older adults' respond to different types of health care practitioner pain communication.

C. Preliminary Studies

In nine studies, the PI has investigated different aspects of practitioner and patient communication that might affect pain management. A summary of the findings from the nine studies includes:

- nurses' administration of opioids after surgery is related to the patients' race and gender;[47]
- some nurses may not attend to their patients' specific pain information, and consequently either omit this pain information or recall it incorrectly;[48]
- many older adults do not plan to talk in the hospital with their practitioners about their pain;[49]
- adults have difficulty communicating their pain to their health care providers after
- surgery;[3]
- postoperative pain after discharge continues to plague many adults and might be decreased if adults understood more about pain management and possessed more effective pain communication skills;[50]
- a majority of postoperative patients used exact Short-Form McGill Pain questionnaire sensory or affective words or synonyms to describe their postoperative pain;[51]
- a slide show teaching older adults about postoperative pain communication and pain management helped decrease postoperative pain;[52]
- a video teaching pain communication and pain management assisted older adults to experience less sensory pain during the early postoperative period;[53]
- a refined video teaching pain management and pain communication skills assisted older adults to experience less pain interference with sleep during the first postoperative day.[54]

The nine studies represent a wide range of methods, including post-test only experiments, patient surveys using audio taped interviews, and content analysis. Five manuscripts,[3,49-50,53-54] contained in Appendix A, provide more detailed accounts of our research.

Summary

The processes used in conducting these studies have provided excellent preparation for the implementation of the proposed research. We have recruited and retained over 320 participants during our previous pain management studies. We have worked exclusively with older adults during four of our recent studies, three of which were randomized controlled trials that provided us with the expertise needed to conduct our proposed experiment. Our experience with refining our video intervention teaching older adults how to communicate with practitioners about pain has prepared us to develop the videos in our proposed study as a way to standardize our experimental manipulations. Our experience in conducting content analyses with participants' responses provides us with the skill required for content analysis of participants' responses in our proposed study. We are well prepared to conduct our proposed study, if the science is deemed sound.

We have established pain communication between the practitioner and patient as an integral part of achieving pain relief. The results from our three pain communication intervention studies indicate that closer scrutiny of pain communication is needed to identify communication strategies that exert the greatest effect on patients and practitioners. We need to directly test specific communication strategies in order to clarify which communication strategies encourage older adults to describe important information, and what important information is missed when health care practitioners use ineffective communication strategies. Research based communication skills provide a more powerful way to help practitioners and older adults communicate about pain problems.

D. Research Design and Methods

Our study takes the novel approach of testing patients' responses to being asked about their pain to determine what important information people communicate. Our innovative use of national osteoarthritis pain management guidelines to analyze the clinical importance of the information communicated by the older adults further strengthens our proposed study. In particular we are interested in knowing whether important pain information is omitted when practitioners use closed ended questions and/or socially phrased questions that might direct responding. Practitioners need to be aware if pain information is gained or lost when different communication strategies are used to talk about pain. The attuning strategies from CAT provides the theoretical framework for our study, allowing us to test two aspects of how well CAT describes the dynamic process of participating in a health care conversation about pain.

Design

A posttest only double blind experiment will test how the phrasing of health care practitioners' pain question, open-ended without social desirability, closed-ended without social desirability, or open-ended with social desirability bias, affects the pain information provided by older adults with chronic osteoarthritis pain. To control for the measurement effect, half of each of the three groups will respond to the Brief Pain Inventory Short Form (BPI-SF) before watching the videos, and the remaining half after responding to the final video. Table 1 depicts the research design.

Sample

Older adults may be even more vulnerable to pain communication difficulties with health care practitioners.[2,49] Inclusion criteria for the sample size of 300 consists of community dwelling adults, age 60 and older who speak, read, and understand English and who have self identified osteoarthritis pain. Exclusion criteria consists of the presence of self identified malignant pain. Older adults with malignant pain might communicate differently due to the life-threatening context of pain associated with a cancer diagnosis. A small effect size is indicated when no previous effect size is available to base the sample size estimate upon.[55] A total sample size of 300 is needed for a multivariate analysis of covariance (MANCOVA) with three groups (open-ended without social desirability, closed-ended without social desirability, or open-ended with social desirability bias), two dependent variables (pain information included and pain information omitted), .05 level of significance, .80 power, and small estimated effect size.[56] Over 20 million Americans have osteoarthritis.[57] More than 80% of older adults over 75 have osteoarthritis.[58] The feasibility is high for recruiting the required sample size.

Table 1
Research Design

	Group		Measurements							
R	open-ended and without social desirability bias (a)	BPI	Xa	O1	X2	O2	X3	O3	
R	open-ended and without social desirability bias (a)		Xa	O1	X2	O2	X3	O3	BPI
R	closed-ended and without social desirability bias (b)	BPI	Xb	O1	X2	O2	X3	O3	
R	closed-ended and without social desirability bias (b)		Xb	O1	X2	O2	X3	O3	BPI
R	open-ended and with social desirability bias (c)	BPI	Xc	O1	X2	O2	X3	O3	
R	open-ended and with social desirability bias (c)		Xc	O1	X2	O2	X3	O3	BPI

R = Random assignment
BPI = Brief Pain Inventory measure for covariates, pain intensity and interference with activities
Xa = Video with open-ended without social desirability bias
Xb = Video with closed-ended without social desirability bias
Xc = Video with open-ended with social desirability bias
O1 = Verbal response to the video clip practitioner pain question
O2 = Verbal response to the video clips about additional information in general
O3 = Verbal response to the video clips about additional information specific to pain
X2 = General additional information question
X3 = Pain specific additional information question

Procedure

We will first describe the overall procedure to provide context for our video experimental manipulation. We will then describe our measures, followed by our plans for content analyses and statistical analyses.

Recruitment.

Eligible older adults will be recruited from independent housing sites in Hartford, Bridgeport, New Haven, and suburban areas of Connecticut. The registered nurse doctoral student graduate assistant (GA) will screen for eligibility, give the older adult an enlarged print copy of the informed consent, and secure informed consent. Screening will include asking participants to self identify if they experience pain from osteoarthritis. To avoid priming participants about how to describe their pain, a yes/no question will be used to screen for osteoarthritis pain, "Do you have pain from osteoarthritis?" Participants will also be asked if they have any cancer pain, "If you have been diagnosed with cancer, do you have any pain from cancer?" Participants with malignant pain will be excluded from the study. Participants will be asked their age. Consenting, eligible participants will be automatically randomized to one of the three conditions by the SuperLab 3.0 computer software program, keeping the GA blind to the condition.

A cover story will be given to each older adult to increase experimental realism and to decrease the introduction of response bias. Participants will be told that the study is testing the feasibility of helping people prepare for their health care office visit while waiting in the office for their appointment. The GA will make the following statement. "We are testing whether asking patients to respond to a video of a health care practitioner asking questions about your health prior to an office visit helps you communicate better during the office visit."

Our cover story provides experimental realism by providing a credible reason for asking older adults to watch and respond to a computer video clip of a health care practitioner. Closely approximating a real life clinical situation increases the likelihood that responses from participants will be similar to their responses to health care practitioners during actual pain communication in the clinical setting. Successful patient coaching interventions prior to office visits have been reported,[24] making the cover story more credible.

Experimental Manipulation and Measurement.

The use of a video clip to provide the experimental manipulation strengthens the study by controlling for differences that occur across repeated live presentations of the same condition, strengthening fidelity[59] to the treatment. The use of video clips controls for any experimenter demand effects by standardizing the way participants are asked about pain in each condition. The use of the health care practitioner title increases the applicability of the findings to both nurse practitioners and physicians. Each of the three video clips will be subjected to a review panel of primary care nurse practitioners and physicians to determine the face validity of the practitioner posed question, and the similarity of other aspects of the clips. The use of the video clip reduces the cost of an additional GA to personally administer the experimental manipulation.

Our method avoids the problem of using patient analogues,[60] people who are asked to imagine themselves as having chronic pain. Responses from patient analogues might not be generalized to people with chronic pain, because patient analogues might not accurately grasp the experience of chronic pain.

The GA will test the audio tape recorder to insure that participants' voices are clearly and completely recorded. The GA will explain that the participant is going to watch three video clips of a health care practitioner on the computer screen and verbally respond to the practitioner's question in each clip before proceeding to the next clip. The participant's response will be audio taped. Participant will be instructed to touch any area of the screen to proceed to the next question, after they have responded to each question. We chose a touch screen for the increased ease of use especially for older adults with osteoarthritis in their hands. The final screen will instruct participants to press the buzzer placed on the table beside the computer to signal the GA to return to the room. After providing the instructions, the GA will use a test video to adjust the sound to a comfortable, audible level for each participant. The GA will start the audio tape recorder, press the computer to start the video clip and then leave the room. There will be a 15 second delay before the video clip begins. During that time, the participant will be randomly assigned to one of the three conditions through use of the SuperLab 3.0 software. The computer software can be programmed to randomly assign treatments to participants, and provide an experimental treatment (the video tape clips). The ability to use video clips as stimuli and randomly assign older adults to condition make the software a valuable resource for our study.

The randomized video clip will begin and the condition will be audio-recorded allowing the PI to later determine the participant's condition. The participant will respond to the practitioner's question about their pain, and the verbal response will be audio taped. The question will consist of one of the following, corresponding to the three experimental conditions.

- Tell me about your pain, aches, soreness, or discomfort. (open-ended and without social desirability)
- What would you rate your pain, aches, soreness, or discomfort on a 0 to 10 scale with 0, no pain, and 10 the worst pain possible? (closed-ended and without social desirability bias)
- How are you feeling? (open-ended and with social desirability bias)

The second part of each practitioner video will consist of the practitioner asking all participants, "What else can you tell me?" The third and final part of the practitioner video will consist of the practitioner asking, "What else can you tell me about your pain, aches, soreness or discomfort?" Responses to all three questions will be audio-recorded. Participants will be instructed by the GA to press the screen to proceed to the next question, after fully responding to each question. The final screen will instruct participants to press the buzzer placed beside the computer after responding to the third and final question. The buzzer will signal the GA to return to the room. A separate audiotape will be labeled for each participant.

Brief Pain Inventory Short Form (BPI-SF) Pain Measure.

The GA will orally administer the BPI-SF to measure participants' pain at the present time. Measuring participants' present pain with the BPI-SF allows us to control for pain differences across participants. Participants might learn how to better describe their pain by responding to the BPI-SF, but might also respond differently to the BPI-SF after viewing and responding to the videos. We will randomly counterbalance the BPI-SF measure to control for these potential learning effects. Fifty participants from each of the three experimental groups will respond to the BPI-SF after responding to the final video. The remaining 50 participants from each group will respond to the BPI-SF prior to watching the first video (experimental manipulation). The PI will randomize timing of the BPI-SF with a computer program for random assignment and compile a list that indicates, by order of entry into the study, whether the BPI-SF will be administered prior to watching the videos or after responding to the third and final video.

Demographic information will be measured last. The GA will orally ask the demographic questions and record responses on a demographic form. The BPI-SF, and demographic form will be coded with the same number used to identify the participant's audiotape.

Upon completion of all of the measures, the following protocol will be followed by the GA for participants who report present pain intensity on the BPI-SF at a level of four or greater. The GA will encourage the older adults to talk with their health care practitioner about their pain problem. If participants state that they do not have a health care practitioner, the name, location and telephone number of nearby accredited ambulatory care clinics will be given in writing to participants, with encouragement to make an appointment. If participants state that they have no health care insurance to pay for an office visit, the name, location and telephone number of a nearby sliding scale community health clinic will be given to them in written form.

Debriefing.

After completing the demographic information, the GA will debrief each participant. Participants will be thanked for their help. The debriefing will first include checking for hypothesis guessing by asking participants what they thought the study was about. Data from any participants guessing what the study was about will be marked and will not be used in the analysis. The study will be completely explained to participants, along with the reason for the deception. Participants will be checked for any concern or distress about the deception used in the study, and reminded that they are free to withdraw from the study. Participants will be asked not to discuss the study with people living in the housing development, because they might participate in the study. Participants will be asked if they have any questions or comments to make about the study. Participants will be thanked for their participation in the study, given a personal copy of the Arthritis Foundation publication, *Managing Your Pain*,[61] compensated for their time with a $20 money order, and informed that their participation has been completed.

Video Clip Experimental Manipulation

A video clip presented on a touch screen equipped laptop computer monitor will be used for the experimental manipulation. Prior to leaving the room, the GA will adjust the sound, using a video clip not associated with the experimental manipulation with the same sound volume of the three experimental video clips. The GA will adjust the sound volume to a level that allows each participant to clearly hear the video.

A brief health care office visit scene will be depicted. The same practitioner will be videoed for each of the three conditions. The conditions will be identical except for how the practitioner asks patients about their pain. Each condition will start out with the practitioner entering the examination room and sitting down in a chair to face the camera (participant). The practitioner will say, "Hello, I am going to ask you some questions about your health." After a slight pause, the practitioner will ask about the participant's pain (the experimental manipulation). The practitioner will use the same volume, voice inflection and nonverbal communication when asking each of the three questions. The three video clips will be reviewed by a group of five primary care nurse practitioners and primary care physicians for face validity and for equality of practitioner nonverbal behavior and verbal behavior such as tone, and voice inflection.

The practitioner will ask only one question in each condition. The three questions representing each of the three conditions are as follows:

- Tell me about your pain, aches, soreness, or discomfort. (open-ended and without social desirability)
- What would you rate your pain, aches, soreness, or discomfort on a 0 to 10 scale with 0, no pain, and 10 the worst pain possible? (closed-ended and without social desirability bias)
- How are you feeling? (open-ended and with social desirability bias)

An alternative approach would be to embed the pain questions within a more prolonged discussion by the practitioner. Further discussion would burden participants with a longer time to complete the study. Additional general health care discussion would also require participants to reveal personal health information unnecessary for the purposes of the study. To increase privacy of health information and decrease burden for participants, we chose to place the pain question at the beginning of the discussion. It would be reasonable for a practitioner to ask older adults with osteoarthritis pain about their pain at the beginning of the visit.

We also chose to leave the health care practitioner credentials ambiguous, rather than specifying the practitioner as a physician or a nurse practitioner. The ambiguity allows us to extend the applicability of the findings to both physicians and nurse practitioners.

Measures

Content Analysis of Included Pain Information.

Participants' verbal response to the practitioner's pain question will be audio taped and transcribed for content analysis. Content analysis for included pain information is described in the section on content analysis.

Content Analysis of Omitted Information.

Two questions will be used to measure additional information that participants communicate, when given the opportunity. After responding to the practitioners' pain question, all of the older adults will watch and listen to a second video clip of the practitioner asking, "What else can you tell me?" Next all participants will respond to a third video clip of the practitioner asking the participant, "What else can you tell me about your pain, aches, soreness or discomfort?" Responses to both questions will be audio taped and transcribed for content analysis. Participant responses to additional information might be increased if measured in a face-to-face interview. Use of the same practitioner video clip format decreases the confounding influence of different measurement methods. Content analysis for omitted pain information is described in the content analysis section.

Brief Pain Inventory Short Form (BPI-SF).

The GA will use the BPI-SF to measure participants' present pain intensity and present pain interference with activities. The BPI-SF was developed to examine the prevalence and severity of pain in the general population.[62] The BPI-SF consists of 15 questions that measure pain location, intensity, pain treatment, and the effect of pain on mood and every day activities. The first question asks if the person has had any pain today. An anterior and posterior body diagram allows the respondent to shade areas where they feel pain and mark with an "X" the area that hurts the most. Respondents rate their worst, least, and average pain in the past 24 hours using a 0 – 10 numeric rating scale with 0, no pain, and 10, pain as bad as you can imagine. They also rate their pain right now. An open-ended question asks what treatments or medications they are receiving for their pain. Respondents then rate the percent of relief they received from the treatments in the past 24 hours. The seven remaining questions evaluate how pain has interfered with activities including general activity, mood, walking, work, relations with others, sleep and enjoyment of life. Anchors for the 0 – 10 scale consist of 0, does not interfere and 10, completely interferes. Zalon[63] compared the BPI-SF with the Short Form McGill Pain Questionnaire (SF-MPQ) with a group of surgical patients. The correlation between the BPI-SF and the SF-MPQ for pain over the previous 24 hours was .61, $p < .001$, supporting concurrent validity. Cronbach's alpha for the overall BPI-SF has been reported as .77 to .87.[54,63] The BPI-SF is in Appendix B.

Demographic Form.

Older adults' demographic information will be measured last. The GA will ask participants to provide the following information: age, gender, race, ethnic group, marital status, highest completed education, if they are currently followed by a health care practitioner for their osteoarthritis and osteoarthritis related pain. The Demographic Form is in Appendix C.

Content Analysis

Krippendorff's[64] components for content analysis will be used to conduct the content analysis of older adults' responses to the practitioner's question about pain and the two follow up questions. The content analysis components include unitizing, sampling, coding, and inferring. The way in which each of the components will be used in the analysis is described below.

Unitizing.

The unit of analysis for the content analysis will be any word or phrase that describes one of the a priori criteria. One point will be given for each word or phrase describing a criterion. Repeated use of the same word or phrase will be counted only the initial time to avoid inflating the communication score. Each distinctly different word or phrase about the same criterion will be credited with one point. The statement, "I start each day off by taking two Tylenol and placing a hot pack on my knee while I eat my breakfast." would be coded for current pain treatments with one point for the Tylenol and one point for the hot pack. One additional point would be coded for the word knee, which addressed the pain location criterion.

Sampling.

All transcripts of older adults' response to the way that the nurse practitioner asked them about their pain will constitute the sample for content analysis of included pain information. The initial practitioner question will be skipped over on the audiotape and omitted from the transcript. The persons conducting the content analysis will remain blind to participants' condition until the content analysis is complete, at which time the experimental condition will be identified directly from the audiotape. Text will be read at the level of words and phrases to identify important content for management of osteoarthritis pain. The same process will be used for responses to the practitioner question asking if there is anything further they want to say (omitted pain information). The same process will be used a third time for responses to the final practitioner question about if there is anything further about their pain that they would like to say (omitted pain information).

Coding.

The American Pain Society (2002) *Guidelines for the Management of Pain in Osteoarthritis, Rheumatoid Arthritis, and Juvenile Chronic Arthritis*[8] will be used to identify important osteoarthritis pain management content included or omitted from older adults' transcribed responses to the practitioner's pain communication question. The Guidelines are the culmination of expert review of the Cochrane Collaboration Reviews, additional published systematic reviews, American Pain Society (APS) commissioned reviews, and reviews conducted by the expert 10 member interdisciplinary panel and APS staff. The a priori osteoarthritis pain management criteria include:

1. Type of pain (nociceptive/neuropathic);
2. Quality of pain;
3. Pain source;
4. Pain location;
5. Pain intensity;
6. Duration/time course;
7. Pain affect;
8. Effect on personal lifestyle;
9. Functional status;
10. Current pain treatments;
11. Use of recommended glucosamine sulfate;
12. Effectiveness of prescribed treatments;
13. Prescription analgesic side effects;
14. Weight management to ideal body weight;
15. Exercise regimen, or physical therapy and/or occupational therapy;
16. Indications for surgery.

QRS N6 (NUD*IST) will be used to manage the content analysis and organize the coded data. The node system will be composed of the a priori codes listed above. Included pain communication content (responses to the first practitioner question) will be coded by highlighting the content and marking the content with a number representing the criterion. The criterion number will be placed at the end of the word or phrase (e.g. pain in my right knee 4; I take Tylenol extra strength10; The Tylenol dulls the pain a little bit 12). A subscript will indicate if the item is the first, second, and so on item for the criterion described by that participant. After coding each participant's responses, the coder will check all coded content on the same criterion to identify repeated instances of coding identical content. Identical content will be coded only one time for each participant. The same procedure will be used to code omitted pain communication content (responses to the second and third practitioner questions). Content will be coded separately for the second question and for the third practitioner question.

Reducing.

Coded data will be entered into an SPSS database. The number of distinct content for each criterion will be entered into the database. Separate sets of variables will be entered for content analyzed from responses to the practitioner pain question, responses to the practitioner's general follow up question, and responses to the practitioner's pain specific follow up question. Frequencies will be used to further reduce the data. The included pain communication score will be calculated by summing all of the important pain content described by participants in response to the practitioner pain question (first question). The omitted important pain information will be calculated by summing all important pain content described by participants in response to the practitioner's two follow up questions.

Inferring.

The American Pain Society (2002) *Guidelines for the Management of Pain in Osteoarthritis, Rheumatoid Arthritis, and Juvenile Chronic Arthritis*[8] provides the research-based criteria for coding the data. The PI will train the GA to conduct the content analysis. The PI and the GA will independently code all of the responses, remaining blind to participants' conditions. The PI and GA will compare the codes. The PI will document each instance of coding disagreement. Disagreements will be resolved through discussion. Inter-rater reliability will be calculated, as described in the analysis section.

Summary of the Methods

Older adults with chronic osteoarthritis pain will be randomly assigned to one of three practitioner pain communication conditions. Participants will watch and verbally respond to a video clip of a practitioner asking them about their pain with either an open-ended question without social desirability bias; closed-ended question without social desirability bias; or open-ended question with social desirability bias. All participants will respond next to a video clip of the practitioner asking them if there is anything further they want to say, and finally to a video clip of the practitioner asking them if there is anything more about their pain that they want to say. The GA will administer the BPI-SF to half of each of the three groups prior to watching the videos, and to the remaining half of each group after responding to the final video, to measure and control for present pain differences in participants across groups, and to counterbalance the effect of the BPI-SF measure. Verbal responses to all three video clips will be audio taped and transcribed. Important included pain information (responses to the first video) and omitted pain information (responses to the second and third videos) will be content analyzed by two trained independent raters, blind to participants' conditions. A priori criteria derived from national osteoarthritis pain management guidelines will be used to code the responses. Our methods provide a context with strong experimental realism to test theory driven pain communication skills for the effect on information included and omitted by older adults important in managing osteoarthritis pain.

Analysis

The characteristics of the sample will be summarized and described with frequencies, (and means and standard deviations for interval level measures) for the descriptive data. These data includes age, gender, race, highest education completed, and if participants are currently followed by a health care practitioner for their osteoarthritis and osteoarthritis related pain.

Inter-rater reliability will be calculated using Krippendorff's alpha to compare the equivalence of coding between the independent raters, the PI and GA. Krippendorff's alpha is calculated by the following formula, $\alpha = 1 - (D_o/D_e)$ where D_o is the measure of observed disagreement and D_e is the measure of the disagreement expected by chance. Krippendorff's alpha corrects for chance, and can be used with large sample sizes.[64]

A check for randomization to condition will be conducted prior to the main analyses to test for significant pre-existing differences between older adult participants in the three conditions:

1. health care practitioner open-ended without social desirability bias pain question;
2. health care practitioner closed-ended without social desirability bias pain question;
3. health care practitioner open-ended with social desirability bias pain question.

Analyses of variance (ANOVA) will test for age differences between the three groups. Cross tabulation using the chi-square statistic will be used to test for differences between the groups for gender, race, ethnicity, highest education achieved, followed/not followed for osteoarthritis by a health care practitioner, and followed/not followed for osteoarthritis pain by a health care practitioner.

The timing effect of the BPI-SF will be tested by ANOVAs on the variables of pain intensity, interference with activities, and responses to practitioner questions about pain (included and omitted information). Each ANOVA will have two factors (groups and timing) and their interaction. Thus, a single ANOVA will test for group differences on a specific dependent variable, timing differences, and the possibility of an interaction, i.e., that one of the groups showed a stronger timing effect than the other. However, a strong interaction is not expected.

Hypothesis

Hypothesis: Older adults asked about their pain with an open-ended question without social desirability bias will describe more important pain information and omit less information than older adults asked about their pain with a closed-ended question without social desirability or an open-ended question with social desirability bias.

The hypothesis will be tested with a multivariate analysis of covariance (MANCOVA). The grouping variable consists of three groups: 1. health care practitioner open-ended without social desirability bias pain question; 2. health care practitioner closed-ended without social desirability bias pain question; 3. health care practitioner open-ended with social desirability bias pain question. The two participant response measures will comprise the input for the multivariate vectors for comparison. The two response measures include: 1. the content analysis summed scores of important osteoarthritis pain information described by the participant in response to the practitioner's pain question; and 2. important omitted pain information measured by responses to the second and third questions about any further information. Present pain intensity and pain interference with activity will be used as covariates to control for pain differences between participants. If timing of the BPI-SF is significant, timing of the BPI-SF will be entered as a covariate. If important pre-existing group differences occur during the preliminary analyses, the variable will also be used as an additional covariate to adjust for the differences. Descriptive discriminant function analysis (DFA) following significant results from the MANCOVA will provide a multivariate way to interpret group differences that result from MANCOVA,[65] maintaining a more rigorous analysis than possible with post hoc univariate analyses. Post hoc DFA involves examination of the correlation between the discriminant function and the pain communication variables, examination of the canonical discriminant function coefficients for lack of redundancy, interpretation of the group centroids, and group membership classification.

Summary of the Analyses

A summary of the data analysis includes: 1) describing and summarizing the participating older adults with descriptive statistics and frequencies; 2) computing the inter-rater reliability for coding participant responses; 3) checking that randomization to condition resulted in no significant differences between the groups; 4) checking that the timing of administering the BPI-SF had no significant effect; 5) testing the hypothesis related to important pain information provided and omitted by participants with a MANCOVA, using present pain intensity and pain interference with activities as covariates, and using DFA as a multivariate technique to interpret the differences if the MANCOVA is significant.

Study Summary

Our study provides an innovative controlled test of how older adults respond to pain communication strategies used by health care practitioners. Following informed consent, older adults with osteoarthritis pain will be randomly assigned to one of three groups. Participants will watch and verbally respond to: (1) one of three video clips of a practitioner asking them about their pain (a. open-ended and without social desirability bias, b. closed-ended and without social desirability bias, or c. open-ended and with social desirability bias); (2) a video clip asking, "What else can you tell me?" (3) a video clip asking, "What else can you tell me about your pain, aches, soreness or discomfort?" All responses to the videos will be audio taped. The GA will counterbalance the BPI-SF measure by orally administering the BPI-SF to a randomly selected half of each of the three groups prior to the videos, or after responding to the final video. The GA will administer the demographic measure as the final measure. The GA will debrief each participant, thank them for their contribution to the study, and compensate each person for their time with a $20 money order and a copy of the Arthritis Foundation *Managing Your Pain* publication. Content analysis will be conducted on the transcribed audiotapes to identify important pain information included in the response to the initial pain question (included information), and important information included in the response to the two follow up questions (omitted information). The summed scores for included and omitted information will be entered into the MANCOVA comparing the three groups for differences in older adult pain communication responses, using current pain intensity and pain interference with activities as covariates. The goal is to identify practitioner pain communication strategies that allow patients to describe pain information important for guiding effective pain management, and to substantiate what pain information is missed when practitioners use less effective pain communication. The results will provide empirically tested theory based communication strategies that can be used in pain communication education for patients. Our study has the potential to inform curriculum across a number of health care practitioner groups, including nursing and medicine. Effective communication between older adults and health care practitioners provides the link for significantly reducing or eliminating pain. Table 2 presents the timeline for completing our study.

Table 2
Study Timeline

Activity	Time 5/1/06	8/1/06	9/1/06	8/31/07	12/1/07	3/1/08	4/30/08
1. Video clips developed, reviewed for face validity, & edited	X_1						
2. SuperLab software loaded & tested		X_2					
3. GA trained, data collected & transcribed			X_3				
4. Content analysis				X_4			
5. Statistical analyses					X_5		
6. Manuscript preparation						X_6	
7. R21 final report							X_7

Note. The time for a listed activity extends from the start date of that activity to the start date of the following activity.

Principal Investigator/Program Director (Last, First, Middle): McDonald, Deborah Dillon

E. Human Subjects Research

Overview

The study involves the participation of community dwelling older adult with osteoarthritis pain but no cancer pain (malignant pain). The risks, adequacy of protection, and potential benefits will be presented, followed by the importance of the knowledge that might be gained. The GA will recruit older adults from elder independent housing sites in Hartford, New Haven, Bridgeport, and suburban areas in Connecticut.

1. Risk to the Subjects

Human Subjects Involvement and Characteristics.

The GA will recruit community dwelling adults, age 60 and older who have osteoarthritis pain but no malignant pain who speak, read, and understand English. Recruitment will be through housing newsletter announcements, posted materials, and direct contact in the public areas of the housing sites. We selected Hartford, Bridgeport, and New Haven as sites for our study to increase representation of Black or African American, Hispanic, and Asian Americans. Older adults interested in participating in the study will be screened for eligibility, receive informed consent, and make an appointment for the GA to conduct the study in the older adults' home. Older adults will be recruited until a total of 300 eligible participants have completed the 15-minute study. The age range is anticipated to be from 60 to 90.

Before beginning the study, the GA will again provide oral informed consent and include written consent with an enlarged print consent form. The GA will instruct the participant to listen and respond in turn to each of three separate video tape clips and press the buzzer after responding to the third and final video clip. Participants will be randomly assigned to one of the three treatment conditions by the SuperLab 3.0 software. All responses will be audio taped. When the participant is ready, and after the video sound level has been adjusted, the GA will start the video clip and leave the room. The first video will begin 15 seconds later. A video clip of a health care practitioner will ask participants about their pain in one of three ways. After responding to the practitioner, participants will touch the screen and view and listen to the practitioner ask them, "What else can you tell me?" After responding to the practitioner, participants will touch the screen again and view and listen to the third and final clip of the practitioner asking them, "What else can you tell me about your pain, aches, soreness or discomfort?" After completing their response, participants will ring the buzzer and the GA will return to the room and turn off the audio tape recorder. The GA will orally administer the BPI-SF to measure present pain, if the BPI-SF was not administered prior to the videotapes, and administer the Demographic Form as the final measure. The GA will then debrief the participant, checking for hypothesis guessing, more fully explaining the study, assessing for any discomfort, and requesting that they do not talk about the study in case others wish to participate. Participation in the study will be complete after the debriefing. Participants will be thanked and given the Arthritis Foundation publication, *Managing Your Pain*,[61] and a $20 money order for participating in the study. Older adults are exclusively studied because they have been identified as having more difficulty in communicating about their pain.[49] The 80% incidence of osteoarthritis in people over 75[58] makes older adults highly vulnerable to pain problems, and a high priority for pain communication studies. Osteoarthritis occurs much less frequently in younger and middle aged adults, and is unlikely to occur in children.

Source of Materials.

Three instruments will be used to gather individually identifiable data for the purpose of the study. The GA will audiotape participants' verbal responses to the three videos which will be content analyzed to extract the two dependent variables, included and omitted important pain information. The GA will orally administer the BPI-SF to measure the two covariates, present pain intensity, and pain interference with activities. The GA will orally administer the Demographic Form to record demographic variables including age, gender, race, ethnic group, marital status, highest completed education, if they are currently followed by a health care practitioner for their osteoarthritis and osteoarthritis related pain. Names will not be linked to the data. A number code will be used to link the audio taped responses and the responses to the BPI-SF and the Demographic Form for each participant. The GA will be absent from the room when participants are audio taped. Only the PI and GA will have access to the data. The audiotapes and the written data will be kept locked in the PI's office at the University of Connecticut. The data will be analyzed on the PI's university office computer, which is secured with password protection. The data will be collected specifically for the proposed study.

Potential Risks.

The intervention involves minimal risk. The practitioner questions comprising the experimental manipulation are commonly used questions about pain that participants have likely responded to before during health care visits. The BPI-SF questions about pain include common areas of pain assessment such as pain intensity, and how the pain interferes with daily activities. The entire study takes approximately 15 minutes to complete. The study will take place in the older adults' homes at a time convenient for them. All participants will be debriefed to check for any psychological discomfort with the study, and to allow participants to withdraw if they so wish. If at any time older adults do feel burdened, they are free to withdraw from the study.

2. Adequacy of Protection Against Risks

Recruitment and Informed Consent.

The GA will recruit participants through housing newsletter announcements, posted materials and direct contact in the public areas of the independent elder housing sites. Older adults interested in participating in the study will be screened for eligibility, receive informed consent, and make an appointment for the GA to conduct the study in their home.

The GA will use the cover story that we are testing the feasibility of helping people prepare for their health care office visit while waiting in the office for their appointment. The GA will make the following statement. "We are testing whether asking patients to respond to a videotaped health care practitioner asking questions about your health just prior to an office visit helps you communicate better during the office visit." The mild deception is warranted to increase the experimental realism and decrease response bias. The GA will explain that the study involves privately watching three brief video clips of a practitioner asking them health questions on a laptop computer screen. Participants will verbally respond after each clip and responses will be audio taped. When they have finished responding to the third clip, the GA will return to the room and ask them questions about pain problems, and general information such as their age and marital status. Their participation will then be complete and no other contact will be requested. The entire study takes about 15 minutes. No names will be linked with any information provided by participants. All information will remain confidential. The information will be kept secure in the University of Connecticut office of Deborah Dillon McDonald. Older adults will be reminded that participation is voluntary. They do not have to be in the study if they do not wish to be. They can withdraw from the study at any time without risk. They will be given an enlarged type copy of the written consent form to keep. The consent form will contain the name and contact office telephone number of the PI and the University of Connecticut IRB, if participants have questions. Older adults willing to participate will be asked to sign the consent form after reviewing the form and receiving informed consent from the GA.

Protection Against Risk.

Several safeguards have been designed into the study to protect participants from risk. The GA will not be present in the room while participants respond to the video clips. After completing the demographic information, each participant will be debriefed by the GA. The study will be completely explained to participants, along with the reason for the mild deception. Participants will be checked for concern or distress about the mild deception, and reminded that they are free to withdraw. No names will be written on any of the collected data. Identification numbers will be assigned by the GA and used to link the three sources of data from each individual. All collected data will be kept confidential and will be locked in the PI's university office.

A referral protocol will be followed in cases where participants describe moderate or greater present pain problems (pain levels of 4 or greater on the 0 to 10 BPI-SF). The protocol will include the registered nurse GA encouraging: (1) the person to contact their primary care provider to assess and treat the problem; (2) if the person has no primary care provider, a list of names and telephone numbers of local accredited ambulatory care clinics will be given if the person; (3) if the person has no insurance, the name and telephone number for a local community health clinic providing sliding scale health care will be given to the person.

3. Potential Benefits of the Proposed Research to the Subjects and Others

Testing how older adults respond to the way health care practitioners ask them about their pain, and whether important information is included or omitted provides a critical starting point for educating patients and practitioners about more effective ways to communicate about pain. Patients who are able to communicate important information about their pain are more likely to be prescribed more effective pain treatments and achieve greater pain relief. Consumer pain management resources such as the Mayday Foundation web site and existing coaching interventions could easily incorporate the communication strategies. The effective pain communication strategies could be incorporated into nursing, medical, pharmacy, and allied health curricula.

Older adults participating in the study might become more aware of the importance of communicating important aspects of their pain to their health care practitioner. The experience of responding to the practitioner might provide a helpful rehearsal for talking with their health care practitioner. The BPI-SF indicates several important components for pain assessment that participants could include when discussing their pain problems. All participants will be given a copy of the Arthritis Foundation *Managing Your Pain* 2003 publication. The publication provides helpful information for decreasing osteoarthritis pain, and has been approved by the American College of Rheumatology. A registered nurse GA will collect the data. The GA will use the referral protocol to encourage participants to get effective treatment for their pain, if participants describe moderate or greater pain intensity.

The risks are minimal for older adult participants. The study takes place in participants' homes at a time convenient to them. We use a mild deception to maintain experimental realism and to avoid response bias. Participants are debriefed and given the opportunity to withdraw from the study at any time, including after the debriefing. The burden for participants is low. The time requirement is 15 minutes, and only verbal responses are required.

Principal Investigator/Program Director (Last, First, Middle): McDonald, Deborah Dillon

4. Importance of Knowledge Gained

Pain communication has been identified as important for effective pain management, but specific communication factors contributing to effective pain management have not been tested. Our study takes the novel approach of testing specific pain communication skills derived from Communication Accommodation theory attuning strategies, for the effect on important included and omitted pain information described by older adults with osteoarthritis pain. Previous pain communication research has generally taken a macro approach, testing general pain communication content and/or increasing patients' confidence in communicating with their health care practitioner. We take a micro approach and link the effect of two specific pain communication strategies, discourse management (open ended/closed ended) and interpersonal control (with social desirability/without social desirability bias), to pain information identified by the American Pain Society[8] as important information in the management of osteoarthritis pain. Our study provides the opportunity to advance our understanding of pain communication by testing Communication Accommodation theory, and improve pain management by incorporating into health care practice the simple strategies tested in our study. The strategies can be taught to health care practitioners and older adults with chronic pain. The results might have implications for acute pain and malignant pain communication.

The risk for older adult participants is minimal. Participation requires only 15 minutes. Older adults are asked to respond to questions similar to those encountered during their usual health care.

Inclusion of Women and Minorities

Selection criteria for our study include women and minorities. Our selection criteria include any community dwelling adult age 60 or older and who have pain from osteoarthritis who can speak, read, and understand English. Osteoarthritis commonly occurs with adults, age 60 and older.[8] People with cancer pain are excluded from the study. Older adults are more vulnerable to problems communicating about their pain. Osteoarthritis is a pain producing condition that crosses gender, racial, and ethnic groups, with high incidence in the older adult population. Women and men will both be recruited for the study. The selection criteria include Hispanics, and also include African or Black Americans, Asian Americans, and members of other minority groups.

In an effort to include more participants from minority groups, independent living housing sites will be included from Bridgeport and New Haven, Connecticut. According to the most recent census data, Bridgeport consists of 30.8% Black or African Americans, and 31.9% Hispanic, and New Haven consists of 37.4% Black or African Americans, and 21.4% Hispanic or Latinos.[66-67] We expect that recruitment in these two cities will increase the ethnic and racial representation of our sample.

pain. *J Holist Nurs.* 1999;17(2);184-196.

17. Zalon M. Pain in frail, elderly women after surgery. *Image J Nurs Sch.*1997; 29, 21-26.
18. Manias E, Botti M, Bucknall T. Observation of pain assessment and management – the complexities of clinical practice. *J Clin Nurs.* 2002;11:724-733.
19. Schumacher K, West C, Dodd M, Paul S, Tripathy D, Koo P, Miaskowski C. Pain management autobiographies and reluctance to use opioids for cancer pain management. *Cancer Nurs.* 2002;25(2):125-133.
20. Ward S, Goldberg N, Miller-McCauley V, Mueller C, Nolan A, Pawlik-Plank D, Robbins A, Stormoen D, Weissman D. Patient-related barriers to management of cancer pain. *Pain.* 52: 319-324.
21. Kemper J. Pain management of older adults after discharge from outpatient surgery. *Pain Manage Nurs.* 2002;3(4):141-153.
22. Closs S, Briggs M. Patients' verbal descriptions of pain and discomfort following orthopaedic surgery. Int *J Nurs Stud.* 2002;39:563-72.
23. Oliver J, Kravitz R, Kaplan S, Meyers F. Individualized patient education and coaching to improve pain control among cancer outpatients. *J Clin Oncol.* 2001;19:2206-2212.
24. Miaskowski C, Dodd M, West C, Schumacher K, Paul S, Tripathy D, Koo P. Randomized clinical trial of the effectiveness of a self-care intervention to improve cancer pain management. *J Clin Oncol.* 2004;22:1713-1720.
25. White M, Bonvicini K. Bayer Institute for Health Care Communication *annotated bibliography for clinician patient communication to enhance health outcomes,* accessed 1/26/05, http://www.bayerinstitute.org/pdfs/biblio/CPC%20Bibliography-2-10-2005.doc; 2003.
26. Beckman H, Frankel R. The effect of physician behavior on the collection of data. *Ann Intern Med.* 1984;101:692-696.
27. Marvel M, Epstein R, Flowers K, Beckman H. Soliciting the patient's agenda have we improved? *JAMA.* 1999;281:283-287.
28. Roter D, Hall J, Kern D, Barker L, Cole K, Roca R. Improving physicians' interviewing skills and reducing patients' emotional distress. *Arch Intern Med.* 1995;155:1877-1884.
29. Roter D, Hall J, Aoki Y. Physician gender effects in medical communication a meta-analytic review. *JAMA.* 2002;288:756-764.
30. Street R. Information-giving in medical consultations: the influence of patients' communicative styles and personal characteristics, *Soc Sci Med.* 1991;32:541-548.
31. Street R. Communicative styles and adaptations in physician-parent consultations. *Soc Sci Med.* 1992;34:1155-1163.
32. Hall, J, Roter D. Do patients talk differently to male and female physicians? A meta-analytic review. *Patient Educ Couns.* 2002;48:217-224.
33. Cegala D, Post D, McClure L. The effects of patient communication skills training on the discourse of older patients during a primary care interview. *JAGS.* 2001;49:1505-1511.
34. Thompson S, Nanni C, Schwankovsky L. Patient-oriented interventions to improve communication in a medical office visit. *Health Psychol.* 1990;9:390-404.
35. Anderson L, DeVellis B, DeVellis R. Effects of modeling on patient communication satisfaction and knowledge. *Med Care.* 1987;25:1044-1056.
36. Robinson E, Whitefield M. Improving the efficiency of patients' comprehension monitoring: a way of increasing patients' participation in general practice consultations. *Soc Sci Med.* 1985;21:915-919.
37. Tran A, Haidet P, Street R, O'Malley K, Martin F, Ashton C. Empowering communication: a community-based intervention for patients. *Patient Educ Couns.* 2004;52:113-121.
38. Kaplan S, Greenfield S, Ware J. Assessing the effects of physician-patient interactions on the outcomes of chronic disease. *Med Care.* 1989;27:S110 – S127.

39. Giamberardino M. (Ed.). *Pain 2002 – an updated review refresher course syllabus 10th world congress on pain.* Seattle, WA: International Association for the Study of Pain; 2002.
40. Turner G, Weiner D. Essential components of a medical student curriculum on chronic pain management in older adults: Results of a modified Delphi process. *Pain Med.* 2002;3:240-252.
41. Roter D, Larson S, Shnitzky H, Chernoff R, Serwint J, Adamo G, Wissow L. Use of an innovative video feedback technique to enhance communication skills training. *Med Educ.* 2004;38: 145-157.
42. Moral R, Alamo M, Jurado M, Torres L. Effectiveness of a learner-centered training programme for primary care physicians in using a patient-centered consultation style. *Fam Pract.* 2001;18:60-63.
43. Ryan E, Hamilton J, See S. Patronizing the old: How do younger and older adults respond to baby talk in the nursing home? *Int J Aging Hum Dev.* 1994;39:21-32.
44. Fox S, Giles H. Accommodating intergenerational contact: A critique and theoretical model. *J Aging Stud.* 1993:7:423-451.
45. Giles H. Accent mobility. A model and some data. *Anthro Ling.* 1973;15:87-105.
46. Coupland N, Coupland J, Giles H, Henwood K. Accommodating the elderly: Invoking and extending a theory. *Lang Soc.* 1988;17:1-41.
Lawrence Erlbaum Associates Inc; 1988.
47. McDonald D. Gender and ethnic stereotyping and narcotic analgesic administration. *Res Nurs Health.* 1994;17:45-49.
48. McDonald D. Nurses' memory of patient's pain. Int *J Nurs Stud.* 1996;23:487-494.
49. McDonald D, Sterling R. Acute pain reduction strategies used by well older adults. Int *J Nurs Stud.*1998;35:265-70.
50. McDonald D. Postoperative pain after hospital discharge. *Clin Nurs Res.* 1999;8: 347-359.
51. McDonald D Weiskopf C. Adult patients' postoperative pain descriptions and responses to the Short-Form McGill Pain Questionnaire. *Clin Nurs Res.* 2001;10:442-452.
52. McDonald D, Freeland M, Thomas G, Moore J. Testing a preoperative pain management intervention for older adults. *Res Nurs Health.* 2001;24:402-409.
53. McDonald D, Molony S. Postoperative pain communication skills for older adults. *Wes J Nurs Res.* 2004;26:836-852.
54. McDonald D, Thomas G, Livingston K, Severson J. Assisting older adults to communicate their pain after surgery. *Clin Nurs Res.* 2005;14:109-126.
55. Cohen J. Statistical Power analysis for the Behavioral Sciences, 2nd ed., Hillsdale, NJ: Lawrence Erlbaum Associates, Inc; 1988.
56. Stevens J. *Applied Multivariate Statistics for the Social Sciences.* Mahwah, New Jersey: Lawrence Erlbaum Associates, Inc; 1996.
57. National Institutes of Health. National Institute of Arthritis and Musculoskeletal and Skin Diseases. *Handout on health: Osteoarthritis.* 2005. Accessed, 4/21/05, http://www.niams.nih.gov/hi/topics/arthritis/oahandout.htm.
58. Sharma L. Epidemiology of osteoarthritis. In Moskowitz R, Howell O, Altman R, Buckwalter J, V Goldberg eds. *Osteoarthritis: Diagnosis and Medical-surgical Management* (3rd ed., pp. 3 – 17). Philadelphia: Saunders; 2001.
59. Resnick B, Inguito P, Yahiro J, Hawkes W, Werner M, Zimmerman S, Magaziner J. Treatment fidelity in behavior change research: A case example. *Nurs Res.* 2005;54:139-143.
60. Roter D. Observations on methodological and measurement challenges in the assessment of communication during medical exchanges. *Patient Educ Couns.* 2003;50:17-21.
61. Arthritis Foundation. *Managing your Pain*. Atlanta, GA: Arthritis Foundation, Inc; 2003.
62. Daut R, Cleeland C, Flanery R. Development of the Wisconsin Brief Pain Questionnaire to assess pain in cancer and other diseases. *Pain.* 1983;17:197-210.
63. Zalon M. Comparison of pain measures in surgical patients. *J Nurs Meas.* 1999;*7*:135-152.

1R21NR009848-01 MCDONALD, DEBORAH

PROTECTION OF HUMAN SUBJECTS UNACCEPTABLE

RESUME AND SUMMARY OF DISCUSSION: The goal of this application is to identify practitioner pain communication strategies that allow patients to describe pain information important for guiding effective pain management and to substantiate what pain information is missed when practitioners use less effective pain communication. This is a very interesting new application form an experienced young investigator using a posttest-only double blind experiment to test type of provider communication on audio taped patient responses. The methods are highly innovative and the application is significant. The design and methods are creative and innovative and the analyses are appropriate to the aims of the project. There may be some introduced bias from the pre-intervention use of the BPI. And, the study protocol could be better presented. The previous work and commitment of this investigator to studying communication about pain and the well-prepared research team and strong environment bode well for the application.

DESCRIPTION (provided by applicant): How practitioners communicate with patients about their pain has been overlooked as a factor contributing to effective pain management. Eliciting important pain information from patients enables practitioners to prescribe more specific pain treatments, and significantly decrease pain. The aim of our study is to test the effect of practitioners asking patients an open-ended question about pain that does not encourage a socially desirable response. A posttest only double blind experiment will test how the phrasing of health care practitioners' pain questions, open-ended and without social desirability bias; closed-ended and without social desirability bias; or open-ended and with social desirability bias, affects the pain information provided by people with chronic pain. Three hundred community dwelling older adults with chronic osteoarthritis pain will be randomly assigned to one of the three practitioner pain communication conditions. Older adults will watch and verbally respond to a videotape clip of a practitioner asking the patient about their pain. The clips will be identical except for the pain question asked by the practitioner. After responding to the pain question, all of the older adults will respond to a second videotape clip of the practitioner asking if there is anything further they want to communicate. The older adults will then respond to a third videotape clip asking if there is anything further they want to communicate about their pain. Responses to the three videotape clips will be audiotaped. To control for pain differences between participants, the Brief Pain Inventory Short Form will be administered to measure present pain intensity and pain interference with functional activities. Participants' audiotaped responses will be transcribed and content analyzed using a priori criteria from national guidelines to identify communicated pain information and omitted pain information important for osteoarthritis pain management. The three groups will be compared for the communicated pain information and omitted pain information while controlling for present pain intensity and pain interference with activities. The goal is to identify practitioner pain communication strategies that allow patients to describe pain information important for guiding effective pain management, and to substantiate what pain information is missed when practitioners use less effective pain communication. The results will provide empirically tested communication strategies that can be used in practitioner and patient pain communication education.

CRITIQUE 1:

Significance: Pain communication between patient and practitioner are crucial if the patientís pain is to be adequately treated. This is particularly the case with conditions characterized by chronic pain such as osteoarthritis. Prior research has indicated that pain control is a problem for patients receiving acute care and for patients with chronic conditions characterized by pain who dwell in the community. This research will test communication strategies that can enhance patient and practitioner communication about pain, which could result in better pain control.

Approach: The aim of the study is straightforward, clear and testable. The importance of clear communication to pain control was highlighted in the background and significance section and prior research evidence supports this view. The principal investigator referenced nine studies focused on communication about pain between providers and patients in the preliminary studies section. A post-test only double blind experiment will be used for this study to test how the phrasing of health care practitionersí pain question (open-ended without social desirability, closed-ended without social desirability, or open-ended with social desirability bias) affects the pain information provided by older adults with chronic osteoarthritis pain. Power analysis supports the projected sample size of 300. The random assignment of subjects to the three conditions that will be assessed is a strength of the study as well as keeping the persons who will do the content analysis of data blind to the condition to which each subject will be responding. Use of video taped provider communication scenarios has the advantage of standardizing provider communication to which the subjects would respond. Audio taping of the participantís responses also will ensure that responses are more accurately captured for later analysis. The second part of each practitioner video as described will ask two open-ended questions ñ one more general and one focused on encouraging discussion about pain. This will allow all subjects to ultimately respond to open-ended without social desirability questions. However, this aspect of the intervention is not fully acknowledged in the discussion of the design and the data analysis. Randomization of the administration of the Brief Pain Inventory Short Form for administration prior to or after the presentation of the videos should control for learning effects. Reliability and validity information for the Brief Pain Inventory Short Form was given. The debriefing session should adequately allow for handling of hypothesis guessing and any distress about deception regarding the focus of the study because of the use of a cover story. The content analysis procedure described follows accepted standards. Use of the American Pain Society's "Guidelines for the Management of Pain in Osteoarthritis, Rheumatoid Arthritis, and Juvenile Chronic Arthritis" for coding data will also help to yield a more reliable content analysis process. The approaches to data analysis are detailed and appropriate the address the research hypothesis. Redundancy and some disorganization of content in the design section was sometimes confusing.

Innovation: Patient and provider communication about pain has been a research concern in health care for many years. The uniqueness of this study lies in its focus on assessing specific communication approaches with older persons suffering with chronic pain in the community. The use of videotaped scenarios to which subjects will respond about their pain is a rather unique methodological approach for collecting this type of data.

Investigators: The principal investigator has a track record of publications focused on pain assessment and communicating pain. She has prior NIH funding for a project focused on post-operative pain. She will collaborate with a psychologist who will assist with statistical analysis and with a computer consultant. The research team has the experience to successfully complete the proposed project.

Environment: The University of Connecticut has the research resources to support this project. Participants will be recruited from seven independent living elder housing sites throughout Connecticut. Letters of support are included from the seven sites. The Seven Seas Film Company will produce the three videotapes required for the study.

Overall Evaluation: The proposed study addresses an important area in health care – control of chronic pain in older adults with chronic conditions. The focus on communication about pain could be a cost-effective approach for helping to address this problem if specific communication strategies are found to aid pain control. The proposed study has many strengths including a straightforward and clearly explicated aim, a background section and preliminary studies supportive of the proposed study, a well designed experimental approach, a well operationalized independent variable, a carefully planned data collection protocol, appropriate content analysis procedures, and detailed plans for statistical analysis which should address the study hypothesis. The description of the study protocol was sometimes confusing due to repetitive content that could have been better organized. This is a relative minor limitation given the many strengths of the proposal.

Protection of Human Subjects from Research Risks: This study will require the participation of 300 community dwelling older adults with osteoarthritis pain who are age 60 and older. Recruitment strategies are described. Procedures for obtaining informed consent and protection against risks are generally adequate. However, participant responses will be audio taped for later analysis. No mention was made if or how these audio tapes would be destroyed after they are analyzed. If they are to be retained for any purpose, permission must be obtained from participants. Potential benefits to subjects and others and the knowledge to be gained also are adequate.

Inclusion of Women Plan: Both women and men will be included in the sample. It is expected that 207 (69%) of the 300 subjects will be women.

Inclusion of Minorities Plan: It is anticipated that 12% of the sample will be Hispanic, 16% African American, and 8% from other minority groups.

Inclusion of Children Plan: Participants will be 60 years of age or older. Older adults have been targeted for the study because they typically have more difficulty communicating their pain than younger persons.

Budget: The budget is justified and appropriate.

CRITIQUE 2:

Significance: This R21 application addresses the problem of inadequate pain communication between patients and health care practitioners that could result in undiagnosed pain due to omission of important information for treatment of pain. If the aims of the application are achieved, practitioners can be taught to use open-ended pain assessment questions such as "tell me about your pain" and not ask: "How are you feeling?" which has social desirability implications. The aims are to determine which communication strategies encourage older adults to describe important information and what information is missed with ineffective communication strategies.

Approach: The review of literature is integrated and organized and the argument for the study is well developed and logical. The Communication Theory Attuning Strategies is described, but more clarity is needed so that concepts of the research are linked to or explained by concepts of the theory. The posttest-only double blind experiment is strong with some ingenious video and software methods planned for randomization to groups and for providing the experimental videotape clips. Blindness of the graduate assistant to computerized random assignment and the method of starting the video after leaving the room are strengths of the innovative methodology.

The previous experience of the PI is varied but fairly strong with 9 studies of practitioner and patient communication that the PI claims prepared the team to conduct randomized controlled trials with older adults, develop standardized intervention videos, and to learn content analysis of participants' responses. Although the findings of the 9 studies are listed, they have not been tied together into a narrative that shows substantive support for conducting this study.

The posttest-only double blind design is strong but a flaw seems to be that half the sample will be randomly assigned to answer the Brief Pain Inventory (BPI) before the experimental test. In doing this they will answer 16 pain assessment questions that could strongly bias the amount of information given in response to the video. Even with randomization of the BPI sequence, it seems that the purpose of the study would be compromised. The investigators do not expect a timing effect (interaction) but responding to the BPI before the test would raise participant awareness of the DV, "important information" when subsequently answering the video questions. Since it seems less likely that they would respond differently to the BPI after the videos and since the BPI is not the major DV, why not simply administer the BPI after the video test for all participants to eliminate the threat introduced by counterbalancing? In addition there is inconsistency in the several reasons given for counterbalancing the assessment of pain intensity and interference with the BPI. These include: to control for present pain differences, for timing of the BPI, for timing differences, for the measurement effect, for the learning effect. On the other hand, counterbalancing would give some exploratory information. The threats to internal validity need to be carefully and consistently identified and minimized

The a prior osteoarthritis pain management criteria from the American Pain Society guidelines need further specification for use in this study. For example, the nociceptive/neuropathic type of pain needs to be operationally defined in terms of what kinds of participant responses will be categorized as each type. Direct questioning by a knowledgeable nurse might more accurately assess that differentiation. In addition, it is not clear what is included in the criterion, current pain treatments.

In general, the analysis procedures seem to answer the research question. However, the multivariate factor is not clear. It seems to be composed of the sum of "important information included" and the sum of "important information excluded," which intuitively may be two sides of the same coin.

Innovation: The study is innovative because it tests patients' responses to different ways of that health care personnel might ask about their pain. There are several very innovative features surrounding the video taped treatment, and the technological methods to randomly assign and maintain blindness.

Investigators: Dr. McDonald is an Associate Professor at the University of Connecticut and holds bachelors and masters degrees in Nursing. Her PhD is in Social Psychology from Columbia University in 1990. She received a pre-doctoral fellowship from the National Center for Nursing Research from 1988 –1990, but does not list the topic, so it is not clear whether the results were published. She also received an R15 award from NINR, 1999 – 2001, and has published the results. She has received two other grants, one from the Donaghu Foundation and one from the University of Athens in Greece with publications. She lists 14 publications that appear to be data based. Dr. Katz is a Professor at the University of Connecticut and has his PhD in Psychology from University of Massachusetts/Amherst. He is a consulting statistician at Mount Sinai Medical School in New York and will consult in Year 2 of this project regarding statistical analyses. Joel Rosiene is an Associate Professor of Computer Science at Eastern Connecticut State University. He will program the laptop computer with the software and insert the healthcare practitioner videotape clips as the experimental manipulation. The research team is well qualified to conduct this study.

Environment: The environment includes seven independent living elder housing sites in Connecticut that will ensure an adequate sample. The study will be conducted in the living quarters of the residents. There is support from University of Connecticut in terms of computer resources, personnel and offices in the school of nursing. As in a previous study, the Pi will work with the Seven Seas Film Company to produce videotapes needed for the study. Support is good for the accomplishment of the aims.

Overall Evaluation: This is a very interesting new application form an experienced young investigator using a posttest-only double blind experiment to test type of provider communication on audio taped patient responses. The methods are highly innovative and the study is very significant. The design and methods are creative and innovative and the analyses are generally appropriate to the aims of the project. The major strengths of the application are the innovative methods for blindness, randomization, and reliability of the intervention; the previous work and commitment of this investigator to studying communication about pain, the well-prepared research team and strong environment. Potential bias from the pre-intervention use of the BPI, lack of operational definitions of the coding criteria, and some inconsistencies are noted. There are some human subjects issues but inclusion of participants is adequate with respect to gender, minority group status and children.

Protection of Human Subjects from Research Risks: The application adequately addresses risks, protection against risks, benefits and importance of the knowledge to be gained. Debriefing the participants is thoughtfully planned, but it seems inappropriate to remind them at the end of the study that if they have distress or concern about the study, they are free to withdraw. Another comment is that the method of contacting the participants is not clear. This is a clinical trial but a data safety monitoring plan is not adequately presented.

Inclusion of Women Plan: The research involves 31% men and 69% women, although rationale was not given.

Inclusion of Minorities Plan: The research involves minorities and non-minorities: 76% white, 16% black, 12% Hispanic, 4% Asian, 2% Native Hawaiian or Other Pacific Islander, and 2% American Indian/Alaskan Native. Recruitment from nearby cities that contain 20% to 30% people of color will increase the ethnic and racial representation of the sample.

Inclusion of Children Plan: The research involves only/adults because osteoarthritis is a painful condition associated with aging and older adults are more vulnerable to problems communicating about their pain. The age range of the sample is 60 and older.

Budget: The requested budget is appropriate for the work.

CRITIQUE 3:

This is a proposal by a new investigator that proposes a novel approach to improving communication between older adults and their health care providers about pain. The design is a post-test only double-blind experiment to test how phrasing of health care practitioners' pain questions affect pain information provided by older adults with chronic osteoarthritis pain. The investigator makes the case for better communication skills on the part of providers. Recent renewed interest by the scientific community and foundations in the effectiveness of provider communication skills, including listening and questioning, in improving health care delivery provides support for a study of this nature. The failure of health care providers to adequately listen to patient's complaints of pain, coupled with known reluctance to adequately treat pain, high light the significance of this study topic. Study outcomes would have immediate application in provider and patient pain communication education. The investigator has experience [including an R15] in studying various aspects of pain and pain communication in a variety of populations. Further, she has amassed a group of collaborators that complement her own skills, including ideography, computerized randomization and experimental manipulation of video clip testing. Adequate resources are described, including agreement from a sufficient number of senior housing units to assure adequate sample size. On page 24 the investigator introduces for the first time the notion of (apriori criteria) for coding the qualitative data and these need more description and clarification; presumably they relate to the American Pain Society Guidelines which appear later. The study design is well developed and described with appropriate rationale for decisions. The need for use of mild deception is adequately addressed in the human subjects section and subjects will be debriefed. There are minimal risks.

THE FOLLOWING RESUME SECTIONS WERE PREPARED BY THE SCIENTIFIC REVIEW ADMINISTRATOR TO SUMMARIZE THE OUTCOME OF DISCUSSIONS OF THE REVIEW COMMITTEE ON THE FOLLOWING ISSUES:

PROTECTION OF HUMAN SUBJECTS (Resume): UNACCEPTABLE. The reviewers noted human subjects concerns because information provided on the Data and Safety Monitoring Plan is insufficient.

INCLUSION OF WOMEN PLAN (Resume): ACCEPTABLE. The reviewers concluded that the degree of inclusion of women is appropriate.

INCLUSION OF MINORITIES PLAN (Resume): ACCEPTABLE. The reviewers concluded that the inclusion of minorities is appropriate.

INCLUSION OF CHILDREN PLAN (Resume): ACCEPTABLE. The reviewers concluded that the exclusion of children is appropriate.

COMMITTEE BUDGET RECOMMENDATIONS: The reviewers recommended no changes in the budget.

NOTICE: The NIH has modified its policy regarding the receipt of amended applications. Detailed information can be found by accessing the following URL address: http://grants.nih.gov/grants/policy/amendedapps.htm

NIH announced implementation of Modular Research Grants in the December 18, 1998 issue of the NIH Guide to Grants and Contracts. The main feature of this concept is that grant applications (R01, R03, R21, R15) will request direct costs in $25,000 modules, without budget detail for individual categories. Further information can be obtained from the Modular Grants Web site at http://grants.nih.gov/grants/funding/modular/modular.htm

appropriate diabetes management program specifically designed for Chinese Americans.

b. This study was quantitative. The investigators collected numeric information about physiologic outcomes (e.g., blood pressure, HbA1c) and psychosocial ones (e.g., satisfaction).
c. The underlying paradigm of this study was positivism/postpositivism.
d. Yes, the investigators gathered empirical information through the senses, facilitated in some cases by the use of special technical equipment (e.g., observing blood pressure and weight).
e. Yes, this study directly addressed a question relevant to the treatment of patients with diabetes. The results of this study, together with those from other similar studies, can contribute to evidence-based treatment decisions.
f. No, this was a primary study, not an example of pre-appraised evidence.

EXERCISE C.2: QUESTIONS OF FACT (APPENDIX F)

a. Yes, this was a systematic study of nurses' experiences with issues relating to social justice. Information was gathered in two countries through in-depth interviews.
b. It was a qualitative study. The researcher used loosely structured methods to capture nurses' experiences.
c. The underlying paradigm was naturalism.
d. Yes, the study involved the collection of information through the senses (e.g., through conversations with nurses).
e. Yes, this study addressed the EBP question described in the textbook as "Meaning and Processes" (i.e., developing an in-depth understanding of nurses' experiences with discrimination and unfairness within their work lives).
f. This was not pre-appraised evidence, it was a primary study.

■ Chapter 3

STUDY QUESTION B.2

a. Independent variable (IV) = participation versus nonparticipation in assertiveness training; dependent variable (DV) = psychiatric nurses' effectiveness
b. IV = patients' postural positioning; DV = respiratory function
c. IV = amount of touch by nursing staff; DV = patients' psychological well-being
d. IV = frequency of turning patients; DV = incidence of decubitus
e. IV = history of parents' abuse during their childhood; DV = parental abuse of their own children
f. IVs = patients' age and gender; DV = tolerance for pain
g. IV = pregnant women's number of prenatal visits; DV = labor and delivery outcomes
h. IV = children's experience (versus nonexperience) of a sibling death; DV = levels of depression
i. IV = gender; DV = compliance with a medical regimen
j. IV = participation vs. nonparticipation in a support group among family caregivers of AIDS patients; DV = coping
k. IV = time of day; DV = hearing acuity among the elderly
l. IV = location of giving birth—home versus hospital; DV = parents' satisfaction with the childbirth experience
m. IV = type of diet in the outpatient setting among patients undergoing chemotherapy; DV = incidence of positive blood cultures

STUDY QUESTION B.5

a. Experimental studies would not be conducted in an ethnographic tradition.
b. In the study described, receipt of relaxation therapy would be the *in*dependent variable, and pain would be the dependent variable.
c. Confounding variables are not controlled in grounded theory studies.

d. In phenomenological studies, there would not be an intervention.
e. In an experimental study, the data collection plan would be developed well in advance of introducing an intervention.

EXERCISE C.1: QUESTIONS OF FACT (APPENDIX E)

a. The researcher was Susan Loeb, who was (when the article was published) an assistant professor of nursing at the University of Delaware. She is an RN who holds a doctoral degree (PhD).
b. The study participants (subjects) were 135 community-dwelling men aged 55 and older.
c. The independent variable in this study was health motivation. The abstract states that health motivation was viewed as a *determinant of* self-rated health and health behaviors. Health motivation is not *inherently* an independent variable. It would be possible to study factors that affect or "cause" health motivation, in which case it would be the dependent variable.
d. The dependent variables were (1) self-rated health and (2) health behaviors. Neither is *inherently* a dependent variable. For example, health behaviors could be studied as the *cause of* health problems, longevity, quality of life, and so on.
e. No, the report did not specifically use the terms independent or dependent variable, as is typical.
f. The data in this study were quantitative. Loeb *measured* her variables in a form that yielded numeric information.
g. Yes, Loeb was interested in a possible cause-and-effect relationship: the relationship between health motivation on the one hand and self-rated health and health behaviors on the other.
h. Loeb's study was nonexperimental—she collected data about her independent and dependent variables without intervening.
i. No, this study did not involve an intervention.
j. Yes, Loeb analyzed her quantitative data statistically.
k. Yes, an IMRAD-type format was followed. The introduction had several sections (Motivation and Attitudes in Relation to Health Behaviors; Self-Rated Health, etc.), followed by methods, results, and a discussion.

EXERCISE C.2: QUESTIONS OF FACT (APPENDIX D)

a. The author of this report is Cheryl Tatano Beck, one of the co-authors of the textbook. She is a professor of nursing at the University of Connecticut and has a doctoral degree (DNSc).
b. No, Beck did not receive funding for this study. There were no end notes or footnotes that acknowledged funding, as would typically be the case if the study had received financial support.
c. The study participants were 38 mothers from four countries.
d. The key concept in this study was post-traumatic stress disorder (PTSD) as a result of a traumatic childbirth.
e. The data in this study were qualitative.
f. Unlike most qualitative studies, this study did not take place "in the field"; the research was conducted over the Internet. The settings, as far as the mothers were concerned, could have been their own homes, although there are other possibilities.
g. No specific relationships were under investigation in this study. The researcher focused on elucidating the PTSD experience, not on relationships between the PTSD and other aspects of the women's lives.
h. Beck's study was a phenomenological study.
i. This study was nonexperimental.
j. There was no intervention in this study.
k. Qualitative researchers do not call their concepts variables, nor are their concepts "measured." Data relating to the key concept in this study were gathered by Internet "interviews" with women who had experienced a birth trauma and subsequent PTSD.
l. The study involved a qualitative (nonstatistical) analysis of the primary data,

although the report did include a few simple descriptive statistics (percentages) that portray participants' characteristics.

m. Yes, the report followed the IMRAD format. There was an introduction, method section, results section, and discussion.

■ Chapter 4

STUDY QUESTION B.4

2a. IV = type of stimulation (tactile vs. verbal); DV = physiologic arousal
2b. IV = infant birth weight; DV = risk for hypoglycemia
2c. IV = use vs. nonuse of isotonic sodium chloride solution; DV = oxygen saturation
2d. IV = fluid balance; DV = success in weaning patients from mechanical ventilation
2e. IV = patients' gender; DV = amount of narcotic analgesics administered
3a. IV = prior blood donation vs. no prior donation; DV = amount of stress
3b. IV = amount of conversation initiated by nurses; DV = patients' ratings of nursing effectiveness.
3c. IV = ratings of nurses' informativeness; DV = amount of preoperative stress
3d. IV = drained vs. not drained with a Jackson-Pratt drain; DV = incidence of peritoneal infection
3e. IV = type of delivery (vaginal vs. cesarean); DV = incidence of postpartum depression

EXERCISE C.1: QUESTIONS OF FACT (APPENDIX A)

a. The first paragraph of this report stated the problem—namely, that adaptation to chronic disease is emotionally challenging and that rural women who are chronically ill have limited access to resources to address their adaptation difficulties.
b. A purpose statement was presented in the last sentence before the "Method" section. Two purposes are stated, the first of which implies a descriptive intent: to *examine* relationships among various psychosocial indicators. The second purpose is consistent with a study using an experimental design, as this study did: to *determine* the effect of the intervention on various outcomes.
c. The report did not explicitly state research questions, although they were implied by the purpose statement. They might be stated as follows: "To what extent are psychosocial indicators such as social support, self-esteem, empowerment, self-efficacy, stress, depression, and loneliness interrelated among rural women who are chronically ill?" and "What is the effect of a computer intervention for chronically ill rural women on these psychosocial indicators?"
d. No hypotheses were formally stated.
e. One hypothesis would be: chronically ill rural women exposed to the computer intervention will have greater improvements to their self-esteem than similar women not exposed to the intervention.
f. Yes, the researchers used hypothesis-testing statistical tests.

EXERCISE C.2: QUESTIONS OF FACT (APPENDIX F)

a. The first paragraph indicated that the research focused on the problem of social injustices within the health care system.
b. Giddings stated the purpose of the study at the end of the first paragraph. The verb used implies an exploratory endeavor: to *investigate* the culture of nursing (about social injustices) by collecting nurses' stories of difference and fairness.
c. The report indicated, near the end of the introduction, that four questions were explored in this study: What happens to nurses who are part of a marginalized cultural or social group? What are their experiences of difference and fairness? What happens to nurses who take a stand on social justice issues? and, Is there a culture of discrimination? These questions provided useful direction to the study and were informative to readers.

d. No hypotheses were stated—nor would one have been appropriate in this exploratory qualitative study.
e. No, no hypotheses were tested. Qualitative studies do not use statistical methods to test hypotheses.

■ Chapter 5

EXERCISE C.1: QUESTIONS OF FACT (APPENDIX J)

a. This was a systematic review—a meta-analysis.
b. Yes, the introduction described a research problem that the researchers addressed. The problem might be stated as followed: Tai Chi exercise has only recently emerged in Western society as an alternative form of exercise, and there is some evidence that Tai Chi can lead to improvements in a number of areas, such as cardiorespiratory function, balance, and muscle strength. However, there is only limited evidence about the aerobic benefits of Tai Chi exercise.
c. Yes, there was a statement of purpose in the last sentence of the introduction: "The purpose of this meta-analysis was to estimate the extent to which Tai Chi exercise affects aerobic capacity."
d. The researchers used seven different electronic databases in their literature search. It does not appear that this computerized search was supplemented by manual methods.
e. The key word was Tai Chi and variations on the English spelling of Tai Chi (e.g., Tai Ji, Tai Chi Quan). The key words used thus related to the independent variable only (i.e., there was no search for *aerobic benefits*, *aerobic capacity*, *peak oxygen uptake*, and so on).
f. No, the researchers included in their search reports written in any language.
g. The researchers originally identified 441 citations.
h. There was some redundancy in the retrieved citations: "Several articles appeared in more than one database."
i. Many articles that were omitted were nonresearch articles, including commentaries, case reports, literature reviews, and so on. Others were excluded because the dependent variables in the study were not related to aerobic capacity.
j. Ultimately, seven studies were included in the meta-analysis.
k. All studies included in the review were quantitative—which is always the case in a meta-analysis.

EXERCISE C.2: QUESTIONS OF FACT (APPENDIX K)

a. Swartz undertook a systematic review of qualitative studies relating to parenting preterm infants (i.e., a metasynthesis).
b. Swartz began with a problem statement that noted the high incidence of preterm births; the risks to which preterm infants are exposed; and the parenting problems faced by parents of preterm infants.
c. According to the report, five electronic databases were searched. If any manual search methods were used, they were not described.
d. The keywords used in the search were "infant, premature," "parenting," and (in CINAHL) "qualitative research."
e. The report did not indicate that the search was restricted to English-language reports, but presumably it was.
f. The search initially identified 68 studies.
g. Ten of the 68 studies were used in the review.
h. All of the studies included in the review were qualitative.
i. The 10 studies in the review included 3 phenomenological studies, three grounded theory studies, and four descriptive qualitative studies.

■ Chapter 6

EXERCISE C.1: QUESTIONS OF FACT (APPENDIX E)

a. Loeb's study used as a conceptual framework the Health-Promoting Self-Care System Model developed by Simmons.

b. Although Simmons' model was not described in the textbook, it represents a synthesis of three nursing models, two of which *were* referenced in the book: Orem's Model of Self-Care and Pender's Health Promotion Model.
c. Yes, a schematic model of the Health-Promoting Self-Care System Model was included as Figure 1.
d. The key concepts in the model are: (1) basic conditioning factors; (2) self-care requisites; (3) therapeutic self-care demand; (4) exercise of self-care agency; (5) health-promoting self-care; and (6) health outcomes.
e. According to the model, the exercise of self-care agency (e.g., a person's motivation and values) is *directly* affected by two sets of factors, as indicated by the arrows pointed directly at this block: therapeutic self-care demand and health-promoting self-care. (Note that the effects are presented as being *reciprocal.*)
f. Health care outcomes are viewed as being *directly* affected only by one set of factors: health-promoting safe-care activities. However, health outcomes are viewed as being *indirectly* affected by all the other factors in the model because health-promoting self-care is affected by exercise of self-care agency, which in turn is affected by therapeutic self-care demand, and so on.
g. The construct "health-promoting self-care" was represented by several variables in this study. Based on information in the abstract (there was more information about this in the method section), we can infer that there was a global measure of health-promoting behaviors, an indicator of health program attendance, and another measure of health screening participation.
h. No, the report did not provide conceptual definitions of key variables. An especially important concept in this study was *motivation*, which was not conceptually defined.
i. Hypotheses based on the model were implied but not articulated. The report suggested that the study was exploratory (". . . the purpose of this study was to *explore* the relationships among health motivation . . ."), and yet the model provides a framework for the development of explicit hypotheses. In the analysis section, hypothesis-testing procedures were used.

EXERCISE C.2: QUESTIONS OF FACT (APPENDIX B)

a. Rew highlighted the framework of Orem's Self-Care Theory. She used this theory as a backdrop for her study because her research question focused on the self-care of homeless youths. (One of the basic underlying theoretical frameworks for a grounded theory study, however, is symbolic interaction, which was not mentioned by Rew.)
b. Yes, Orem's Self-Care Theory was cited in the textbook, and symbolic interaction was also briefly discussed.
c. Yes, Figure 1 of the report was a schematic model depicting Rew's grounded theory. The figure was a good way to illustrate the three categories of taking care of oneself in a high-risk environment. The schematic model was concrete and helped to summarize the major findings for readers.
d. The three key concepts in Rew's grounded theory were: Staying alive with limited resources; Becoming aware of oneself; and Handling one's own health. Rew tied these findings back to Orem's Self-Care Theory (e.g., she stated in her discussion section that ". . .becoming aware of oneself through the processes of gaining self respect and increasing self reliance support Orem's (2001) conceptualization of functioning with integrity")
e. Inasmuch as this was a grounded theory study, no hypotheses were tested. The end point of a grounded theory study often is the identification of hypotheses that can be tested in a future quantitative study.

■ Chapter 7

EXERCISE C.1: QUESTIONS OF FACT (APPENDIX C)

a. Yes, in the "Procedures" subsection, the researchers indicated that human subject approval was received from the university's IRB.
b. No, study participants would not be considered "vulnerable subjects."
c. There is no reason to suspect that participants were subjected to any physical harm or discomfort or psychological distress.
d. It does not appear that participants were deceived in any way. They were recruited through community outreach efforts, were told about the purpose of the study, and were encouraged to involve family members in the learning process.
e. There is no reason to suspect any coercion was used to force unwilling people to participate in the study.
f. The report indicated that written consent was obtained. Presumably, given the IRB review, the consent form stated that participation was purely voluntary. It is not possible to determine the extent to which disclosure was "full," but there does not appear to be any reason to conceal information in this study.
g. There was no specific information about privacy and confidentiality issues–which, of course, does not mean that the participants' privacy was violated.

EXERCISE C.2: QUESTIONS OF FACT (APPENDIX B)

a. Yes, the report indicates that approval for the study was granted by the IRB of the university with which Rew was affiliated.
b. The study participants would be considered "vulnerable" in terms of their adverse circumstances, and certainly extra precautions would be needed in conducting a study with a group that may have experienced various forms of exploitation and abuse. Whether the study participants are also "vulnerable" in terms of traditional criteria is a bit tricky. The average age of the youth was 18.8, and all but one out of the 15 participants were 18 years old or older at the time of the study (Table 1). Thus, 14 participants would not be considered minors. The 16-year-old was technically a minor, and some might consider it appropriate to obtain consent of parents or guardians—which would be impossible in this situation because the youth were living on the street. Most jurisdictions would probably conclude that the 16-year-old was an "emancipated minor" who would have some of the rights of an adult, including the right to sign a consent form.
c. The participants were not subjected to any physical harm or discomfort. It is possible that they experienced some psychological distress in describing their situations—but it is more likely that they found the interview pleasant and possibly even therapeutic. The researcher was expressing interest in them and asked questions that were respectful and that assumed that the youth had autonomy and self-direction. The interviews were conducted in a pleasant and private environment.
d. It does not appear that the participants were deceived.
e. It does not appear that any coercion was involved. The report specifically noted that the participants volunteered. The cash incentive was not so large that this could be construed as a coercive device. It is possible—but only remotely—that the youth felt some pressure to participate because of their reliance on the street outreach program from which they were recruited.
f. Rew indicated that participation in the study was voluntary: "Fifteen youth . . . volunteered to participate . . ." (There was no information about whether some youth who were asked to participate refused to do so.) The report stated that Rew obtained written consent. The report also stated that the investigator "described the purpose of the study in . . . detail," suggesting full disclosure.

g. Yes, Rew indicated that the interviews took place in a private setting. She did not explicitly discuss who had access to the audiotaped interviews or the transcripts, but it seems safe to presume that they were safeguarded. Rew stated that "pseudonyms were used to protect the identity of all participants."

▪ Chapter 8

EXERCISE C.1: QUESTIONS OF FACT (APPENDIX C)

a. Yes, the study involved a culturally tailored education intervention for Chinese Americans with type 2 diabetes.
b. Yes, the investigators compared values on several outcomes (e.g., DQOL scale scores, HbA1c levels) before and after the intervention.
c. The design for this study was a within-subjects design. There was not a second group *not* receiving the intervention to whom program participants were compared.
d. This study was longitudinal. Data were collected from study participants three times: before the intervention, immediately after the intervention, and then 3 months after the intervention.
e. The study was prospective; the intervention (the independent variable) was administered, and then outcome data were gathered subsequently.
f. It does not appear that any blinding was used in this study.
g. The educational intervention was administered at a clinic in Chinatown in Hawaii. Baseline data and data immediately after the intervention were gathered at the clinic. The report did not say where the 3-month follow-up data were collected, but presumably this also occurred at the clinic.

EXERCISE C.2: QUESTIONS OF FACT (APPENDIX D)

a. No, this study did not involve an intervention.
b. No explicit comparisons were reported in this descriptive study. However, although this was not mentioned in the published article, Beck did compare the stories of mothers who had cesarean deliveries vs. vaginal deliveries, mothers who were induced and those who were not, and primiparas vs. multiparas. None of these comparisons suggested variation in the themes revealed in her study.
c. The study was cross-sectional. Participants provided data about their experiences at one point in time.
d. Qualitative studies are not typically described as being prospective or retrospective, but it could be said that the data represented retrospective descriptions of the mothers' experiences.
e. No, no blinding of any type was used in this study.
f. In an Internet study, there is no designated "location." Study participants could have answered the questions from anywhere—e.g., from their homes, public libraries, Internet cafés. Data were gathered from women in four countries.

▪ Chapter 9

STUDY QUESTION B.1

a. Grounded theory
b. Ethnography
c. Discourse analysis
d. Phenomenology

EXERCISE C.1: QUESTIONS OF FACT (APPENDIX B)

a. Rew's research was a grounded theory study. No ideological perspective was expressed in the report.
b. Rew used the Strauss and Corbin approach.
c. The central phenomena were the self-care behaviors and attitudes of homeless youth.
d. No, the study was not longitudinal. All study participants were interviewed at a single point in time.

e. The setting was a street outreach program for homeless youth in a church basement in central Texas.
f. Yes, in the data analysis subsection, Rew stated, "The constant comparative method was used to develop open coding, analytic memos, and categories." She also indicated later in the same section, "Each interview was analyzed by comparing it to all previous interviews for preliminary conceptualizations."
g. Yes, Rew needed to use a qualitative approach to get a rich, holistic understanding of the lifestyles and experiences of the homeless youth, and of their approaches to taking care of themselves. Grounded theory was an appropriate strategy for discovering fundamental processes.

EXERCISE C.2: QUESTIONS OF FACT (APPENDIX D)

a. Beck's study was phenomenological. It did not have an ideological perspective.
b. This study was descriptive.
c. The central phenomenon under study was women's experience of posttraumatic stress resulting from childbirth.
d. No, this study was not longitudinal.
e. Yes, Beck specifically noted that her inquiry was guided by the work of the phenomenologist Colaizzi, whose method begins "by carefully questioning presuppositions about the phenomenon under investigation." Such questioning represents researchers' efforts to bracket preconceived views.
f. Yes, the research question is completely congruent with a qualitative approach—specifically with phenomenological methods.

EXERCISE C.3: QUESTIONS OF FACT (APPENDIX F)

a. Giddings' study used a cross-cultural life history approach, which is allied with narrative analysis. The study was informed by feminist theory and critical social theory.
b. The central phenomenon under study was nurses' experiences with social injustices in the health care system.
c. Although the study participants were interviewed on multiple occasions, this study could not be described as longitudinal. The purpose of having more than one interview was not to gather information about changes, or about the evolution of a phenomenon over time. Multiple interviews were likely necessary, in part, because of how much information Giddings wanted to gather from each participant, which would have been unwieldy in a single session. Moreover, as explained in the report, the follow-up interviews gave the nurses an opportunity to listen to and reflect upon the first interview.
d. The interviews were conducted both in New Zealand and the United States. The specific settings where data gathering occurred were not specified.
e. This study could not have been conducted as a quantitative inquiry—it is well-suited for an in-depth inquiry, and using a life history approach was totally congruent with the study aims. Giddings provided excellent examples of how an ideological perspective influenced the conduct of the study.

■ Chapter 10

EXERCISE C.1: QUESTIONS OF FACT (APPENDIX A)

a. Yes, the purpose of the study was to evaluate the effects of a computer-delivered intervention for chronically ill rural women.
b. The design for this study was experimental.
c. The experimentally manipulated independent variable was participation versus nonparticipation in the special intervention. The dependent variables included several measures of psychosocial health, including social support, self-esteem, empowerment, self-efficacy, depression, loneliness, and stress.

d. Yes, randomization was used, but the report did not provide much information about the actual randomization procedure. It appears that a basic randomization process was used (i.e., not a Zelen approach, PRPP, etc.).
e. The counterfactual in this study was the absence of a special intervention.
f. In this study, data were collected from experimental and control group members twice—at baseline and at some point after the intervention. Thus, the specific design was a before–after experimental design.
g. The design is a between-subjects design because the intent was to compare outcomes for the experimental and control group members, who were not the same people.
h. It does not appear that any masking/blinding was used in this study.
i. Although data were collected twice (before and after the intervention), the study would not be called longitudinal. If Hill and colleagues had collected another round of follow-up data 3 months later to ascertain long-term effects of the intervention, then the study would be described as longitudinal.
j. The authors cited previous work of their own dating back to 2000, so it is possible that there was a pilot study for this project. Pilot work was not specifically noted, however.

EXERCISE C.2: QUESTIONS OF FACT (APPENDIX E)

a. No, there was no intervention in this study.
b. The study design was nonexperimental.
c. It is not straightforward to ascertain the independent and dependent variables in this study. The abstract indicated that the focus of the study was on "health motivation as a *determinant* of self-rated health and health behaviors." This implies that health motivation is the independent variable and self-rated health and health behaviors are dependent variables. There is a bit of ambiguity, however, because the stated purpose of the study was to "explore the relations among health motivation, self-ratings of health, and various health behaviors. . . ." This exploratory intent suggests that the researchers did not specifically conceive of the variables of interest as *independent* or *dependent*. The ambiguity is further compounded by the conceptual model (Figure 1), which suggests that perceived health status (under "basic conditioning factors") is an antecedent or determinant of motivation (under "exercise of self-care agency"). Nevertheless, we suspect that health motivation was considered an independent variable, and engaging in health-promoting activities was considered a key dependent variable.
d. None of the variables in the study could be experimentally manipulated.
e. No, randomization was not used.
f. This is a descriptive correlational study. It could also be described as retrospective: Loeb was interested in retrospectively identifying correlates of the study participants' health behaviors.
g. No, masking/blinding was not used in this study.
h. No, this study was cross-sectional.

■ Chapter 11

EXERCISE C.1: QUESTIONS OF FACT (APPENDIX A)

a. Hill and colleagues used two methods to control confounding variables, the most important of which was randomization to treatment groups. Another method (although this method was undoubtedly not explicitly used as a control method) was homogeneity. All of the study participants were women (not men), lived in rural areas (not urban or suburban areas), and had a chronic (not acute) illness.
b. Through randomization, virtually all subject characteristics (e.g., age, income, marital status, type of chronic illness, etc.)

would have been controlled. Through homogeneity, gender, area of residence, and acute vs. chronic illness were controlled (i.e., held constant).

c. Yes, there was attrition. As shown in Figure 1, 17 members of the experimental group (28%) did not receive the intervention, and 18 did not complete the follow-up data collection forms. Additionally, 2 control group members (3%) did not provide follow-up data.

d. In this study, it would have been difficult to achieve constancy of conditions. The intervention itself was delivered in a manner that made it possible for women in the treatment group to "participate at any convenient time" (or to *not* participate). Researchers had no control over such factors as privacy, comfort, time of day, etc. Data were collected by self-administered questionnaire, and again there would have been no opportunity to ensure that conditions were constant or even similar. On the other hand, by having a standardized Internet-based program, the researchers had control over some aspects that would be difficult to achieve if the intervention had been delivered "live" in various community settings.

e. As noted in the previous question, the researchers did not have much control over the intervention, except to offer it to those in the experimental group and withhold it from those in the control group. It would have been possible for those in the treatment group to get virtually no intervention, and it might have been possible for those in the control group to get alternative (and varying) forms of social support and health-related information. Given the decentralized nature of the intervention, this was not an aspect over which researchers had much control.

EXERCISE C.2: QUESTIONS OF FACT (APPENDIX C)

a. The design for this study was quasi-experimental.

b. The independent variable for this study was participation versus nonparticipation (i.e., before participation) in the diabetes education program. The dependent variables included quality of life, body weight, blood pressure, and HbA1c levels.

c. No, randomization was not used, but it would have been possible to use a true experimental design for this study, i.e., to randomize participants to the intervention or to a control group condition.

d. The researchers used a counterfactual strategy that involved a comparison of outcomes before and after subjects were exposed to the intervention.

e. The researchers used a one-group pretest–posttest design.

f. It could be said that the researchers used homogeneity—all of the subjects were Chinese Americans diagnosed with type 2 diabetes and were middle-age to older-age adults. Other strategies discussed in the chapter (e.g., randomization, matching) are not appropriate with a one-group design. A crossover strategy was also not possible—once the subjects had been exposed to the program, they could not be "unexposed." Statistical controls also were not used.

g. The only confounding variables relating to subject characteristics that were controlled in this study were racial/ethnic background, residence in Hawaii, and, to some extent, age. Extraneous variables relating to the intervention and setting were, however, controlled (see Question h).

h. Yes, there is an explicit reference to the researchers' efforts to maintain constancy of conditions in the subsection *Setting and Sample*: "Information presented in each session strictly adhered to a predetermined agenda and was delivered in a standardized manner to minimize variations between different sessions."

i. Yes, in the second paragraph of the results section, the researchers indicated that 33 of the 40 recruited participants completed the 10-session program, for an attrition rate of 17.5%.

■ Chapter 12

EXERCISE C.1

a. Mixed method research:
   - The Hill et al. study in Appendix A is quantitative, but the authors mentioned (in the design subsection) that they gathered "illustrative comments from the women's online conversations," suggesting a qualitative component. Data from this component were not presented in this report.
   - Forchuk and colleagues (Appendix G) administered an instrument that gathered both qualitative and quantitative data, the Family Stressor Inventory. They also solicited qualitative feedback about the intervention.
   - The Johnson and Rogers study (Appendix I) could be considered mixed method, in the sense that quantitative methods were used to test an instrument that included items generated on the basis of an in-depth qualitative inquiry.

b. A clinical trial:
   - The Hill et al. study in Appendix A could be described as a clinical trial—a randomized design was used to test an innovative intervention.
   - The Wang and Chan study in Appendix C might be considered a Phase II clinical trial because it was a pilot test of an intervention and information was sought about its acceptability as well as its potential for effectiveness in improving important health outcomes.
   - The Forchuk et al. study (Appendix G) could be described as a clinical trial—it involved a randomized design to test the efficacy of the postoperative massage intervention.

c. Outcomes research:
   - None of the studies in the appendices would be considered outcomes research.

d. Survey research:
   - The Loeb study (Appendix E) involved a survey.

EXERCISE C.2: QUESTIONS OF FACT (APPENDIX I)

a. No, the study by Johnson and Rogers would not be considered a clinical trial or nursing intervention research.

b. This study *evaluated* the Medication-Taking Questionnaire with regard to its adequacy as a useful instrument, but this would not be considered evaluation research as the term is usually used.

c. This study is not an example of outcomes research.

d. This study is not specifically a survey, although it could be said that a survey-type approach was used to gather data for Phase II and Phase III.

e. Yes, this study is a good example of methodologic research. The purpose of the study was not to gather evidence relating to a substantive problem, but rather to design and test an instrument that could be used in substantive research and in clinical settings.

f. The study was nonexperimental. The researchers did not introduce an intervention or manipulate an independent variable.

g. As noted earlier, this study could be considered mixed method. Sophisticated quantitative methods were used to test the adequacy of the Medication-Taking Questionnaire. However, items for the instrument were generated on the basis of an in-depth qualitative inquiry by one of the investigators. The design for this study might be considered a sequential, component design. This design could be symbolized as follows: *QUAL* → *QUAN*.

■ Chapter 13

STUDY QUESTION B.4

a. Multistage (cluster) sampling
b. Convenience sampling
c. Systematic sampling
d. Quota sampling
e. Simple random sampling
f. Purposive sampling

EXERCISE C.1

a. None of the studies used probability sampling.
b. Almost all of the studies used convenience sampling, at least initially, although the sampling in the qualitative studies in Appendix B and D evolved into other forms of sampling. In the ethnographic study in Appendix H, Walsh purposively sampled all of the *comadronas* with busy practices to serve as key informants.
c. None of the studies used quota sampling.

EXERCISE C.2: QUESTIONS OF FACT (APPENDIX E)

a. The target population in Loeb's study could be described as community-dwelling men aged 55 and older in the United States. The accessible population was older men living in both urban and rural areas in a Mid-Atlantic state who participated in various social activities in their communities.
b. The eligibility criteria for the study included (a) male gender; (b) age 55 or older; (c) ability to read, understand, and write English; and (d) absence of obvious cognitive impairments.
c. Loeb's sampling method was nonprobability, specifically, sampling by convenience.
d. Loeb used a wide range of recruitment strategies. She recruited in locations where she knew older men would be present, such as in senior exercise classes, at restaurants, at a drivers' safety class, and through her own network of friends.
e. Loeb recruited in both rural and urban areas to increase the likelihood that her sample would be ethnically diverse.
f. The total sample size was 135.
g. Yes, the report indicated that Loeb performed a power analysis to estimate her sample size needs. The power analysis suggested that the minimum number needed was 130 to achieve desired statistical criteria.

EXERCISE C.3: QUESTIONS OF FACT (APPENDIX B)

a. Rew stated that the eligibility criteria for the study included the following: (a) 16–20 years of age; (b) ability to understand and speak English; and (c) willingness to volunteer for an interview. Note that an implicit criterion was that study participants were not living at home with parents or other family members.
b. Study participants were recruited through a street outreach program that offered services to homeless youth.
c. The report indicated that theoretical sampling was used, which is the appropriate approach for a grounded theory study. Unfortunately, the report did not provide a specific example of how the emerging theory helped to shape sampling decisions. Also, although this is not stated, it seems likely that Rew *began* with a volunteer sampling—theoretical sampling is appropriate after data are obtained from early participants, whose information helps to shape a developing theory and drive subsequent sampling decisions.
d. There were 15 homeless youth in the sample.
e. The report indicates that data saturation was achieved at the end of 12 interviews.
f. Rew's sampling strategy did include 3 cases that were "confirming cases," i.e., the three cases over and above the 12 needed to achieve saturation.

■ Chapter 14

EXERCISE C.1

a. None of the studies in the appendices relied on data from records.
b. Wang and Chan (Appendix C) gathered biophysiologic data (e.g., blood pressure).
c. Rew (Appendix B) and Walsh (Appendix H) gathered unstructured observational data. Forchuk et al. (Appendix G) used structured observational methods (not biophysiologic instrumentation) to

measure swelling, range of motion, and shoulder function.

EXERCISE C.2: QUESTIONS OF FACT (APPENDIX A)

a. Hill's data collection methods were high on all four dimensions. The instruments were highly structured, yielded numeric information, were obtrusive to participants, and could be objectively scored.
b. The researchers used instruments and scales that had been developed by others.
c. Yes, this study used self-report measures. The self-report data were recorded by subjects themselves—that is, they completed self-administered questionnaires. A range of psychosocial variables were measured, including social support, self-esteem, empowerment, self-efficacy, depression, loneliness, and stress.
d. No, none of the variables was measured through observation. Technically, it would be possible to operationalize some of the variables through observation. For example, respondents could be observed as they engaged in certain activities, and psychosocial concepts such as depression could be inferred. However, this would not typically be the best approach to operationalizing the variables in this study.
e. There were no biophysiologic measures in this study, nor could such measures have been used to capture the outcomes.
f. Records were not used in this study, nor could they have been.
g. Hill and colleagues described, in greater detail than is typical, the criteria they used to select instruments in the subsection labeled "Measures." The article stated that instruments "were selected based on the strength of their psychometric properties, prior use in research with chronic illness, conceptual fit, use by the research team, and because there is evidence in earlier work and the literature that they are amenable to change. . . ."
h. There were no data collectors (e.g., interviewers) in this study because the data collection instruments were self-administered. Thus, training was not needed.

EXERCISE C.3: QUESTIONS OF FACT (APPENDIX D)

a. Beck's data collection methods were low on structure. Aspects of the narratives *could* have been quantified (e.g., what percentage of participants experienced terrifying nightmares), but they were not. Data were collected obtrusively, i.e., participants knew that they were providing data for the study. Beck's methods were not high on objectivity, as is typical in qualitative research in which the subjective judgments of the researcher are considered an important tool.
b. Yes, Beck's study involved self-report data, recorded by study participants themselves in the form of written narratives that were sent to the researcher by e-mail or regular post.
c. No, data were not collected through observation. Observation could potentially have been used to supplement the self-reports (e.g., through observation of women participating in a support group meeting).
d. This study did not collect any biophysiologic measures. The concepts being studied were not physiologic in nature.
e. Beck did not seek to use records, documents, or artifacts in this study. It would have been possible, however, to request study participants to maintain a diary over a certain period, or to send her any relevant diaries or letters written during the period immediately after childbirth.
f. Beck herself conducted all of the Internet "interviews." Beck's extensive experience with mothers during the postpartum period made study-specific training unnecessary.

▪ Chapter 15

EXERCISE C.1: QUESTIONS OF FACT (APPENDIX B)

a. Yes, Rew collected self-report data. The homeless youth in her study talked about their self-care attitudes and behaviors.
b. Unstructured interviews were used to collect data.

c. Yes, Rew's report indicated that the interviews were guided by two main tour questions: What helps you remain healthy living as you do? and What would you like to tell me about how you take care of yourself?
d. Rew reported that the interviews lasted an average of 30 minutes.
e. The interviews were tape-recorded, and then transcribed by a professional transcriptionist.
f. Rew made observations of the homeless youth during the interviews. There is no information about the specific behaviors or characteristics that were the focus of Rew's observations. The report indicated only that Rew made notes about the youths' "appearance and gestures."
g. Rew kept field notes in a journal.
h. Rew collected all the data in this study.

EXERCISE C.2: QUESTIONS OF FACT (APPENDIX F)

a. Yes, Giddings collected self-report data. The nurses in her study described their experiences of fairness and injustice in their nursing careers.
b. Giddings collected data by life history interviews—interviews in which respondents were encouraged to tell their life stories in their own words. Giddings described the interviews as "semistructured." The report indicated that "The interviews. . .were structured so the women could reflect on their lives in relation to issues of oppression, power, and social action that may have led to personal and social change."
c. The report provided an example of a broad question used early in the interviews ("What has it been like for you to be a nurse?"). Examples of more focused questions were not reported.
d. Each participant was interviewed two or three times, and interviews lasted 45 to 90 minutes each.
e. Interviews were recorded in duplicate. Each participant listened to their own tape-recorded interview before subsequent interviews. The taped interviews were transcribed.
f. It does not appear that observational data were collected in this study. It might have been possible to observe nurses in their practice settings and wait for situations in which social justices arose, but self-reports were undoubtedly the most expedient method of collecting data on this topic.
g. Not applicable.
h. Giddings collected the data in this study.

▪ Chapter 16

STUDY QUESTION B.2

Score of Y = 11; score of Z = 26

EXERCISE B.3

A = acquiescence; B = none; C = extreme response set; D = nay-sayers' bias

EXERCISE C.1: QUESTIONS OF FACT (APPENDIX C)

a. Yes, there were self-report measures in this study. The variables measured through self-reports included diabetes-related quality of life and satisfaction with the intervention. (Presumably demographic information was also obtained by self-reports.)
b. Three specific questions about participant satisfaction were described in the report, but there were no examples of the questions on the Diabetes Quality of Life (DQOL) survey.
c. The researchers' instruments appear to have included only closed-ended questions. Satisfaction was measured using two rating-scale–type questions and a dichotomous (yes/no) question. The DQOL was described as a 42-item multiple-choice instrument. It does not appear that other specific types of questions (e.g., a VAS or event calendar) were used.
d. Yes, the DQOL was a composite scale, and it probably was a Likert-type scale,

but this was not specifically noted. The three questions relating to satisfaction were also apparently combined into a scale, but there is some ambiguity about this because results were reported for individual questions and not for scale scores.

e. Self-report data were gathered by self-administered questionnaires.
f. The researchers apparently developed their own measure of participant satisfaction with the program, but the DQOL was an existing instrument, adapted for use with elderly Chinese by Cheng and colleagues.
g. The researchers did not offer a rationale for selecting the DQOL, but presumably the fact that it had been culturally adapted for the population under study played a prominent role.
h. No, the report did not mention the readability level of self-report instruments.
i. No, time required to complete the self-report instruments was not mentioned.
j. No, observational data (e.g., degree of active participation in the classes) were not gathered.
k. Several outcome variables were biophysiologic measures, including blood pressure and HbA1c levels.
l. Yes, the report provided a fair amount of information regarding how the biophysiologic measurements were made and standardized. For example, the specific test kit for the HbA1c values was mentioned, and the conditions under which blood pressure was measured were described.
m. The report did not specify who collected the data, nor how they were trained.

EXERCISE C.2: QUESTIONS OF FACT (APPENDIX E)

a. Yes, Loeb gathered data on a range of variables by self-report, including health motivation, perceived health status, engagement in health-promoting activities, satisfaction with health behaviors, barriers to and benefits of health promotion behaviors, participation in health screenings and programs, and demographic characteristics such as age and ethnicity.
b. The exact wording of questions was not indicated for any of the measures, although in some cases, the descriptions were fairly detailed. For example, one of the questions of the Older Men's Health Program and Screening Inventory asks respondents to "rate how satisfied they are with their health-promoting behaviors (never satisfied to always satisfied)" on a 4-point scale. By contrast, there were no examples of items used to measure health motivation.
c. Closed-ended questions were apparently used exclusively. No specific question types were mentioned, but it appears that most were multiple choice and rating-scale type questions.
d. Yes, there were several Likert-type scales in this study, such as the Health Self-Determinism Index (HSDI) and the Health-Promotion Activities of Older Adults Measure (HPAOAM).
e. The self-report data were gathered by self-administered questionnaire, but the researcher was always present to answer questions.
f. Loeb developed the Older Men's Health Program and Screening Inventory, but also used two existing scales, the HPAOAM and the HSDI.
g. Loeb indicated that she chose the HPAOAM specifically because it was designed to measure health-promoting lifestyle practices of older adults. No other selection criteria were mentioned. Loeb did not provide a rationale for selecting the HSDI.
h. Yes, it was noted that the required reading levels for the instruments ranged from a grade of 5.7 to a grade of 7.9. The report also indicated that a large font was used in printing the questionnaires to enhance readability.
i. No, there is no information about how much time was needed to complete the questionnaires.
j. No, data were not collected through observation. Self-reports were the only viable method of gathering relevant data in this study.

k. No, none of the variables were biophysiologic in nature.
l. Loeb apparently collected all of the data for this study.

■ Chapter 17

EXERCISE C.1: QUESTIONS OF FACT (APPENDIX A)

a. All of the scales used in the Hill et al. study were assessed for internal consistency reliability using Cronbach's alpha. The reliability coefficients were all presented in Table 2. As computed using study data, the values of alpha were as follows: The Personal Resource Questionnaire (PRQ2000): .90; Self-Efficacy Scale: .88; Self-Esteem Scale: .87; Perceived Stress Scale: .90; CES-D Depression Scale: .90; and UCLA Loneliness Scale: .94
b. The researchers selected instruments that have a strong reputation, but no specific information about validity was provided in the report.
c. Hill and colleagues reported reliability assessments from other researchers, but they also computed Cronbach's alpha using data in their own study. There was no documentation of validity, either in this study or in earlier research.
d. No, there was no information about the specificity or sensitivity of any of the instruments used in this study.

EXERCISE C.2: QUESTIONS OF FACT (APPENDIX E)

a. Reliability information in Loeb's study is as follows:
    - The demographics instrument: no information on reliability
    - Older Men's Health Program and Screening Inventory: reliability was assessed for the final three questions (the Likert items) only; the Cronbach alpha method was used (alpha = .78).
    - Health-Promotion Activities of Older Adults Measure: the Cronbach alpha method was used (alpha = .91).
    - Health Self-Determinism Index: the Cronbach alpha method was used (alpha = .61 in the current study).
b. Validity information was not provided for any of the instruments in this study.
c. The reliability of the scaled items of the "Older Men's Health Program and Screening Inventory" was assessed by Loeb, but it is not clear whether the assessment was done with the present study sample or with a different sample. There is a citation to a 2003 publication by Loeb, which could have been an earlier study with a different sample, or a prior publication using data from the present sample. The reliability of the HPAOAM and the HSDI was assessed with the study sample, as well as with samples in other studies.
d. No, information about the specificity or sensitivity of the instruments was not reported.

■ Chapter 18

EXERCISE C: QUESTIONS OF FACT (APPENDIX I)

a. The Medication-Taking Questionnaire: Purposeful Action (MTQ) was based on a model developed by Johnson and colleagues and is referred to as the Medication Adherence Model or MAM.
b. The items that were initially developed were "based on the statements given by participants in a qualitative study" that was conducted by Johnson and colleagues.
c. The MTQ was a 7-point Likert-type scale, with the following response options: 7 = always agree, 6 = very frequently agree, 5 = usually agree, 4 = occasionally agree, 3 = rarely agree, 2 = almost never agree, and 1 = never agree. In this scale, there was no neutral midpoint.
d. Higher scores on the scale represent greater intent to take prescribed medications.

e. Yes, readability was assessed. The reading level for individual items ranged from grade level 1.0 to 6.2, and the average grade level for the instrument was 3.5.
f. It does not appear that the instrument was formally pretested, although members of the target population were involved in the content validity effort. It does not appear that cognitive questioning was used.
g. Yes, the content validation involved both experts and the target population. Five experts in hypertensive treatment served on the expert panel; two were physicians, and three were nurses with relevant clinical and research experience. The experts were asked to rate items on relevance, on a standard 4-point scale. If a CVI was actually computed, which would have been possible, its value was not reported. The content validity effort did, however, result in the elimination of 1 of the initial 20 items.
h. A total of 229 people from 7 different sites served as participants in the psychometric study. The participants were adult hypertensive patients who lived in situations in which they managed their own medications.
i. Yes, internal consistency of the scale, as revised on the basis of preliminary analyses, was assessed. The coefficient alpha for the Benefits subscale was .90, and alpha for the Safety subscale was .80. According to Table 2, alpha for the overall scale was .88, although the text indicated that total alpha was .87, so perhaps there was a typographical error.
j. The test–retest reliability of the scale was assessed, using a randomly selected subsample of participants who were administered the scale 1 week after the initial administration. For the overall scale, the test–retest reliability coefficient was .80.
k. Yes, an EFA was undertaken. Principal axis factoring with oblimen (oblique) rotation was used. The EFA yielded two interpretable factors—even though the MTQ had been conceptualized as having three subscales. The first factor (Benefits), with 9 items, had an eigenvalue of 5.5 and explained 46% of the variance. The second factor (Safety), with 3 items, had an eigenvalue of 1.9 and explained 16% of the variance. Six items were deleted because their loadings on the two factors were less than .40.
l. Yes. The inter-item correlations for the Benefits subscale ranged from .25 to .72—only one was less than .30. For the Safety subscale, the inter-item correlations ranged from .57 to .58.
m. Yes, a CFA was performed. According to the authors, "The CFA supported the hypothesis that benefits and safety underlie the cognitive component of medication taking in hypertensive medications."
n. The authors assessed construct validity by examining correlations between MTQ scores with scores on other theoretically relevant instruments.

■ Chapter 19

STUDY QUESTION B.3

a. A grounded theory analysis would not yield themes—a phenomenological study involves a thematic analysis.
b. Texts from poetry are used by interpretive phenomenologists, not by ethnographers (unless the poetry is a product of the culture under study, which it is not in this case).
c. Phenomenological studies do not focus on domains, ethnographies do.
d. Grounded theory studies do not yield taxonomies, ethnographies do.
e. A paradigm case is a strategy in a hermeneutic analysis, not in an ethnographic one.

EXERCISE C.1: QUESTIONS OF FACT (APPENDIX B)

a. There were 193 pages of transcribed interviews. The report did not describe the extent of the field notes.
b. Yes, the report indicated that "the constant comparative method was used to develop open coding, analytic memos, and categories."
c. It does not appear that Rew created conceptual files.

d. Yes, a computer program (called NUD*IST Q5) was used to manage the data and help with the analysis.
e. Rew did a kind of qualitative "accounting" that implies a quantitative intent—although whether this was intentionally a form of quasi-statistics is difficult to determine. For example, she wrote in the first paragraph of her results section, "For the majority of street youths in this sample, this process begins with an awareness that life at home was intolerable. . . ." The term *majority* means "more than half," which suggests at least a loose numeric calculation.
f. Rew used the Strauss and Corbin approach to grounded theory analysis.
g. Yes, the report indicated that Rew prepared analytic memos. For example, she wrote, "These early conceptualizations were recorded in analytic memos that were used in an iterative process of rereading and recoding."
h. Rew did not give specific examples of open coding. She said that constant comparison was used to develop open coding, and that all 15 interviews were analyzed line-by-line during open coding.
i. Rew indicated that "axial coding produced categories in terms of causes, dimensions, and context." No specific illustrations were provided (which is not unusual, but such illustrations are extremely helpful to readers).
j. Initially, 12 categories emerged.
k. Ultimately, three major categories were refined. They were: Becoming aware of oneself; Staying alive with limited resources; and Handling one's own health.
l. The BSP was "Taking Care of Oneself in a High Risk Environment." According to Rew, taking care of oneself among homeless youth is a process of deciding and acting in ways that enhance basic self-respect and that promote health.

EXERCISE C.2: QUESTIONS OF FACT (APPENDIX D)

a. The report did not specifically mention that Beck used computer software to organize and manage her data. However, Beck (co-author of this book) does not use computer software in her analyses, but rather uses a file card system. She puts each significant statement on a file card and then sorts the file cards into the themes.
b. It does not appear that Beck calculated any quasi-statistics.
c. Beck reported that she used Colaizzi's descriptive phenomenological approach.
d. The report did not state whether Beck created analytic memos.
e. Beck discussed the analytic process in terms of the steps outlined by Colaizzi. After reading and rereading the participants' descriptions of their experiences, Beck extracted "significant statements that pertain directly to the experience of PTSD and formulating their meanings." Then these meanings were categorized into theme clusters.
f. Beck's analysis revealed five themes: "Going to the movies: Please don't make me go"; "A Shadow of myself" ;"Seeking to have questions answered and wanting to talk"; "The dangerous trio of anger, anxiety, and depression"; and "Isolation from the world of motherhood"
g. Yes, Beck provided rich supportive evidence for her themes, in the form of direct quotes from the women's narratives.

■ Chapter 20

EXERCISE C.1: QUESTIONS OF FACT (APPENDIX B)

a. Rew used method triangulation—that is, interview data were triangulated with observational data.
b. Regarding methods used to enhance credibility:
   - There is not much information about this in the report, but it does not appear that prolonged engagement or persistent observation were strategies that Rew adopted. Indeed, one potential problem is that Rew's interviews were relatively

brief (only 30 minutes, on average). Such a short interview raises concerns about the depth of information obtained.

- Peer debriefings were not mentioned. It appears that Rew collected and analyzed all data herself.
- Rew did use member checks, which are one of the most widely used methods of enhancing credibility. She indicated that "member checks were conducted with three participants who agreed that the interpretations were accurate."
- There is no indication that Rew undertook a search for disconfirming evidence.
- There is little explicit information about Rew's background and experience, although the introduction cited several of Rew's prior studies with homeless youth.
- Other aspects of the study could be described as enhancing the study's credibility. For example, Rew indicated that she was reflexive before going into the field, and kept a journal about initial preconceptions and beliefs about homeless youth. She also maintained personal impressions of the youth in a journal, in addition to purely descriptive observational notes. A professional transcriptionist was used to transcribe the interview data to ensure high quality. Finally, manual methods of coding the data were verified with coding based on a computer program for analyzing qualitative data.

c. Regarding other methods to enhance study quality:
   - The only information in the report relating to the issues of confirmability and dependability is the notation that Rew maintained an audit trail, and that her journal was part of that audit trail.
   - Rew did not specifically address transferability—but we can to some extent consider the transferability of her findings by looking at her sample. All the participants in this study were recruited from youths seeking health and social services from a street outreach program in central Texas. Thus, caution is needed in transferring these findings to homeless youths who are not part of an outreach program. Rew displayed the demographic characteristics of her sample in Table 1. One strength of Rew's sample with regard to its potential for transferability of the findings is its ethnic and gender diversity. Out of the 15 youths who participated in the sample, 7 were minorities. The sample was almost equally divided between males and females.
   - The vignettes of individual youth, and the quotes that Rew used extensively throughout the report, enhanced the authenticity of the study.
   - Rew did a reasonably good job with regard to the criterion of explicitness. She provided more information than is typical regarding her methods and her efforts to enhance the integrity of this study, and thus documentation could be described as very good. Rew further enhanced the rigor of her study by audiotaping her interviews, transcribing them verbatim, maintaining a reflexive journal, and maintaining an audit trial.

EXERCISE C.2: QUESTIONS OF FACT (APPENDIX F)

a. Giddings used time triangulation as a strategy to enhance credibility. Participants were interviewed on multiple occasions, not so much as a strategy for collecting longitudinal data (i.e., she was not capturing information about how a process unfolded or changed), but in an effort to get the story right. Participants listened to their earlier interviews and were encouraged to reflect on and enhance their stories. Giddings also used analytic triangulation. The report explicitly noted that there were four levels of analysis of the data.

b. Regarding methods used to enhance credibility:
   - Giddings used both prolonged engagement and persistent observation as

strategies to enhance the quality of the study. She went back to participants multiple times, both in individual interviews and in focus group interviews. Although Giddings did not specifically mention observation as a data collection strategy, she clearly attended to what happened to the women during the interviews and during focus group sessions.

- It appears that Giddings collected and analyzed her data single-handedly, without getting feedback from any peers.
- Giddings went back to study participants multiple times, and made explicit effort to have participants validate her interpretations.
- A potential weakness of this study is that Giddings does not appear to have made any effort to look for disconfirming evidence. She encouraged participants to think about injustices (as is often the case in critical research), and did not seek evidence that phenomena that could be considered social injustice were exaggerated or misinterpreted. Nor did she include in her sample nurses who said that they never encountered social injustices in their work life. In fact, there was no information in the report about how study participants were recruited.
- Giddings spoke in considerable detail about her own professional and personal background, and how she disclosed extensive information about herself to her study participants.

c. Regarding other methods to enhance study quality:

- Although Giddings specifically indicated that dependability was a standard of rigor that she applied to this study, the strategies that are most commonly associated with dependability (e.g., maintaining an audit trail) were not described. Member checking does enhance the dependability of data, however, and member checking in this study was extensive. Moreover, the fact that Giddings' analysis and interpretations withstood the test of time (i.e., over multiple interviews) suggests a fair level of dependability.
- Audit trails and peer reviews are the most frequently cited strategies for enhancing confirmability, neither of which appears to have occurred in this study.
- Commendably, Giddings undertook this study in two different countries and with participants who varied in age, experience, specialty area, sexual orientation, and cultural backgrounds—all of which can contribute to transferability. Unfortunately, though, Giddings did not describe the kinds of settings in which the nurses practiced, which could be highly relevant to the issue of transferability.
- Giddings gathered rich life history information from participants in multiple sessions. The report, with rich stories and quotes from the interviews, provided a strong sense of authenticity.
- As with the Rew report, the amount of information that Giddings provided about how the study was conducted and how rigor was enhanced was unusually good. More information about the auditability of her decisions could have enhanced explicitness, but explicitness was attained through her use of thick description throughout the report.
- There is considerable evidence of Giddings' sensitivity to her study participants. She explicitly stated that the interviews were structured so that women could reflect on their lives, and she encouraged them to become "active subjects in their own stories." Participants were encouraged to "follow their own thoughts and tell the stories that mattered."

■ Chapter 21

STUDY QUESTION B.1

a. Interval
b. Ordinal
c. Ratio

d. Ratio
e. Nominal
f. Ratio
g. Interval
h. Nominal
i. Interval
j. Ratio

STUDY QUESTION B.2

Unimodal, fairly symmetrical

STUDY QUESTION B.3

Mean = 81.8; median = 83; mode = 84

STUDY QUESTION B.4

a. 45
b. 3
c. 27.8%
d. 2.2%
e. 66.7%

STUDY QUESTION B.7

Absolute Risk, exposed group (AR_E) = .60; Absolute Risk, nonexposed group (AR_{NE}) = .90; Absolute Risk Reduction (ARR) = .30; Relative Risk (RR) = .667; Relative Risk Reduction (RRR) = .333; Odds Ratio (OR) = .167; Number Needed to Treat (NNT) = 3.33

EXERCISE C.1: QUESTIONS OF FACT (APPENDIX C)

a. Referring to Table 2:
    - Nominal-level: gender, native language, and preferred medical treatment
    - Ordinal-level: Length of time in U.S. (as presented in groups of years)
    - Interval-level: None
    - Ratio-level: Length of time in U.S., duration of diabetes management, age
    - Descriptive statistics: percentages, means, SDs, and ranges
    - The mode for length of time in the U.S. was 11 to 20 years
    - The distribution of values for duration of diabetes management was skewed positively
b. Several demographic characteristics of the sample members were described in the text but not in Table 2, including marital status, retirement status, educational level, and income.
c. Referring to Table 3:
    - All four variables were measured on a ratio scale.
    - Average weight decreased over the three measurements; variability increased from baseline to the two follow-ups.
    - Both diastolic and systolic blood pressure decreased, on average, and variability increased over time.
    - Changes in weight and blood pressure measures were changes most pronounced between baseline and the first measurement after the program.
    - Values for HbA1c at baseline were positively skewed.
d. The text described a crosstabulation between subjects' initial weight on one dimension (through categories with those in the upper third weighing 148 pounds or more), and ability to lose 5 pounds or more on the other dimension.

EXERCISE C.2: QUESTIONS OF FACT (APPENDIX G)

a. With regard to sample characteristics in this study:
    - Yes, Forchuk and her colleagues presented descriptive statistics about the characteristics of their sample members.
    - Descriptive statistics about the sample were presented in the text.
    - The levels of measurement included nominal level (e.g., type of procedure, marital status) and ratio (age).
    - The descriptive statistics used included percentages and one mean
b. Referring to Table 2:
    - Yes, this table presented information about study outcomes.

- Women in the intervention group got the highest average number of massages on Day 3.
- There were some people in the intervention group who got *no* massage on any of the three days.
- Not everyone in the sample got pain control from medication. On Day 1, at least one person in the intervention group reported no pain control from medication.

c. Referring to Table 3:
- Yes, this table presented information about study outcomes.
- The descriptive statistical indexes presented in this table include means and standard deviations.
- Control group members had more difficulty, on average, washing their backs.
- Control group members were more variable than intervention group members in terms of difficulty removing something from their back pocket.
- The most difficult task for those in both the intervention and control groups was placing an object on a high shelf.

■ Chapter 22

STUDY QUESTION B.3

a. Chi-square test (also possible: Fisher's exact test or the phi coefficient)
b. *t*-test for independent samples
c. Pearson's *r*
d. ANOVA

STUDY QUESTION B.4

a. 958
b. .113
c. Yes, it is significant at $p < .02$.
d. $p = .002$ (2 in 1000)
e. Depression, physical health, and mental health scale scores
f. The correlation between the two variables (−.643) indicates a fairly strong and statistically significant relationship between the two variables. Respondents who had high depression scale scores tended to have low mental health scores (i.e., the scale is a measure of *positive* mental health. The probability is less than 1 in 1000—actually less than 4 in 10,000—that the correlation is spurious).

STUDY QUESTION B.6

a. Approximately 500 in all, 250 per group
b. Approximately 165

EXERCISE C.1: QUESTIONS OF FACT (APPENDIX A)

a. Pearson's *r* and RM-ANOVA
b. There was information relating to hypothesis tests, but confidence interval and effect size information was not presented (except that the Pearson *r*s are also ES estimates).
c. Referring to Table 3:
   - Correlation between depression and self-efficacy scores = −.586.
   - All variables *except* depression were negatively correlated with loneliness.
   - Stress scores were significantly correlated with all other variables.
   - The correlation between stress and loneliness was the strongest (.716).
   - The correlation between self-esteem and empowerment was the weakest (.354).
   - *All* of the correlations were statistically significant at or beyond the .05 level.
   - Pearson's *r*
d. Referring to Table 5:
   - The independent variable is treatment group status.
   - There are both between-subjects tests (for treatment group) and within-subjects tests (across time).
   - There was a significant main effect for time (i.e., overall, empowerment levels improved over time for the sample as a whole) and a significant interaction effect (i.e., the improvement was significantly greater for the intervention group).

- Neither the main effect nor the interaction effect for self-efficacy was significant; neither group had a significant change in self-efficacy.
- Changes over time differed significantly for the two groups with regard to self-esteem, social support, and empowerment.
- Significant changes over time were observed for empowerment, depression, loneliness, and stress.
- RM-ANOVA

e. No, the report did not indicate that a power analysis was done to estimate sample size needs.

EXERCISE C.2: QUESTIONS OF FACT (APPENDIX E)

a. Pearson's *r* and *t*-tests
b. There was information relating to hypothesis tests, but confidence interval and effect size information was not presented (although the Pearson *r*s are also ES estimates).
c. Referring to Table 1:
   - The correlation between the men's Healthiness of lifestyle scores and Health-promoting behaviors (HPAOAM) scores was .368.
   - Variables that were negatively correlated with the variable "total screenings" include health motivation, personal evaluation of health, and healthiness of lifestyle.
   - There was a statistically significant correlation between HSDI scores and the following variables: Personal evaluation of health; Healthiness of lifestyle; Satisfaction with health behaviors; and Total benefits. (Note, however, that Loeb made an adjustment—a Bonferroni correction—to account for the fact that she was performing multiple tests with the same subjects. When this correction is applied, only two variables met this higher standard: Personal evaluation of health and Healthiness of lifestyle.)
   - The strongest correlation in the matrix was between Satisfaction with health behaviors and Healthiness of lifestyle, $r = .665$, $p < .001$.
   - The weakest correlation in the matrix was between Total programs and Personal evaluation of health, $r = .005$, $p = .957$.
   - The statistics are Pearson's product moment correlation coefficients (r).
   - No, none of the variables in the table was a nominal-level measure.
   - In this study, the men who attended more health-promoting programs were not significantly more likely than other men to participate in appropriate health screenings ($r = .156$, $p = .071$).
d. Referring to Table 3:
   - Race was the independent variable.
   - The statistical tests were *t*–tests.
   - Whites had higher average scores on the HSDI than nonwhites, but the difference was not statistically significant. This means that the racial differences are likely to be spurious (i.e., not likely to be true in the population of older men).
   - The two racial groups were significantly different with regard to three outcome variables: Total benefits, Total health conditions, and Total screenings. The test results suggest that the racial group differences are "real"—would likely be found again in another sample of older men.
e. Referring to Table 4:
   - Urban versus rural residence was the independent variable.
   - The title should be "Comparison of Older Men from Urban and Rural Areas."
   - *t*-Tests were used.
   - Men from urban areas had significantly higher HPAOAM scores than men from rural areas.
   - Men from different residential areas differed with regard to HPAOAM, total benefits, and total screening, if the traditional $p < .05$ is used as the criterion for significance.
f. Yes, Loeb stated that she did a power analysis to estimate sample size needs.

■ Chapter 23

STUDY QUESTION B.2

a. Logistic regression (or discriminant analysis)
b. ANCOVA
c. MANOVA
d. Multiple regression

EXERCISE C.1: QUESTIONS OF FACT (APPENDICES A, C, AND G)

a. None of these studies used multiple regression analysis.
b. None of these studies used ANCOVA.
c. No multivariate analyses of any type were used in these three studies.

EXERCISE C.2: QUESTIONS OF FACT (APPENDIX E)

a. Stepwise regression was used.
b. Referring to Table 2:
   - The dependent variable was health-promoting behaviors, i.e., HPAOAM scores.
   - The variable most strongly correlated with HPAOAM scores entered the regression equation first, i.e., Satisfaction with health-promoting behaviors. Table 1 shows that the correlation between these two variables was .564.
   - After the Satisfaction variable was in the regression, the value of R^2 was .298.
   - There were only two predictor variables in the final regression equation, Satisfaction and Total anticipated benefits of health-promoting behaviors.
   - Loeb used 8 potential variables as predictor variables (urban/rural site, age, and 6 of the variables from Table 1). However, the other variables added no explanatory power (i.e., did not significantly improve the prediction of HPAOAM scores beyond what was achieved with Satisfaction and Benefits) and so did not get included in the final regression equation.
   - The final value of R^2 was .414.
c. Yes, the authors assessed the risk for multicollinearity for their regression analysis. They found a low level of collinearity, with a high tolerance value of .916.

■ Chapter 24

EXERCISE C.1: QUESTIONS OF FACT (APPENDIX A)

a. There was no information about how missing data were handled.
b. Yes, in the Results section, there was a sentence indicating that the researchers assessed whether their data met assumptions for ANOVA.
c. Baseline values on the dependent variables were presented in Table 4 for both experimental and control group members, but there was no indication about whether group differences were statistically significant. For some outcomes (e.g., loneliness), the groups may have differed significantly at the outset.
d. More than one fourth of those in the intervention group dropped out of the study, compared with fewer than 4% of those in the control group. Hill and colleagues appeared not to have tested for attrition biases.
e. No, the analysis was not intention to treat.
f. Hypotheses relating to Aim #1 were not formally stated, although the implication was that intercorrelations among psychosocial variables were expected. A statement that the correlations were "in the anticipated direction" (first paragraph of the Results section) confirms this inference. All of the correlations were statistically significant.
g. Hypotheses with regard to the effects of the intervention were not formally stated, although they were certainly implied. Results were mixed—there were intervention effects for some outcomes (self-esteem, social support, and empowerment), but not for others.

h. No, confidence intervals were not presented.
i. Effect size estimates were not calculated, although the authors used language relating to effect magnitude (e.g., toward the end of the Results section, the authors said that "These results suggest that the intervention had an appreciable effect on self-esteem, social support, and empowerment. . . .")
j. There was no explicit discussion about internal validity in the Discussion section.
k. In the subsection labeled "Strengths," the researchers noted that the external validity of the study was strengthened by the fact that the intervention was tested among women with a variety of chronic illnesses.
l. Yes, in the subsection labeled "Limitations," the authors noted a potential problem with regard to statistical power as a result of attrition. Other factors that might have reduced statistical conclusion validity, however (e.g., a treatment that was insufficiently powerful, problems with intervention fidelity), were not mentioned.
m. Yes, considerable space in the Discussion section was devoted to discussing the findings within the context of earlier research.
n. Yes, there was a section on study limitations, although it did not mention several important ones, such as the possible risk for attrition or selection bias, possible problems with intervention fidelity, etc.

EXERCISE C.2: QUESTIONS OF FACT (APPENDIX C)

a. There was no information about how missing data were handled.
b. No, the report did not mention assessments for congruence with assumptions for parametric tests such as *t*-tests. In fact, the report indicated that scores on the DQOL were ordinal measures. Strictly speaking, this is likely to be true, but the authors did not indicate why they opted to use paired *t*-tests for their ordinal scores rather than a nonparametric test such as the Wilcoxon signed ranks test.
c. Seven of the 40 study participants did not attend all of the sessions, for an attrition rate of 17.5%. These 7 program drop-outs did, however, return for the 3-month postprogram evaluations. There was no information about how the 7 drop-outs differed from the 33 full participants.
d. The report indicated that pretest/posttest differences on DQOL scores were analyzed using a paired *t*-test, yet the test results (i.e., statistical significance) were not reported. There is no information about whether a *t*-test (or RM-ANOVA) was used to analyze changes over time with regard to physiologic measures such as blood pressure and HbA1c levels.
e. No confidence intervals were reported.
f. No effect size estimates were reported.
g. Yes, the Discussion section considered findings within the context of results from earlier research.
h. The purpose of a pilot study is to gain insights that can be applied to a larger endeavor, and commendably, the Discussion section of this paper did describe some "lessons learned" about how to improve the intervention.
i. Yes, some limitations of the study were explicitly noted in the Discussion section. The limitations were not so much about study methods as they were about the intervention and efforts to implement it.

■ Chapter 25

EXERCISE C.1: QUESTIONS OF FACT (APPENDIX J)

a. The stated purpose of this study was to estimate the effect of Tai Chi exercise on aerobic capacity.
b. Seven electronic databases were searched. There does not appear to have been a special effort to identify relevant "grey literature."
c. A total of 441 citations was originally obtained. Fifteen citations were reviewed in-depth, and 7 met all criteria for inclusion in the meta-analysis.

d. No, studies were included only if aerobic capacity was an outcome variable.
e. Four of the studies in this meta-analysis involved an intervention, and these studies used a quasi-experimental or true experimental design. Three studies were nonexperimental and involved observations of existing groups of people, some of whom had engaged in Tai Chi exercise.
f. Each primary study was given a quality assessment score. The section "Development of Study Quality Scoring Tool" indicated that 16 study elements were critically appraised. The highest possible score on the scale was 32 (a maximum of 2 points for the 16 elements). The Results section indicated that quality scores ranged from 22 to 28; the average score was 25.1. There is no information about who scored the studies for quality, nor whether inter-rater agreement was assessed.
g. The researchers decided to exclude a study if the quality score was below 21, but no study had such a low rating, and therefore none was eliminated.
h. The standardized mean difference (*d*) was used as the effect size measure. Effect sizes were weighted by (a) sample size and (b) pooled variance. These adjustments were made to give more weight to (a) studies with a larger number of subjects and (b) studies with a more heterogeneous sample.
i. Across all 7 studies, data from a total of 344 subjects were included in the meta-analysis.
j. Regarding information in Table 1:
   - The citations for the two experimental studies (i.e., the RCTs) are Brown et al., 1995 and Young et al., 1999.
   - In two studies (Brown et al., 1995 and Lan et al., 1998), the control group was sedentary, whereas in the other two, there was an alternative treatment—a walking program and aerobic exercise.
   - The effect size was largest among female subjects in the Lan et al. (1998) study: 1.334. Effect size is not statistically significant if the lower and upper bounds of the confidence interval—the LBCI and UBCI—include zero. In this case, the lower bound was 0.3809 and the upper bound was 2.307, indicating a significant effect size because zero is not included between these two confidence limits.
   - The effect of −.1598, favoring controls, was smallest in magnitude; it was not significant.
k. Regarding information in Table 2:
   - The average age of subjects in the Tai Chi and comparison group was most discrepant in the Schneider et al. study: those in the Tai Chi group were more than 5 years *older* than those in the comparison group (35.5 versus 30.0, respectively). This suggests a selection bias because age is related to the key outcome variable, aerobic capacity.
   - Aerobic capacity was greatest, on average, among subjects in the Tai Chi group in the Schneider et al. study.
   - The effect size was largest among the women in the Lan et al. study—1.3965. This effect size was statistically significant.
l. Forest plots were constructed, but it does not appear that formal statistical tests for heterogeneity were done.
m. The report did not specifically indicate which model was used, but we assume that it was a fixed effects model.
n. Regarding Figures 1 and 2:
   - Figures 1 and 2 are forest plots.
   - The effect size for both RCTs (Brown et al. and Young) was negative, indicating higher values for control group members than for those in the Tai Chi groups.
   - The average ES for the experimental studies was .33 (see Table 3). The 95% CI was (−.41, 1.07) and thus not significant. The average ES for nonexperimental studies was 1.01, which was significant, with a 95% CI of (.37, 1.66).
   - Heterogeneity was fairly high, with some studies favoring controls and others showing large, positive effects for those in the Tai Chi group.

o. Yes, subgroup analyses were performed. These analyses examined methodologic features of the studies (e.g., effects for experimental versus nonexperimental studies), as well as subject characteristics (e.g., effects for men versus women). The subgroup analyses also tested for features of the intervention (e.g., effects for subjects exposed to the longest form of the Yang style of Tai Chi versus those exposed to other types of Tai Chi).
p. The average ES was positive and significant (1.10) for the classical Yang style of Tai Chi, but was negative and nonsignificant (−.17) for other types. The average effect size across studies was modestly higher for women (0.83) than for men (0.65).
q. It does not appear that a meta-regression was performed.
r. Strictly speaking, the researchers did not do a sensitivity analysis—for example, they did not compute average effect sizes separately for studies with a low quality rating versus high quality ratings. However, the comparison of effect sizes for experimental and nonexperimental studies (which almost certainly had lower quality ratings) could be considered a type of sensitivity analysis.
s. It does not appear that this meta-analysis addressed the issue of publication bias.

EXERCISE C.2: QUESTIONS OF FACT (APPENDIX K)

a. The stated purpose of this metasynthesis was to synthesize the findings from qualitative studies focused on parenting preterm infants.
b. Five bibliographic databases were searched. There was no indication that efforts were made to locate "grey literature."
c. Initially, 68 studies were identified, but only 10 that met the inclusion criteria were chosen for the metasynthesis.
d. Swartz did not formally state her position, but she used studies from three traditions (grounded theory, phenomenological, and descriptive), suggesting her stance was that integration across traditions is acceptable.
e. There is no mention of appraising the primary studies for quality, and so this presumably was not done.
f. Swartz's report did not indicate the data collection strategies of the primary studies, although in Table 1, there are a few notations about participants being interviewed. It seems likely that interviews were the primary mode of data collection in these studies.
g. At least in some primary studies, both mothers and fathers were interviewed (e.g., Casteel, Murphy). In the Miles et al. study, 4 grandmothers with legal custody of infants were interviewed.
h. The metaethnographic approach of Noblit and Hare was used.
i. No, a meta-summary was not performed.
j. If it can be assumed that a "set of parents" (e.g., in Jackson et al.) means that both parents were *always* included, the total number of participants in the 10 studies was 243.
k. There were five shared themes: (1) adapting to risk; (2) protecting fragility; (3) preserving the family; (4) compensating for the past; and (5) cautiously affirming the future.
l. Yes, Swartz included many verbatim quotes to support her thematic integration.
m. No, study limitations were not mentioned for the metasynthesis nor for the primary studies.

▪ Chapter 26

EXERCISE C: QUESTIONS OF FACT (APPENDICES A–K)

a. The articles in Appendices A through F were published in *Nursing Research,* which had an impact factor of 1.528 in 2005. The article in Appendix G was published in *Cancer Nursing,* which had an impact factor of .823 in 2005, and the one in Appendix I was published in *Western*

Journal of Nursing Research, whose impact factor was .745. Articles in the remaining appendices (H, J, and K) were in journals whose impact factor in 2005 was not available.

b. With some minor variations (especially in the introduction and method sections), all of the reports followed a traditional IMRAD format.

c. Five of the articles (Appendices A, C, G, I, and J) were multiply authored, and in only one of them (the report by Johnson and Rogers, Appendix I) were the authors listed alphabetically.

d. None of the reports used first-person narratives. The authors used third-person narrative to describe their own actions ("The researchers administered . . ."), or used the passive voice ("Study participants were asked . . .").

▪ Chapter 27

EXERCISE C.1: APPENDIX L

a. No, this program announcement (PA) funded projects through the R01 and R21 mechanisms, as described in the section "Mechanisms of Support."

b. For R01 applications, this PA expired July 30, 2006 (unless it was reissued after this book went to press).

c. Nine other institutes within NIH, besides NINR, participated in this PA.

d. Yes, the PA specifically indicated that research on behavior-related interventions was being sought.

e. Yes, the PA specifically mentioned an interest in studies that explored "basic mechanisms of the conscious perception of pain and the affective responses to pain."

f. For this PA, the four major sections of the grant application were restricted to 15 pages.

EXERCISE C.2: QUESTIONS OF FACT (APPENDIX L)

a. Total direct costs = $175,000; Total requested funds: $259,000

b. May 1, 2006 to April 30, 2008

c. Five people were listed as key personnel. The PI (McDonald) was proposed at a 20% level for two academic years, and at a 50% level in the summers.

d. Yes, the Specific Aims section started on page 14, and the Research Design and Methods section ended on page 28, for a total of 15 pages.

e. McDonald presented her hypothesis in the Specific Aims section, which is consistent with guidelines.

f. McDonald described her own prior research on pain communication in the Preliminary Studies section. She mentioned 9 prior studies.

g. McDonald's Research Design and Methods section had the following subsections: Design; Sample; Procedure; Video Clip Experimental Manipulation; Measures; Content Analysis; Summary of the Methods; Analysis; Hypothesis; and Summary of the Analyses.

h. McDonald proposed a double-blind random assignment (experimental) design.

i. McDonald proposed a total sample of 300 participants, and based this estimate on a power analysis.

j. Blinding was proposed for study participants, the graduate assistant administering the "treatment," and the people doing the content analysis of participants' responses.

k. Yes, it was proposed that participants be compensated with a $20 money order, and a publication about pain management.

l. Yes, multivariate analysis of covariance was proposed.

EXERCISE 3: APPENDIX L

a. R21

b. Nursing Science: Adults and Older Adults (NSAA)

c. 167

d. The study section had human subjects concerns. Two reviewers requested a data and safety monitoring plan, and another had concerns about future use of the project audiotapes.

Answers to Crossword Puzzles

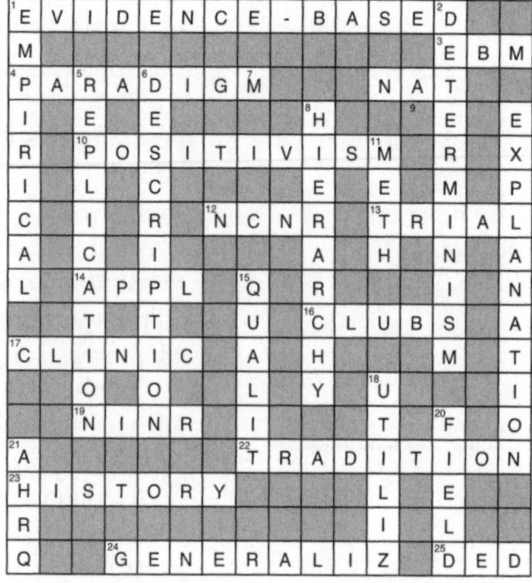

Chapter 1

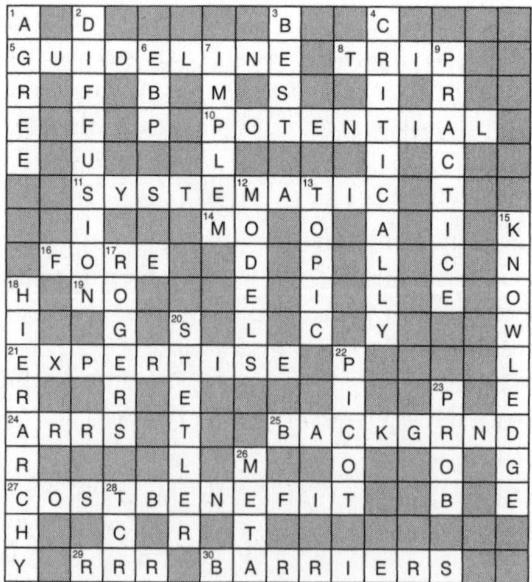

Chapter 2

				P		D	E	P	E	N	D	E	N	T			S
		S		H		I						T					E
	G	A	T	E	K	E	E	P	E	R		H		G	R	A	M
		T		N		T		O				N		R			E
		U			C			P	R	O	T	O	C	O	L		H
		R	A	D	O	N		U						U		E	T
		A			N			L			S	I	G	N	I	F	
D	A	T	A		S		R	A	W			V		D		F	
I		I			T			T			C			E		E	
S		O	P	E	R	A	T	I	O	N	A	L		D	I	C	H
C		N			U			O			U					T	Y
R					C	L	I	N			S		L				P
E					T				S	T	A	T	I	S	T		O
T	I	P							T		L	I	T				T
E	M	E	R	G	E	N	T		E			M					H
	R	E		O			E	X	P	E	R	I	M	E	N	T	
J	A	R	G	O	N		S					N				W	
	D			D		S	T	U	D	Y		G	N	I	D	O	C

Chapter 3

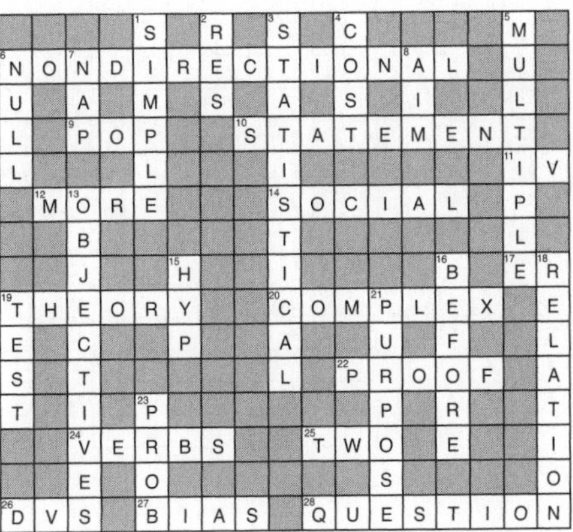

Chapter 4

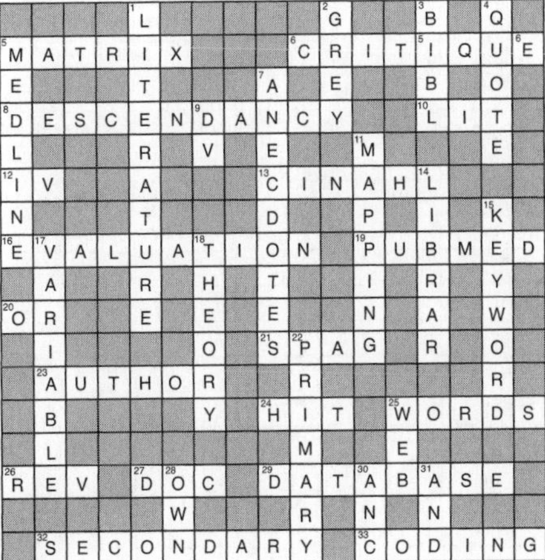

Chapter 5

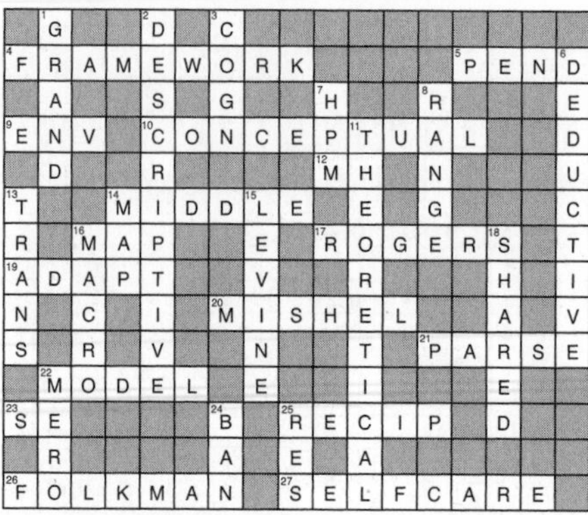

Chapter 6

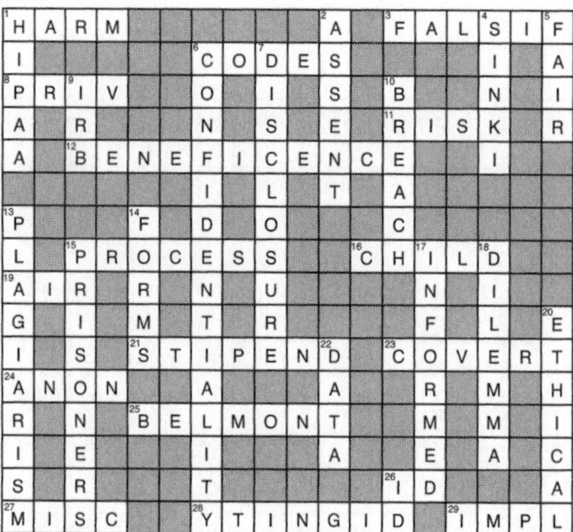

Chapter 7

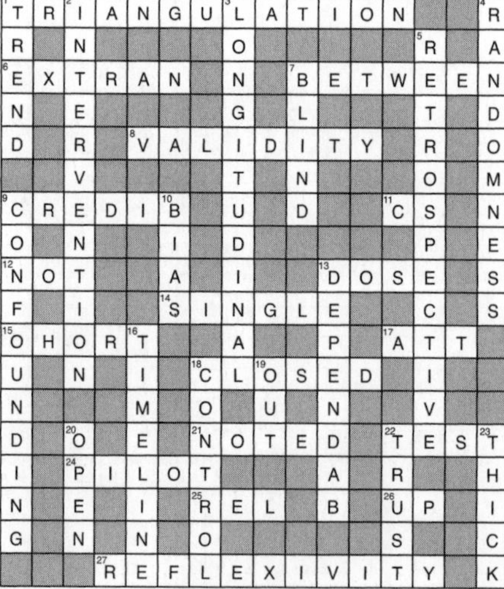

Chapter 8

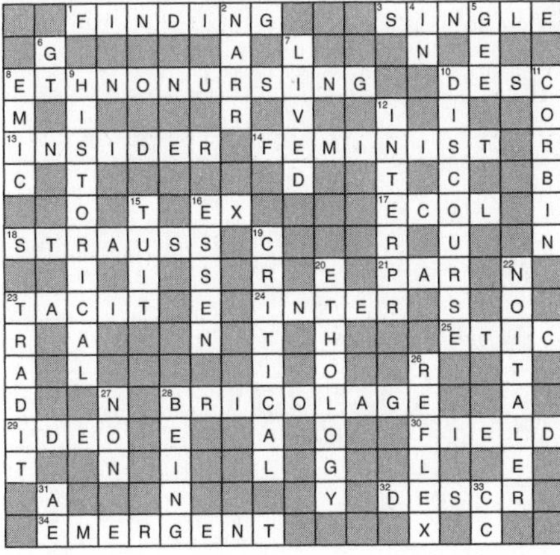

Chapter 9

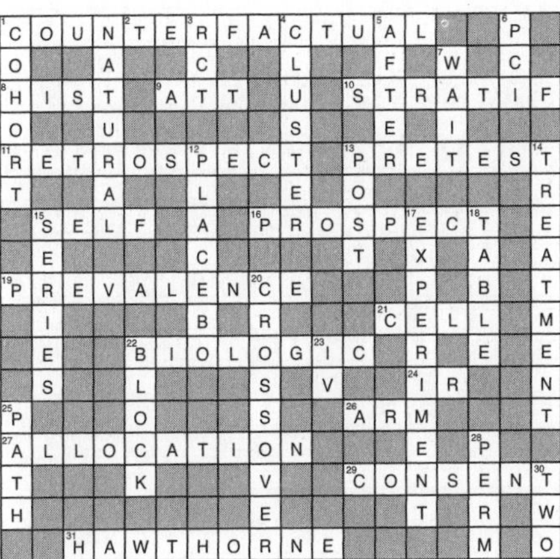

Chapter 10

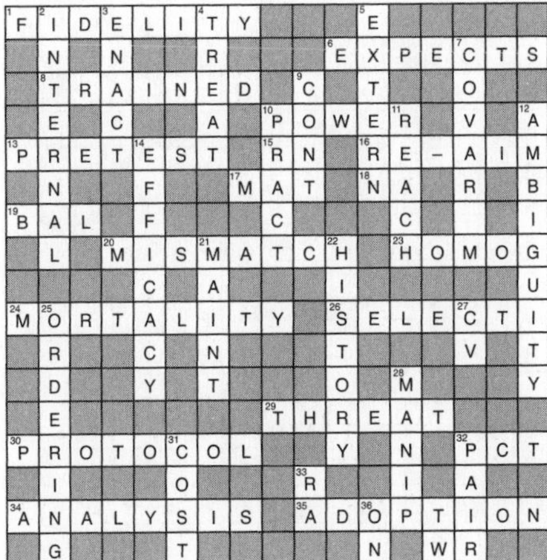

Chapter 11

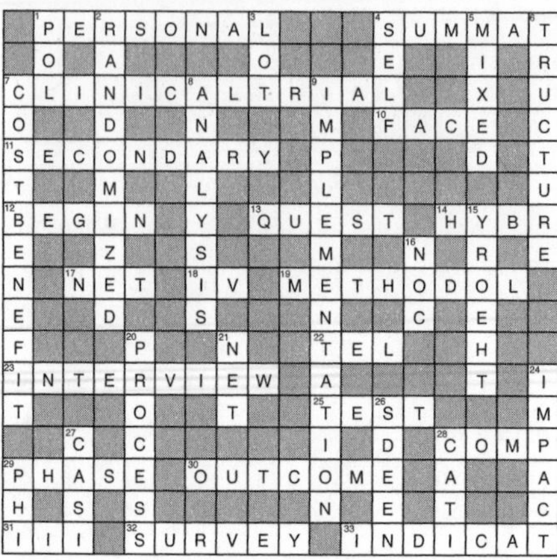

Chapter 12

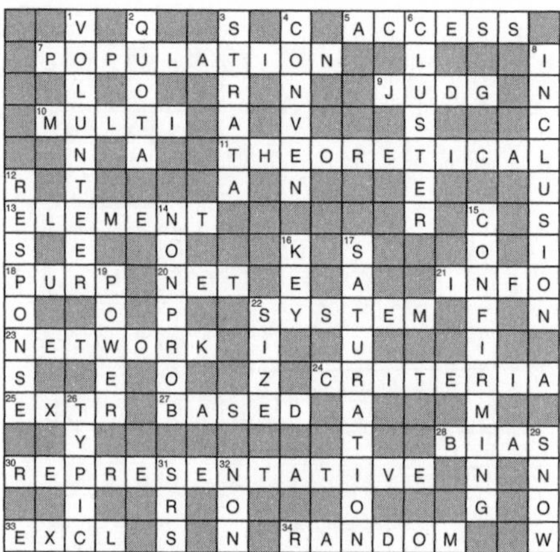

Chapter 13

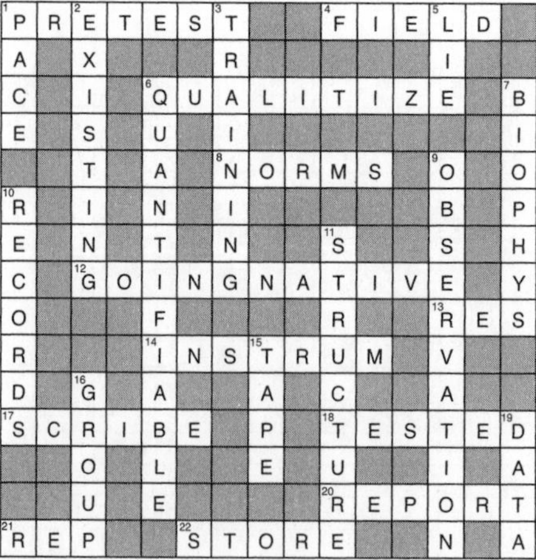

Chapter 14

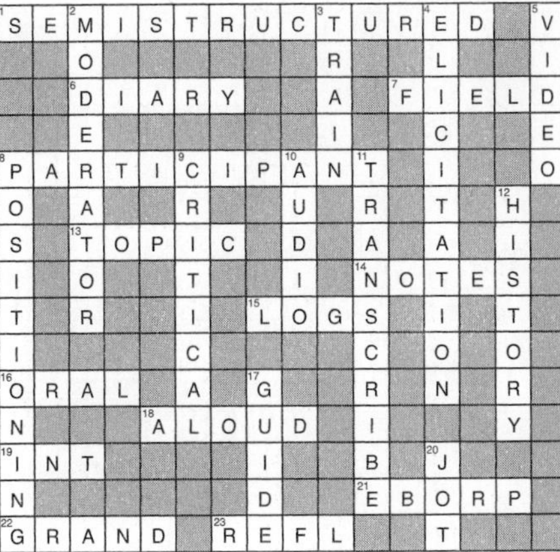

Chapter 15

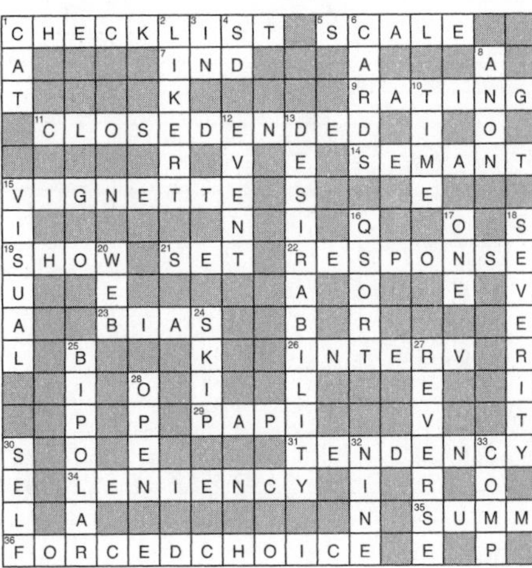

Chapter 16

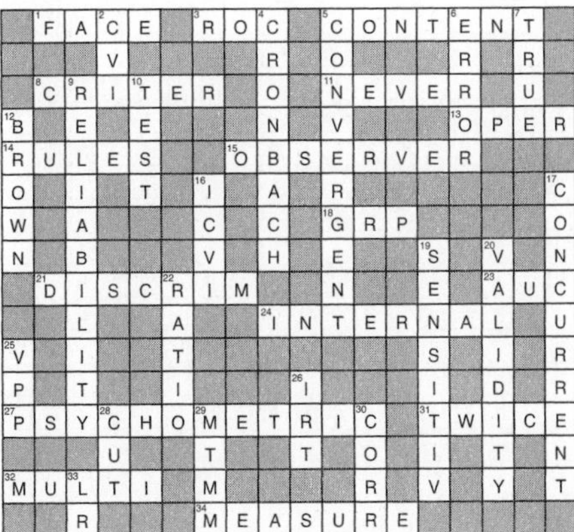

Chapter 17

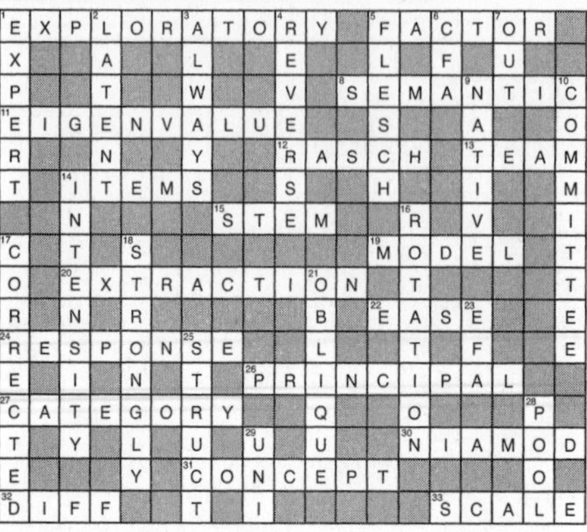

Chapter 18

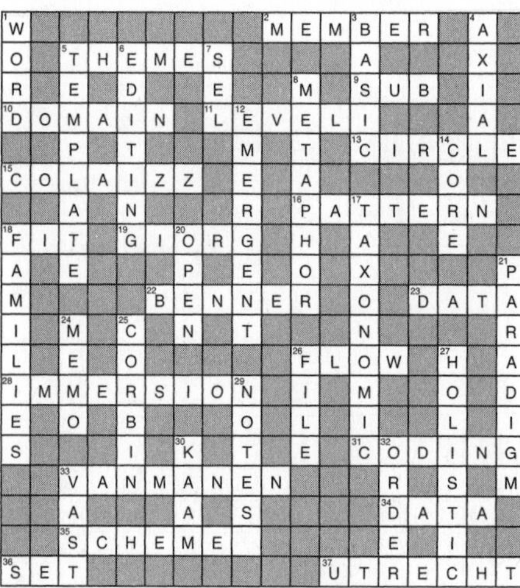

Chapter 19

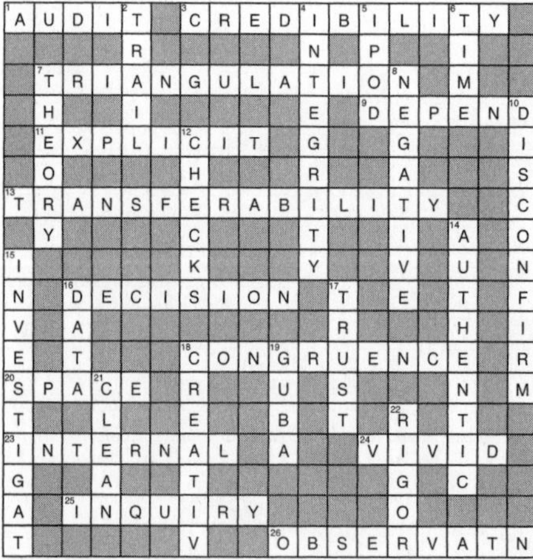

Chapter 20

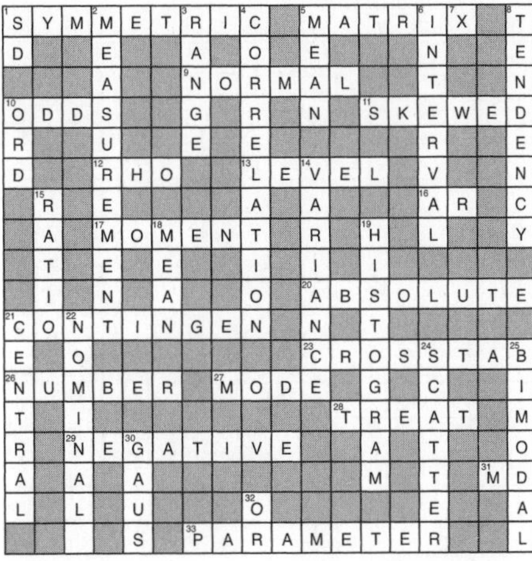

Chapter 21

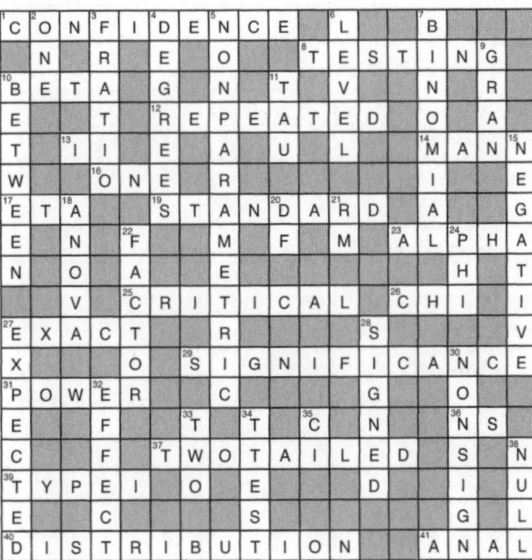

Chapter 22

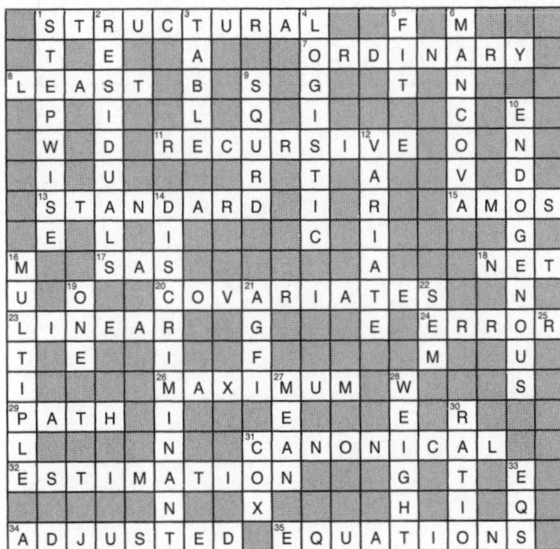

Chapter 23

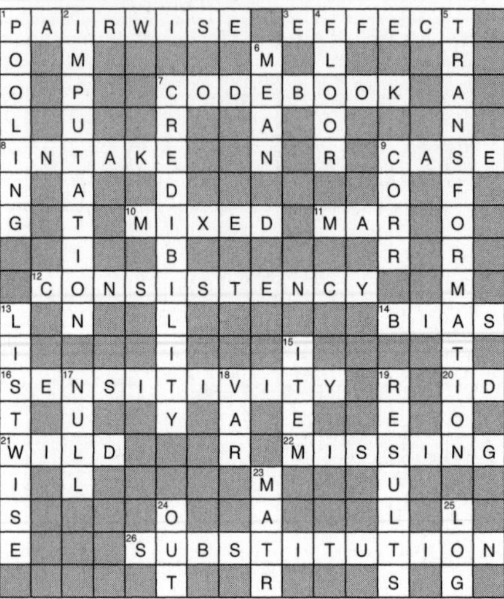

Chapter 24

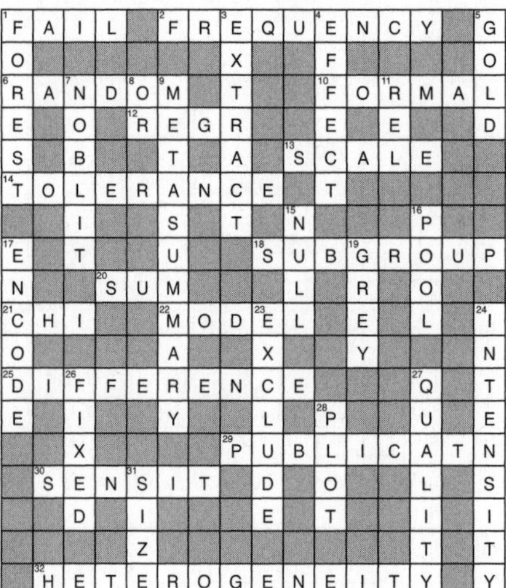

Chapter 25

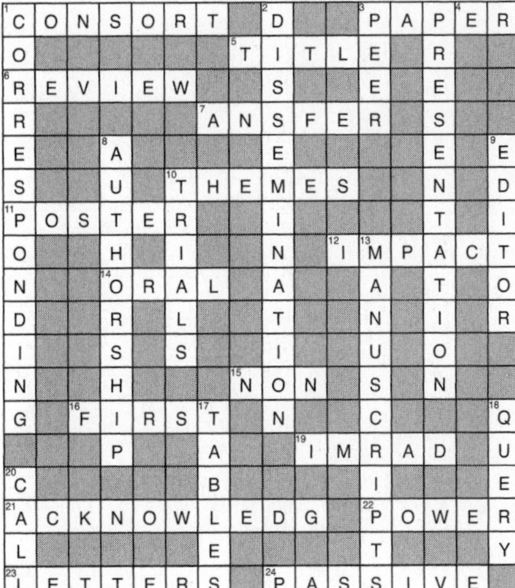

Chapter 26

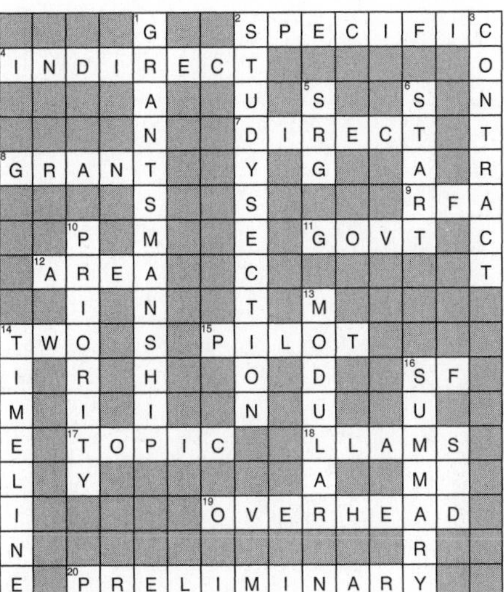

Chapter 27